Health Promotion

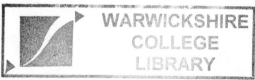

Health promotion is central to current public health and health care delivery. Emerging at the close of the last century, it unified diverse disciplines and fields of study with a single focus. This book provides an introduction to the multidisciplinary roots of health promotion and examines how different disciplines inform current research and practice.

The first edition of the book, published in 1992, was the first to examine this important aspect of health promotion and public health discourse. The second edition takes into account developments over the last ten years and adds three new disciplines: politics, ethics, and genetics.

In this book, leading authors outline the individual contributions of their disciplines to health promotion and the past and current concerns that are influencing developments today. Included are disciplines that have made a major contribution to the field, such as psychology, sociology and epidemiology, as well as those that have made an important, if lesser, contribution, such as social policy, economics and, more recently, genetics.

Health Promotion: Disciplines, diversity, and developments offers an excellent up-to-date introduction to the field of health promotion. Its multidisciplinary and theoretically grounded approach makes it appropriate for a broad range of academic and professional courses concerned with the study of health.

Robin Bunton is Professor of Sociology, University of Teesside. **Gordon Macdonald** is Senior Research Fellow and Principal Lecturer at the University of Glamorgan. Both have previously worked as researchers and practitioners in health promotion and have published widely in the field of health.

Health Promotion

Disciplines, diversity, and developments

Second edition

**Edited by Robin Bunton
and Gordon Macdonald**

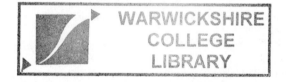

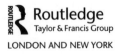 Routledge
Taylor & Francis Group

LONDON AND NEW YORK

First published 1992
by Routledge
11 New Fetter Lane, London EC4P 4EE

Simultaneously published in the USA and Canada
by Routledge
29 West 35th Street, New York, NY 10001

Reprinted 1993 (twice), 1995, 2002

Second edition first published 2002

Reprinted 2004

Routledge is an imprint of the Taylor & Francis Group

Editorial matter and selection © 1992, 2002 Robin Bunton
and Gordon Macdonald
Individual chapters © 1992, 2002 the contributors

Typeset in Sabon by
Keystroke, Jacaranda Lodge, Wolverhampton
Printed and bound in Great Britain by
Biddles Ltd, King's Lynn, Norfolk

British Library Cataloguing in Publication Data
A catalogue record for this book is available from the British Library

Library of Congress Cataloguing in Publication Data
A catalog record for this book has been requested

ISBN 0–415–23569–3 (Hbk)
ISBN 0–415–23570–7 (Pbk)

Contents

Foreword

I've always had great difficulty in explaining to my mother what I do for a living. The term *health promotion* has little currency in everyday language, and my mother's eyes quickly glaze over as I try to explain the subtle ideology that distinguishes health promotion from health education and preventive medicine, terms that are marginally more self-evident. As I struggle on I find I revert to simple slogans – helping people to improve their health, making healthy choices easy choices, and so on – generally to no avail. As a last resort, I try the Ottawa Charter definition – a process of enabling people to exert control over, and to improve their health. Personally, I still find this definition very helpful. It highlights the facts that health promotion is a process (i.e. it involves doing something!) that is enabling and empowering (i.e. done *for* and *with* people, not *on* or *to* people), and that it is directed towards *changing* health status (it is outcome focused). However, the conversation with my mother generally ends around this stage.

The subtlety and complexity inherent in the Ottawa Charter definition are both a strength and weakness of contemporary health promotion, as is superbly illustrated in this book. Although I could not recommend it to my mother, it is an excellent resource for students with an interest in strategies to improve the health of whole populations. It explores the complexities of this disarmingly simple definition, digging deep beneath the surface to examine the tangled roots of contemporary health promotion. The editors dare to suggest that from these tangled roots a distinctive discipline is emerging, with a unique contribution to make to the theory and practice of public health.

This is audacious behaviour/thinking from a field of study that is still only 20 years young. However, the editors have chosen their authors exceptionally well. The individual chapters in the book offer insightful, free-standing analyses of the diverse range of perspectives and disciplinary roots of health promotion. By bringing these perspectives together, the book as a whole offers a compelling case for the emergence of a genuinely different perspective on public health practice, and a strong case for an emerging discipline. At the heart of the debate and discussions emerging from these chapters is the differentiation between method and outcome. On the one hand, health promotion can be seen as part of a natural progression and extension of learning from experience in public health interventions, embracing the lessons of the past concerning the need to combine the actions of individuals with those of society to achieve optimal health. The focus is on taking the best combination of actions to achieve the best possible health outcomes for the community and the individual. Identifying scientifically sound solutions to measurable health problems is the base on which such action is built.

On the other hand, health promotion may be seen as having more complex and radical roots, representing a reaction to the medically dominated, individually-focused health systems that evolved in recent decades. In this context a wider set of goals which emphasize the achievement of equity, social justice, participation, and self-determination are seen as being the essential elements of health promotion.

In this context, the method of intervention in which action is taken becomes at least as important as the outcome to such action, and the outcomes themselves may not be as simply utilitarian as the greatest health gain for the greatest number – the distribution of benefit is also important.

Like all good texts, these chapters find the right balance between communication of the information that forms the knowledge base of contemporary health promotion, and an invitation to further debate and investigation of the subject. This makes the text ideal as a primary resource for students, as well as a source of inspiration and discussion for academics and practitioners and a prompt for future investigation. The revised text, with the three additional chapters, has ensured the freshness of the content and the continued relevance of the debates that are prompted by that content.

Don Nutbeam
Department of Health, London

Contributors

Amanda Amos is Senior Lecturer in Health Promotion in the Department of Community Health Sciences at the University of Edinburgh. She is Director of the MSc in Health Promotion and Health Education. Her main area of research is in smoking and tobacco control. Originally trained as a geneticist, from 1994–7 she was co-grantholder with Dr S. Cunningham-Burley of an ESRC funded study on the social and cultural impact of the new genetics.

Paul Bennett is Senior Lecturer at the University of Wales College of Medicine. He has published over 100 articles and chapters, and three books, including *Psychology and Health Promotion* (with Simon Murphy). His present research interests include the social impact of the new genetics and the use of new technology in the prevention of CHD.

Robin Bunton is Professor of Sociology at the University of Teesside. He has previously worked as researcher and practitioner in health promotion and public health fields and published widely in sociology of health. He was co-editor of the books: *The Sociology of Health Promotion: Critical Analyses of Consumption, Lifestyle and Risk* (Routledge, 1995) and *Foucault, Health and Medicine* (Routledge, 1997); and co-author of *The New Genetics and Public Health* (Routledge, 2001). He is Editor of the international journal *Critical Public Health* (Carfax).

David Cohen is Professor of Health Economics and Head of the Health Economics Unit at the University of Glamorgan. After receiving a degree in economics in 1972 from McGill University in his native Canada, David undertook postgraduate study at Edinburgh University. His interest in the economics of health began at Aberdeen University where he worked for five years as a Research Fellow at the Health Economics Research Unit. He has published widely on a variety of issues in health economics and worked on a number of committees and working parties, including the Royal College of Physicians Working Party on Preventive Medicine and the Department of Health Working Group on Cancer Genetics Service. He has acted as specialist adviser to the World Health Organization and to the House of Commons Select Committee on Welsh Affairs.

Alan Cribb is Director of the Centre for Public Policy Research, King's College London. He previously worked as a Fellow of the Centre for Social Ethics and Policy, and in the Department of Social Oncology, University of Manchester. His interests are in applied philosophy and health policy, and he is editor of *Health Care Analysis: An International Journal of Health Care Philosophy and Policy*.

Sarah Cunningham-Burley is Reader in Medical Sociology at the Department of Community Health Sciences, University of Edinburgh and Co-Director of the newly established Scottish Centre for Research on Families and Relationships (CRFR). Her research interests span the areas of the sociology of health and illness and the family, with a particular focus on lay perspectives on health, qualitative research methods, family sociology; children; young people; disability; the social context of the new genetics; the familial and relational impacts of genetic technologies and knowledge. Some of her recent publications include: Cunningham-Burley, S. and Watson, N. (eds) (2001) *Exploring the Body*, Palgrave, Basingstoke; Cunningham-Burley, S. and Kerr, A. (1999) 'Defining the Social: towards an understanding of scientific and medical discourses on the social aspects of the new genetics', *Sociology of Health and Illness*; Pavis, S., Cunningham-Burley, S., and Amos, A. (1998) 'Health Related Behavioural Change in Context: young people in transition', *Social Science and Medicine* 47 (10): 1407–18; Davis, J., Watson, N. and Cunningham-Burley, S. (2000) 'Lives of Disabled Children: A Reflexive Experience', in James, A. and Christensen, P. (eds) *Researching Children*, Falmer, Hampshire.

Peter Duncan is Director of the Postgraduate Programme in Health Education and Health Promotion, Centre for Public Policy Research, King's College London. He has worked in both academic and professional contexts, including as a Health Service Manager. His main research interests are in health promotion, ethics, and medical education. He is co-author (with Alan Cribb) of *Health Promotion and Professional Ethics* (Blackwell Science, 2002).

Janine Hale After completing an MSc in Health Economics at York University in 1994, Janine Hale joined the Health Economics Unit at the University of Glamorgan. In July 1997, she was seconded to Health Promotion Wales, with responsibility for looking at the role that health economics could play in health promotion. Janine has been the Chair of the UK Health Promotion and Health Economics forum since 1998 and has published an article looking at the potential for health economics and health promotion to work together in Health Promotion International. Since May 2001, Janine has been working in the Health Promotion Division of the National Assembly for Wales.

Dominic Harrison is the Deputy Director of the Public Health and Health Professional Unit at the University of Lancaster. He works for the Health

Development Agency (HDA) as the Regional Health Development Specialist in the North West of England. The views expressed in this article are his own and do not necessarily reflect those of the HDA or the University of Lancaster.

Craig Lefebvre received his PhD in Clinical Psychology from North Texas State University, and has held post-doctoral fellowships in behavioural medicine at the University of Virginia Medical Centre and in cardiovascular behavioural medicine research at the University of Pittsburgh. He is an Associate Professor (Research) in the Department of Community Health, Brown University, and has been the Intervention Director of the Pawtucket Heart Health Program since 1984. He has written and lectured widely on social marketing approaches to public health interventions.

Gordon Macdonald has spent 20 years in health promotion as a manager of a local service, and in management in a national agency before becoming an academic. He has published widely in the field, including co-editing *Quality, Evidence and Effectiveness in Health Promotion* (Routledge, 1998). He is Regional Editor (Europe) of *Health Promotion International* and an editorial board member of two other international health promotion journals. He has undertaken a range of consultancies for the EU, WHO and the World Bank and is currently a visiting Professor at the Karolinska Institute in Stockholm.

Simon Murphy is Principal Lecturer in Health Psychology at the Department of Psychology, University West of England and a member of the Centre for Appearance and Disfigurement Research. His research interests include explaining and predicting health-related behaviour and behaviour change, the application of psychological theory to the design and evaluation of health promotion, and public health initiatives and health inequalities.

Don Rawson was Principal Lecturer in Health Education Research at the Southbank Polytechnic, London. His interest in health promotion emerged from his research on the social psychology of decision making. At the time of writing this chapter he was studying the social representation of health actions.

Andrew Tannahill trained in community medicine (now public health medicine) in the East of Scotland before setting up a Department of Health Promotion at East Anglian Regional Health Authority. His contribution to this book was made while he was Senior Lecturer in Public Health Medicine at the University of Glasgow with teaching responsibilities in both epidemiology and health promotion. He has since worked as General Manager of the Health Education Board for Scotland.

Nicki Thorogood has worked as a Senior Lecturer in Sociology in the Health Promotion Research Unit of the London School of Hygiene and Tropical Medicine since November 1999. Prior to this she was Lecturer in Sociology at Guy's, Kings' and Thomas's Dental Institute for eight years. Her research interests are aspects of 'identity', e.g., ethnicity, gender, disability, and sexuality, particularly in relation to public health and health promotion, and in the sociology of the body. She is also currently working on the uses of everyday technologies in oral health (electric toothbrushes) with Simon Carter and Judith Green and on a multi-disciplinary project exploring 'lay' participation in food policy making processes funded by the Food Standards Agency. She is joint author, with Judith Green, of *Analysing Health Policy: Sociological Approaches* (Longmans) and they have a further book forthcoming on *Qualitative Methods for Health Research* (Sage).

Katherine Weare is a Reader in Education in the Research and Graduate School of Education. Her interests include research and development on 'settings' approach to education: she has been heavily involved in the 'Health Promoting School' movement in Europe, where she has carried out research and run training courses in over 30 countries. Her most recent work has been in Russia, helping to develop healthy school networks. She is also particularly interested in the centrality of mental health and emotional and social issues in education. She is currently carrying out a research project for the Department of Education and Skills investigating what works in promoting emotional and social competence in schools, and is writing a book on *Developing the Emotionally Literate School*, to be published by Sage in August 2002. Recent books include *Promoting Mental, Emotional and Social Health: A Whole School Approach* (Routledge, 2000).

Acknowledgements

Since the first edition of this book was published, a number of people have made helpful comments and suggestions. Students and colleagues have provided us with ideas and criticisms in the years since 1992. We are grateful to all those who have encouraged us to continue with this second edition. In particular we would like to thank Heather Gibson, previously commissioning editor at Routledge, and more recently Edwina Wellham who took over the responsibility for this project through to publication. Thanks also to colleagues at Teesside and Glamorgan Universities. Particularly, to Barbara Cox and Radha Sing who provided vital administration support and to Paul Crawshaw, Neil Meikle and others in the School of Social Sciences at Teesside for their continued support. Thanks too to Lesley Jones for reading various drafts of these re-worked chapters. Thanks also to Gina Dolan at Glamorgan who updated the glossary, and to all other colleagues who provided useful support. We would like to thank again a number of people who helped at various stages in the production of the first edition of this volume including: Lesley Jones, Sally Baldwin, and Simon Murphy for commenting on early drafts; Jenny Saunders for helping to compile the original glossary to the text. Thanks also to Jane Bennett and Eiluned Williams for their diligence and patience in typing much of the first edition. Finally, thanks to Elisabeth Tribe for her support in the production and editing of the first edition.

Introduction

Robin Bunton and Gordon Macdonald

Health promotion emerged in the 1980s and 1990s amidst considerable ferment and debate within the public health field. Debate was so intense that a new title 'the new public health' emerged to distinguish it from what went before. In one sense, it looked 'back to the future' by drawing upon the spirit of the birth of the modern public health movement in the 1840s. The last decade has seen health promotion come of age, not simply as a standardized term in academia and academic publishing but also as a practice and area of expertise within public and community health. Debate over the definition and scope of health promotion continues, but few today would challenge its centrality in public health practice or its contribution to the development of thought and theory in an evolving social model of health.

The term 'health promotion' has meant many different things to different people. To many social and political activists working to combat the social organization of ill health, it was akin to a new social movement, and a rallying point around which to fight for better health. Development was such that the 'movement' possessed significant moral force and ideological support with its catch phrases, language and values, as some critics pointed out (Stephenson and Burke 1991). To others health promotion represented a new way of addressing contemporary health and social care policy needs, and provided a strategy for health at the turn of the twenty-first century which suited new global 'neo-liberal' forms of economic organization. Many of the founding concepts in health promotion grew out of international dialogue and collaboration and the subsequent strategies were intentionally global in vision.

For yet others, health promotion was an exciting intellectual development that presented new theoretical challenges drawing upon a social, as opposed to bio-medical model of health. The possibilities for empowerment, participation, capacity building, and enhancing social capital were not simply a theoretical, values-driven endeavour, but one that had implications for methodology, research, and professional practice. Health promotion promised, uniquely, to make links between environments and behaviour, policy and participation, lifestyle and social organization, and public policy and health. This multi-focused approach was truly multi-disciplinary in nature and called for a wider cross-disciplinary and cross-professional imagination than could be found in much of the discourse on health and welfare. As key texts of the 1970s and 1980s pointed out, health and health outcomes bore little relation to the number of health professionals employed (Lalonde 1974) or the amount of services provided. The effective interventions were truly multi-sectoral. It was appropriate then, as it is now, to reflect on the intellectual and disciplinary context of health promotion.

Debate continues over definitions of health promotion, public health and population health, and the relationships between these fields. This discourse inevitably leads one to consider the origins of health promotion and its theoretical and disciplinary base. Which older, more established disciplines have had the greatest impact on theory and practice? Which sub-disciplines or fields of study are important to health promotion? Can we argue, as we do in the next chapter, that health promotion is developing into a discipline in its own right? Such questions have remained important throughout the last decade since the first edition of this text in 1992. This new edition continues to ask these questions by bringing together contributions from other disciplines to illustrate the theoretical and disciplinary roots of health promotion. The debate on the theoretical bases for health promotion interventions is now also regularly covered in relevant books and periodicals (Glanz *et al.* 1997; Macdonald 2000; McQueen 2000), but linking this to disciplinary development is the unique feature of this text.

The academic roots of health promotion lie in a variety of disciplines, some having had more influence than others. Psychology, education, epidemiology, and sociology to date have had perhaps the greatest influence on health promotion theory and practice, and might be thought of as *primary feeder disciplines*. Other disciplines such as social policy, politics, economics, ethics, philosophy, and communications have made substantial contributions but may be viewed as *secondary feeder disciplines*. An underlying and pervasive influence on health promotion development is medical science. However, we have not included this discipline in this text, apart from the chapter on epidemiology, for several reasons. One reason is that the medical contribution is acknowledged in many of the chapters, particularly the contribution of 'social medicine'. Another reason is that the place of medicine in health promotion has often been problematic and much of health promotion thinking has developed in reaction to, rather than in collaboration with, what has been depicted as the 'bio-medical model'. As health promotion enters medical curricula, this perspective may change and subsequent disciplinary collections may include such contributions.

The book's approach is designed to lay out relevant theories from all feeder disciplines and relate these to health promotion concepts, planning, and practice. In some cases the contribution to the field is more self-evident than others. Psychology's contribution is widely acknowledged, particularly as applied to health behaviour. Other disciplines have a less discernible influence, such as politics. Yet other disciplines, such as ethics and genetics, are only just beginning to influence health promotion. These three areas are included here as additions to the second edition. We have not been able to include all the disciplines that have made a contribution to health promotion development in this one volume, though we believe the more substantial ones are included. Apart from the three new chapters, most (but not all) original chapters have been updated for this edition. The complete text represents a robust collection of the disciplinary contributions relevant to current theory and practice. The book is designed to lay out some of the sources and types of theory that can be drawn upon by practitioners and researchers. We are aware that health promotion practitioners also contribute to the theory base. Such work is represented here, implicitly, in disciplinary contributions.

We have placed the contributing disciplines into parts representing *primary* and *secondary feeder* disciplines, with a third part on *reflection and developments*. The third and final part is an addition to the original text, and reflects the rapid growth within and across disciplines that informs the knowledge base to health promotion and public health. The order of these contributions is to some extent arbitrary, but roughly reflects the contribution to the field to date. We anticipate that this contribution will change over time. The current political and policy rhetoric, certainly in the UK, places emphasis on public health (as opposed to health promotion) in broad focus, and includes geographical information systems and mapping, globalization and sustainability, health consumption, social inclusion, and health impact assessment methods. Undoubtedly, such developments will have an impact on the disciplinary development of health promotion in the future.

Our discussion of the development of health promotion and the consideration of it as an emergent discipline opens this second edition. We trace the history and development of health promotion within broader public health. This development can be understood, we argue, as something similar to the broader development of disciplines, and a wider paradigm shift associated with the movement or progress of scientific knowledge more generally.

In Chapter 11 of the book however, *Rawson* argues that there is insufficient evidence to support the case for a disciplinary paradigm shift and development. Rawson is more interested in how health and health promotion relate to the philosophical understanding of scientific method, epistemology, and the search for truth. He discusses the need to ask certain fundamental questions about the development of theories in health promotion, such as how far they provide better, or more adequate 'truths' or epistemologies, as the means to improve health. In his (unrevised) paper, Rawson concludes that, even if no ready answers can be found to such questions, 'The asking will help define the subject matter and create the discipline to discover the true potential of health promotion'. This statement reflects our desire to contribute to the 'asking' and is illustrated in this second edition.

Chapter 2 by *Murphy and Bennett* examines the contribution of psychology. This chapter updates that of Bennett and Hodgson and draws upon their work which has contributed to the field (Bennett and Murphy 1997). They acknowledge the huge contribution this discipline has made and argue that psychology continues to play an important role in identifying relevant aims and objectives for health promotion and suggesting effective approaches. Traditionally, psychology has helped guide health education methods that target individuals, increasing our understanding of how effectively to influence their behaviour or behavioural change. They argue for a more sophisticated social-psychological theory, with a broader focus, that attempts to create supportive environments, develop healthy public policy, increase personal resources, and strengthen community action. A theory which acknowledges social exchange, community involvement, a holistic view of health, as well as the psychosocial aspects of health. The chapter provides a historical overview of the main psychological theories that have informed health promotion initiatives and suggests potential future developments for the application of theory to practice.

Thorogood (Chapter 3), considers the contribution of sociology to both the theory and the practice of health promotion. She points out that many sociological categories are implicit in the work of health promotion and that articulation of these will assist in making that work more effective. After a short introduction to the main sociological theoretical approaches and their key concepts, she illustrates how the sociology of health and illness continues to contribute to the field as well as providing a critique of contemporary medicine. She makes the distinction between *sociology applied to health promotion*, that is the ways in which a sociological perspective can aid the work of health promotion, and the *sociology of health promotion*, which can provide a critique itself. This enables a critical analysis to be made of such aspects of health promotion as its norms and values, its ideological underpinning and its propensity to act as social regulation.

Tannahill's chapter on epidemiology's contribution (Chapter 4), has not been revised but it still retains its originality that argued for an approach we now call social epidemiology. The first part of the chapter is devoted to more traditional epidemiological methods and ideas, but the second half critiques this tradition and argues for a more social model of disease, that firmly roots the epidemiology of health, as opposed to disease, in the health promotion camp.

In Chapter 5 *Weare* introduces the disciplinary contribution of education. She suggests that education has a central role in the realization of modern health promotion principles and goals. Education is presented as more than a mere communication of facts about health; it must also involve emotional involvement, relationships and social contexts. Education is crucial to the achievement of a reflective and empowering health promotion model, and is central to the notion that health promotion should avoid coercion. She illustrates the wide range of educational approaches and strategies and their use by health promoters and health educators. She also notes health promotion's contribution to the development of mainstream education.

In Chapter 6, *Bunton* examines the contribution the study of social policy can make to health promotion. Professing to be centrally concerned with the social policy process, most definitions of health promotion place notions of social structure and policy process at the centre of their concerns. To promote health, we need to be able to understand, analyse, and ultimately influence social and health policy. More than this, the study of social policy also contributes to our understanding of the emergence of health promotion itself. Health promotion is shown to be a response to the social and political developments of the late twentieth century and at the forefront of social and cultural change. Like sociology, as Thorogood argues in Chapter 3, social policy is a critical discipline that provides critique of health promotion and public health. Bunton points out how healthy public policies may have unintended consequences. By creating new forms of communication, co-ordination, inter-sectoral and inter-agency liaison may also introduce new types of social regulation, citizenship, and governance, bringing dangers of manipulation and social control.

Harrison in Chapter 7 introduces us to health promotion and the discipline of politics and highlights the case that politics itself is subject to the very act of defining itself. This chapter explores the broad domains of contemporary political concern as applied to health promotion and public health. The central argument here is that the political process has been transformed by globalization to the point where progressive social change is only possible through governance. In its broadest sense, this will involve alliances within civic society. Harrison argues that it is no longer tenable to view health promotion and public health as distinct territories and that health promotion, which might be placed within the broader field of health development disciplines, be located within wider concerns for 'sustainable human development'. He concludes by arguing for a 'politics of integration'. The chapter illustrates how politics – a discipline not commonly drawn upon by health promotion professionals – can help frame and shape its broader concerns.

Chapter 8 is devoted to the application of economics to health promotion and *Cohen and Hale* argue that economics can help us understand how efficiently health promotion achieves its objectives and how we might use resources in the most cost-effective manner. They point out that the economic term 'utility' can have an effect on human health behaviour, by developing a kind of individual cost-benefit approach to action. This is similar to the metaphorical way psychologists suggest we weigh up options for behaviour change through theories of planned behaviour (see Chapter 2). Alternatives to traditional cost-benefit analyses are posited but with the conclusion that economics can offer health promotion a means of determining the best cost-effective use of resources to achieve maximum health gain.

In Chapter 9 *Macdonald*, after describing aspects of communication theory more generally, concentrates on innovation diffusion theory more particularly. The principal concepts are discussed with appropriate health promotion examples. He highlights the fact that many contemporary innovation diffusion studies are concentrated in the United States and around school-based curricula take-up. Consequently much of the research and publication in this area, one that does provide health promotion with a sound and applicable theory, is somewhat culture-bound. The chapter concludes with a critique of diffusion theory, which has research method faults and which tends to implicitly fail to address issues related to equity.

Lefebvre, in Chapter 10, considers the contribution of social marketing to health promotion. In this unrevised chapter, Lefebvre discusses the role social marketing plays in organizing programmes to meet consumer needs and organizational objectives. He describes the eight characteristics of social marketing and emphasizes the point that it is not about social control, but is a tool to help problem solving during the life of a community-based programme. Through careful planning and implementation social marketing can, he argues, be a powerful strategy for social change.

The final section of the book is devoted to, in part speculation, and in part reflection. *Rawson's* Chapter 11 (discussed earlier) is perhaps more reflective and philosophical, whereas the other two chapters in this section are concerned with the growing influence ethics should have and genetics will have on health promotion and public health. *Cribb and Duncan*, in Chapter 12, point out that ethics is essentially a form of academic enquiry into what is good and right, and helps set out a form to help guide the way we ought to live. By initially setting out the key features of mainstream Western thought, deontology, and consequentialism, they provide a good basis for the rest of the chapter. They provide ample case study examples of how ethics can inform health promotion practice and decision making, and urge health promoters to feel able to justify their actions. This is particularly the case if health promotion is concerned with minimizing harm. The chapter then focuses on the principal tenets of academic writers in this field and concludes that health promoters must be able to appreciate various moral philosophical views in order to justify action. They need to appreciate that different value bases between them and their clients can lead to 'unethical interventions' and that each intervention needs to be based on sound ethical principles.

The subject of the 'new' genetics has been hotly debated across a range of health fora and also in broader public discourse. Controversy and hype surrounded the Human Genome Project at the turn of the new century. Popular media coverage heralded scientific 'breakthroughs' and explored complex moral issues which these new technologies raised for individuals and society. Whilst public health more generally has begun to engage with the broader debate, health promotion more specifically has yet to engage seriously with the issues raised by the new genetics, at the level of research, theory, and practice. *Cunningham-Burley and Amos's* chapter begins such engagement by exploring the nature of the 'new' genetics and some of the ways developments in this body of knowledge and technique are affecting our conceptions of health promotion and public health.

Since the discovery of recombinant DNA in the 1970s, interest in research into the genetic components of a range of disease, illness, and behaviour has been considerable. Prior to these developments, the application of genetics to medicine was restricted to a narrowly focused concern for relatively rare, single-gene disorders such as sickle cell disease and phenylketonuria. More recently, new technologies have led to identification of genes or markers of genes for a range of disorders. With recent improved detection and surveillance facilities, there are now opportunities to extend concerns to the 'genetic basis' of common, adult-onset disorders and more mainstream public health disease targets, potentially 'revolutionizing' public health. Recent discoveries, contingent on the ability to produce and manipulate DNA in the laboratory, has quickly led to the development of genetic tests for a range of diseases. These developments are also leading to different understandings of disease, and knowledge of the genotypes associated with specific diseases is leading to reclassifications of some diseases, such as diabetes and the promise of treatment of others. Cunningham-Burley and Amos argue that the new genetics is moving the focus from 'clinic to community', or from those in families known to be at high risk of inherited disease, to wider populations and to mainstream health care. They point out, however, that there are mixed views on the extent of the influence of the new genetics on matters of health, illness, and well being.

Although the new genetics may not yet touch health promotion practice, other than tangentially through issues relating to genetic screening for disease or disease susceptibility, it certainly raises issues that are fundamental to the core values and practices of health promotion. Health promotion, it is argued, must begin to tackle these issues for two main reasons. First, by attempting to place health promotion firmly within these recent developments, and second, by exploring potential issues for theory and practice.

This new edition of *Health Promotion* has added three new emergent disciplines to health promotion as a *developing* field of study or discipline. These three new chapters represent emerging critical themes contributing to the continued evolution of health promotion in the twenty-first century. Whilst the nomenclature of health promotion still remains contentious, there is little doubt that its contribution to wider public health developments has been substantial. It would be surprising if debate and development in this area ceased in the coming decades. For our part, we hope to continue to contribute to this exciting, dynamic, and diverse disciplinary development.

References

Bennett, P. and Murphy, S. (1997) *Psychology and Health Promotion*, Buckingham: Open University Press.

Glanz, K., Lewis, F., and Rimer, B. (1997) *Health Behaviour and Health Education: Theory Research and Practice*, San Francisco, CA: Jossey-Bass.

Lalonde, M. (1974) *A New Perspective on the Health of Canadians*, Ottawa: Information Canada.

Macdonald, G. (2000) 'A new evidence framework for health promotion practice', *Health Education Journal* 59 (1): 3–11.

McQueen, D. (2000) 'Perspectives on Health Promotion; theory, evidence, practice and the emergence of complexity', *Health Promotion International* 15 (2): 95–7.

Stevenson, H. M. and Burke, M. (1991) 'Bureaucratic logic in new social movement clothing: the limits of health promotion research', *Health Promotion International* 6: 281–96.

1   Health promotion: disciplinary developments

Gordon Macdonald and Robin Bunton

Health promotion emerged in the 1990s as a unifying concept which brought together a number of separate, even disparate, fields of study and has become an essential part of the contemporary public health. Regarded by some as the delivery vehicle or mechanism for public health, health promotion now forms an important part of the health services of most industrially developed countries and is the subject of a growing number of professional training courses and academic activities. The implications of this growth have concerned many of those involved in health and health care delivery. Some of the initial momentum for its development sprang from dissatisfaction with what was typified as the bio-medical model of health associated with focus on disease, aetiology, and clinical diagnosis. More recently, health promotion appears to be addressing the mainstream health care issues of the twenty-first century by contributing to newer approaches to health improvement, whole population programmes, health impact assessment, investment for health projects, capacity building, community planning and involvement, and perhaps most importantly, evidence-based practice. Less effort has been made, however, in considering the nature of this new form of knowledge and practice, its salient features and the likely constraints on, and possibilities for, its development. Such reflection continues to be useful for facilitating and development in the field.

This chapter is concerned with the rapid development of discourse on health promotion as a field of study and practice. It asks whether or not health promotion can legitimately be thought of as a discipline and whether we can make sense of recent changes and conceptual ferment in terms of its emergence as a discipline. Though we argue that this question is far from answered, we suggest that recent changes in the knowledge base and the practice of health promotion are characteristic of paradigmatic and disciplinary development. The process and direction of development may not always be clear. Like the development of other bodies of knowledge, it can be complex and subtle. What is clear is that a broader range of theory is being drawn into the health promotion arena and new alliances of theoretical approaches are being made. Different theories are being drawn upon in a variety of different practical orientations to produce a more varied practice. The knowledge base of health promotion would appear to be growing more multi-disciplinary, as the professional background of health promoters is becoming more varied. We might then conceive of this diversity and change as disciplinary and/or multi-disciplinary development. Before considering this, it is valuable to review the nature of health promotion, its history, and how it relates to health education and public health.

What is health promotion?

Stated simply, health promotion is a strategy for promoting the health of whole populations. This is true whether one adopts a structuralist or individual approach. Most definitions of health promotion (Tones 1983; WHO 1984; Tannahill 1985; Kickbusch 1997; Bracht 1999; Griffiths and Hunter 1999) accept that both individual (lifestyle) and structural (fiscal/ecological) elements play critical parts in any health promotion strategy. These two elements in health promotion can be divided into a number of subordinate themes. Lifestyle approaches are concerned with the identification and subsequent reduction of behavioural risk factors associated with morbidity and/or premature death. A number of the themes within it can be grouped around the idea of education in its broadest sense. Education involves the transfer of knowledge and skills from the educator to the student or learner. Knowledge improvement and attitude shift (cognitive and conative changes), health skills (behavioural changes), and the development of self-esteem are all constituent parts of these educational sub-themes. School health education curricula, stop-smoking clinics, and assertiveness training are all examples where these three educational methodologies are used in a lifestyle approach to health promotion.

Structuralist approaches to promoting health which focus on macro-social and political processes can also be divided into several sub-themes. These often centre around fiscal and legislative measures aimed at building healthy public policies, such as alcohol and cigarette taxation policies; progressive taxation policy to reduce inequalities in health, transport and agricultural policies; and ecological or environmental measures, such as waste disposal policies and urban planning. Health protection measures such as screening and immunization programmes lie between the lifestyle approach and the structuralist approach, since both service provision and behaviour change are involved. Community approaches to health promotion may, similarly, be placed between lifestyle and structuralist approaches. Health promotion is concerned then with two principal themes and a number of subordinate themes, all ultimately directed at reducing ill health and premature death.

Although having common themes, and with perhaps signs of conceptual convergence (Anderson 1984), conventional definitions of health promotion seem likely to continue to be characterized by diversity. Definitions of health promotion, like health itself, are subject to social and political influence and are, therefore, likely to vary across organizations and social contexts, making universal definition almost impossible. It might be preferable to allow a certain elasticity of definition such that each approach makes explicit its assumptions and distinguishes itself from its competitors (Simpson and Issaak 1982). Different definitions can represent different options or types of health promotion available to the health promoter according to the task or programme in hand, reflecting the variety of health promotion goals, target populations, as well as the focus and type of intervention (Rootman 1985; Raeburn and Rootman 1998). In this volume different versions of health promotion are assumed to be representative of current, and probably continued diversity in the field, rather than any inherent flaw. We feel it inappropriate in such a volume as this to attempt definitive definition. Any eventual consensus on such matters will be the outcome of developments within the field and the allied disciplines we draw together here. Attempts at definitive definition are likely to anticipate the outcome of this disciplinary process or knowledge system development, which is something we wish to avoid.

Health promotion and public health

Health promotion did not grow in a vacuum but developed largely out of health education and in tandem with the development of the 'new public health' movement of the late twentieth century. We are not concerned here with a strict chronological development of health education since that is covered more than adequately elsewhere (e.g. Sutherland 1979). Our focus is the evolution of health promotion, and the ways in which theory has emerged and interacted with practice. We refer to the different ways scientific knowledge and disciplines are developed, and relate these to recent shifts in theoretical reasoning underpinning public health debate. In order to find the conceptual roots of health promotion, we must look to the roots of public health more generally.

Dating the origins of public health is difficult, as specifying health domains by place – 'public' and 'personal' or 'private' – is a fairly recent preoccupation relating to the last 300 years or so of the rise of modern bio-medicine. Early systems of medical thought, such as those codified by Galen, linked health to the flows of humours and were closely tied to the public realm, including the movement of forces of the seasons and the universe in general. It is difficult to place notions of personal or 'private' health within such systems of thought. Movement of the cosmos was directly related to our 'internal' health and was deemed integral to the substance of our 'individual' bodies. There are, however, some precursors in early Greek and Roman thought to the distinctions now routinely made between public and personal health. For example, Hippocratic notions of endemic (always present diseases) and 'epidemic' (occasional and excessive disease) qualities are direct ancestors of the concepts used in contemporary public health and epidemiology (Porter 1998); indeed, such ideas were drawn upon in the first attempts to deal systematically with the plague. In ancient times and throughout the Middle Ages in Europe, isolation was deemed an appropriate way to regulate diseases that were seen to spread through contact. The use of the *cordon sanitaire* in seventeenth-century Europe, and much older *lazaretto* or 'pest house', became an institutionalized strategy which foreshadowed later developments in the government of health and interventions in the health of populations. The newer preventative methods of sanitation and immobilization for use in public health fit within the development of the new discourse of the Enlightenment and liberalism (Porter 1998). Contemporary concepts of public health would appear to owe much to the early modern period.

Whilst most commentators date modern public health by the first UK Public Health Act of 1848, they would also acknowledge developments in Germany and France at that time. Moreover, the early development of the field was associated with the health problems of newly industrialized cities in Northern Europe much earlier. Health in the public sphere can be related to the idea of 'social medicine', which has been closely tied to the development of greater state intervention under the doctrine of mercantilism. The early history of public health is linked to the ideas of social medicine, health administration, medical policing (*Medizinalplizie*), and social reform (Rosen 1958). More recent attempts at definition have tried to account for public health as a field of knowledge. Frenk (1993) argues that the discipline (or field of study) has constructed two major objects of analysis: the epidemiological study of the health conditions of populations, and the study of the organized social responses to these conditions. These foci correspond to two main currents of thought with their roots in the worship of Hygeia and Aesculapius (Dubos 1959). They also provide taxonomy with an analytical focus, which allows us to subdivide health research into bio-medical research (sub-individual level), clinical research (the individual level), and public health research (the population level).

Modern public health legislation in the UK emerged in the aftermath of the Poor Law Amendment Act of 1834. Edwin Chadwick was appointed to administer the new scheme and soon became aware that there was a relationship between poverty and ill health. Sickness and ill health were largely the result of bad sanitation at home (and work) and filth and poor ventilation at work. As a result, Chadwick propounded his 'sanitary idea', which was in effect the beginning of a national public health service, and gave rise to the first Public Health Act in 1848. John Simon took up Chadwick's ideas and as the first full-time salaried medical officer of health, he was instrumental in getting the second Public Health Act passed in 1872; this created local medical officers of health and led essentially to the medicalization of the public health movement. Although initially these doctors had a broad remit that included sanitation and housing, increasingly through the last quarter of the nineteenth century and the first quarter of the twentieth, their focus began to narrow as a technologically focused, hospital base gained ascendancy. The work of the Central Council for Health Education, founded in 1927, was the education arm of a service that primarily dealt with illness and disease.

Public health went through periodic reorganization in the twentieth century. Whereas nineteenth-century public health directed interventions, in the main, at environmental infrastructures that affected health, by the early twentieth century the focus had begun to shift towards individual health, with the development of comprehensive vaccination and immunization programmes. Changing social conditions at that time, as Turner has observed (1992, 1995), supported the growth of hospital-centred, specialist medicine, based upon an individually focused, fee-for-service, largely led by a growing middle-class demand for health care. This emergent health care challenged the social interventionism preferred by 'social medicine' of the turn of the twentieth century. A belief in technological progress was implicit in this period, following several major technological advances in science and medicine and improvements in surgery, drug treatments, and hospital procedures. Anaesthesia and germ theory were making advances, as were antiseptic procedures based on the work of Lister and Pasteur. There is a sense in which social medicine and the concerns for public health in the late nineteenth and early twentieth centuries were at odds with the development of scientific or 'techno-medicine'.

The so-called 'golden age' of scientific, techno-medicine is normally dated to the period 1910–50. This was a period in which the rising fortunes of the medical profession were instituted in university systems of Europe and the USA, in increasingly specialized medical education and research institutes along the lines recommended in the influential Flexner Report (1910). This golden age was substantially to influence the development of public health over the period. Interestingly, developments in micro-biology during the same period, for some leading public health progressives, heralded a 'New Public Health,' as practitioners appeared to recognize a shift in the paradigm away from the environmental or 'social' focus (Porter 1998). This earlier claim to being 'new' was in contra direction to the now more familiar 'New Public Health' movement of the late twentieth century, which advocated a renewed focus on the environment (Draper 1991).

The second half of the twentieth century, then, witnessed a return to the more traditional nineteenth-century public health approaches with concerns about structure, environment, and ecology, which rather ironically, became known again as 'the new public health'. A broader focus became apparent within clinical medicine, where the focus has been on the individual within his or her psycho-social context (Arney and Bergman 1984). Lifestyles and health behaviour became concerns of public health and clinical medicine. Patients began to be drawn into the diagnosis and treatment of disease. They became not just consumers of health services but also quasi-producers of their health status. A theoretical shift reflecting these changes can be identified which undermines more traditional oppositions between health and illness (Armstrong 1988). Health promotion has emerged against this changing theoretical backdrop.

Health promotion first appeared as a term and concept in 1974, when the Canadian Minister of National Health and Welfare, Marc Lalonde, published *A New Perspective on the Health of Canadians* (Lalonde 1974). It introduced into public policy the idea that all causes of death and disease could be attributed to four discrete and distinct elements: inadequacies in current health care provision; lifestyle or behavioural factors; environmental pollution; and finally, big physical characteristics. The basic message was that critical improvements within the environment (a structuralist approach) and in behaviour (a lifestyle approach) could lead to a significant reduction in morbidity and premature death. As a result of this report, the Canadian government shifted its emphasis in public policy away from treatment to prevention of illness, and ultimately to the promotion of health. The Lalonde report echoed the concerns of many who had become critical of a narrow view of health associated with the 'medical model'. Basaglia has expressed such sentiments, arguing that the medical model somehow separates the 'soma' from the 'psyche', the disease from the patient, and the patient from the society in which he or she lives (Basaglia 1986). The roots of this model are said to lie in scientific explanations, aetiologies, clinical diagnoses, and prognoses that ignore the far more complex social issues facing individuals in the world, such as employment (or unemployment), housing (or homelessness), and low income, or cultures engendering behaviour harmful to health.

The Lalonde report prompted a series of initiatives principally by the World Health Organization covering the next 15 years or so and beginning with the Alma Ata declaration in 1977. This declaration, by the World Health Assembly at Alma Ata in the Soviet Union, committed all member countries to the principles of Health For All (HFA 2000). Although the principal thrust of the declaration was primary health care, it incorporated a commitment to community participation and inter-sectoral action, which are now accepted elements within any serious health promotion programme. Implicit in the HFA strategy was this new vision of health promotion combining both lifestyle and structuralist approaches. WHO (Europe) launched its formal programme on health promotion using these twin supporting themes or pillars in 1984 (WHO 1984) and this programme gave rise to the first international conference on health promotion held in Ottawa, Canada, in November 1986.

The Ottawa conference concluded with the production of a charter which outlined five principal areas for health promotion action: building healthy public policy, creating supportive environments, strengthening community action, developing personal skills, and reorientating health services. These five action areas provide a useful framework for the delivery of health promotion programmes. The Ottawa Charter also included three process methodologies – mediation, enablement, and advocacy – through which people could begin to take control over their own health.

The second international conference on health promotion was held in Adelaide, Australia, in April 1988 and it concentrated more on healthy public policy as an arm of health promotion and delineated certain policy priorities.

These were policies supporting the health of women, nutrition policies, policies on alcohol and tobacco, and policies concerned with the environment. Underpinning these priority areas were the twin concepts of health equity and policy accountability but also an implicit assumption that somehow only central government policy making had any real effect on measures for health promotion (WHO 1988).

The third international conference in Sundsvall, Sweden, in June 1991, focused on 'Supportive Environments for Health'. Specifically, it attempted to find practical ways to create physical, social, and economic environments for health compatible with sustainable development. It produced a handbook on action to improve public health and the environment (WHO 1991).

The fourth WHO international conference on health promotion was held in Jakaarta in 1997. It recognized the need to bring 'new players' into the health promotion arena in order to rekindle thinking and the theory base for practice. However, the 'Declaration' made plain health promotion's continued commitment to alliances for health but at the global level, arguing that many health issues such as tobacco, HIV, environmental pollution, and food safety – recognize no national boundaries and need international alliances to address them (WHO 1997).

The fifth and most recent conference in Mexico City in 2000 issued a Ministerial Statement (Editorial, *Health Promotion International*, 2000) which reiterated health promotion's role in tackling health improvement and development but added both a call for research to demonstrate effectiveness dimension and a call for UN agencies to attempt health impact assessment in their development agenda.

The work of WHO has paralleled attempts of policy makers, practitioners, and researchers to develop newer models of achieving health symbolized by the launch of the Verona Initiative in Europe (WHO/EURO 1998). Initiatives have also been taken outside the World Health Organization (e.g. within the World Bank). Alongside these international developments, individual countries appear to have been shoring up the health promotion and public health arms of policy making in the 1990s and early twenty-first century. In the UK, for example, the Labour government has pursued a policy direction that has privileged public health initiatives. A series of policy statements and discussion documents have recognized that health is dependent upon social, economic, and environmental factors as well as lifestyle factors (White Papers on the future of the NHS in the UK [DoH 1997; SODH 1997] and Green Papers on health improvement, *Our Healthier Nation* [DoH 1998] and *Working Together for a Healthier Scotland* [SODH 1998]). Policy initiatives (such as Health Action Zones) have attempted to redress inequalities in health and tried to develop intersectoral collaboration and community participation (Judge and Bould 2001). The focus on health improvement, rather than illness prevention, is significant in this respect.

Health promotion then probably preceded the late twentieth-century 'new public health' movement etymologically, though development in the two fields are inextricably linked. Health promotion in the UK grew out of the legacy, albeit a narrow one, of health education. Sutherland (1979) points out that health education in the UK really started with the establishment of the Central Council for Health Education in 1927. This body had two principal functions or aims:

> First to promote and encourage education . . . in the science and art of healthy living [and, second], to coordinate the work of all statutory bodies in carrying out their powers and duties under the Public Health Acts . . . relating to the promotion . . . of Public Health.

Unfortunately, health education confined itself in the main to the first, largely lifestyle, function and neglected the second, largely structuralist, issue. Health promotion in the last 20 years or so has attempted to fill that gap. It is worth noting, however, that health education in turn did not develop in a vacuum but emerged as a consequence of the public health measures of the late nineteenth and early twentieth centuries.

Health promotion has, then, developed alongside public movements – old and new. Health promotion contributed to, and formed part of the late twentieth-century 'new public health' movement and continues to contribute to national and international development in the related fields of public health and healthy public policy. Health promotion, characterized as a new body of expertise or 'new science' (McQueen 1988), was been informed by concepts and principles, largely, but not exclusively derived from the social and behavioural sciences. Just as health education has been integrated and brought into health promotion (Downie *et al.* 1996), it is suggested here that health promotion contributes to and becomes a part of the new public health. This 'new science' might continue to develop and identify diverse approaches to aetiology, assessment formulation, intervention, evaluations, and the analysis of the process of behavioural change. The growing influence and contribution of other disciplines within health promotion will contribute to the broader concerns of public health. Both individualist and structuralist perspectives within health promotion will also contribute to these broader concerns. This account of conceptual development draws largely upon developments in Europe and North America. Clearly, concepts of health promotion in other parts of the world, and the south in particular, will vary (Morley *et al.* 1986), and some commentators have criticized the 'eurocentric' nature of much health promotion thinking and practice (MacDonald 1998). Discursive development in health promotion can be seen to be heavily dependent upon work in the northern hemisphere.

Disciplinary development and change

Dictionary definitions of disciplines refer to their function to train or discipline scholars, introducing them to the 'proper action by instruction, exercising them in the same method and moral training' (*Shorter Oxford Dictionary*

1985). A discipline then involves an ordered area or field of study, and it is this definition we use when we refer to disciplinary contributions to health promotion. In this book we use the term 'discipline' to refer to bounded groups or federations of theories, perspectives, and methods associated with an area of study. Our concern is how disciplines or bodies of knowledge develop and change, and how their development takes place alongside other disciplinary developments. The nature of the development and change in bodies of knowledge and disciplines has become an identifiable field of study in itself which should be referred to here.

The work of Thomas Kuhn has often been used as a starting point to describe the ways in which scientific bodies of knowledge change, using the notion of a paradigm or disciplinary matrix. Kuhn's concept of scientific paradigm – a kind of licensed way of seeing, describing, and acting upon the world – provides an image of the subject matter of a discipline and levels of agreement on how scientific study should proceed. Such a notion has been described by others using the terms 'epistemic communities' (Holzner and Marx 1979) or 'thought collectives' (Fleck 1979). Like others, Kuhn has emphasized that the ideas, concepts, and theories of a scientific community are the outcome of collective effort and therefore subject to social and cultural influence. They will change and be transformed according to changes elsewhere in society. The routine grounds of scientific procedure are subject to change and modification. Kuhn draws our attention to periods of revolution and change, when the main features of the paradigm – those that order and organize a body of knowledge – undergo change.

Kuhn described three basic stages of scientific development: a pre-paradigm stage in which several theories compete for dominance; a period of 'normal' science, when a single paradigm has gained wide acceptance and provides the primary structuring of the field; and a crisis stage during which one paradigm is replaced by another. The development of physics can been used to illustrate this. Prior to Newtonian physics, there existed several competing systems of thought – the pre-paradigmatic stage. Newtonian thought provided a paradigm that replaced previous thought and provided an extended period of 'normal science'. This stage entered a period of crisis followed by the emergence of a new paradigm influenced by Einstein and Bohr (Kuhn 1962, 1970).

Kuhn's account suggests that once a revolution in thought has been achieved, it is followed by a more stable period in which the incremental growth typical of normal science is more usual. However, it is likely that the development of bodies of knowledge is more complex than this, involving, simultaneously, incremental growth as well as searches for new ordering principles that would restructure a paradigm. Moreover, many sciences or disciplines lack a single overarching paradigm and may be more accurately seen as multi-paradigmatic fields (Ritzle 1975). It is apparent that new ways of thinking frequently run alongside older systems, with a branching or segmented development (Holton 1973; Bucher and Stelling 1970). As different branches continue to develop, the boundaries of disciplines are permeated and new disciplines emerge.

More recent studies in the sociology of scientific knowledge have paid attention to the broader social and technical infrastructures of disciplinary development, as well as the 'interests' involved in knowledge system development (Latour 1986, 1993). Such work has highlighted the ways in which scientific and technical knowledge systems are situated within broader networks of actors, involving for example: funding bodies, academic institutions, professional associations, private industry sponsorship, government bodies, scientific governance procedures, ethical committees, community groups, and pressure groups. Though there is great variety in the study of scientific and technological innovaton and change, most contemporary approaches agree that the introduction of new knowledge technology involves social, economic, political, as well as technological processes and that technology develops hand in hand with new sets of social relationships. Similarly, health promotion and public health knowledge systems form part of a complex network of relationships, crossing the public and private realms and involving the state, citizen and corporate actors, as well as constituting an academic discipline and a field of practice. Disciplines, scientific knowledge, and techniques often make these relationships appear fixed beyond question – even natural to a point where one can forget the social context that supports a particular knowledge system.

The recent development of newer geno-technologies illustrates the potential complex negotiation between large numbers of actors in one field. Private industry and academics are working alongside national and internal government bodies to map the human genome – sometimes in competition, sometimes in co-operation. Private interests and those of consumers may collide as governments, patenting authorities, and others respond to issues of ethics (Nielson 1999). Resulting development in knowledge, research, and practice is having an effect on the conception of fundamental aspects of public health, including the nature of the environment, the host, and agent (Zimmern 1999; Petersen and Bunton 2002) and the disciplinary structure itself (Kerr *et al.* 1997). Knowledge and technique developed in this are raising critical questions for health promotion too, as Amos and Cunningham-Burley illustrate in this volume. Development of health promotion and the new public health can be seen to have occurred within larger global socio-political networks. More traditional concerns of public health and health education have run alongside the emergence and development of health promotion and 'the new' public health. New objects of study, such as health behaviour, have emerged, whilst more traditional health education research has continued. New types of theories have been developed, drawing on different combinations of disciplines, or even new ones, whilst more traditional theory is still being used.

In recent years, there has been increasing debate about the theoretical roots of health promotion (McQueen 2000; Poland *et al.* 2000; Macdonald 2000), about the evidence base underpinning practice (Perkins *et al.* 1999; Speller *et al.* 1997; Nutbeam 1999), and a concern for quality assurance (Davies and Macdonald 1998). Such debate might be indicative of the growth of health promotion as a field for study for academics and practitioners from diverse disciplinary backgrounds. We could argue that this is also evidence of an emerging discipline. Recent years have witnessed increasing work building the disciplinary infrastructure, directed at ordering the principles of public health and of health education/promotion. This work has resulted in considerable conceptual development characteristic of periods of paradigm change and revolution. It is probably also fair to say that this period of rapid theoretical and conceptual change is not yet over.

In referring to these developments, we are not suggesting that such bodies of knowledge are sciences, but merely that they show some similarities in their development and production. Knowledge production relating to areas of systematic organized enquiry has become increasingly important in the latter part of the twentieth century. The complex manner in which forms of knowledge are produced, organized, distributed, and applied are key features of what has been characterized as 'post-modern society' (Holzner and Marx 1979). Marked advances in information-handling capability, advanced communication techniques, and in particular the development of electronic information systems, have changed the nature of social and institutional organization and have had a profound influence on our cultural system. The institutionalizing of technological knowledge and professional expertise has become a key social policy issue (Burrows and Pleace 2000, Keble and Loader 2001).

Nowhere is this more apparent than in health care where dependence upon highly differentiated specialized bodies of knowledge and specialized occupations or professions is at a premium. Health promotion has developed within the post-war period when the institutional structure of the health care delivery system, in the West at least, has grown dramatically in size and complexity. The development of bodies of knowledge surrounding health promotion should be seen within this development and within the tendency towards systematizing of professional knowledge in general.

It may be possible to draw a distinction between the scholarly or scientific bodies of knowledge and the practising disciplines (Freidson 1970) as well as the professional groups that staff them. Most professional groups have made efforts to systematize, codify, and organize their bodies of knowledge. Not all would be considered as 'scientific' disciplines, though a move towards this hallowed status is discernible. The professional production of knowledge has developed hand in hand with the organization into disciplines within the university system, along with the production of a series of disciplinary ideologies. The health disciplines are no exception to this and their development may be viewed from within this system. Foucault's work has shed light on the history of human sciences, including medicine (Foucault 1970, 1973) and can be usefully drawn upon here. Analysing the emergence and development of a number of bodies of knowledge or 'discursive formations', he has identified a tendency towards systematization and self-reflection (Foucault 1973).

Disciplinary and scientific development

Some bodies of knowledge discursive formations achieve what Foucault (1970) has called 'scientificity'. There is no inevitability about development towards this, and other types of systematized knowledge have emerged without subsequent development, yet still involving degrees of codification and formalization. There is no uniform, simple trajectory or evolutionary system as suggested by Kuhn (the authors' epistemological assumptions are in fact fundamentally different). Development is characterized by discontinuity and irregularity, dependent upon a number of social, political, and organizational forces. Forms of knowledge, Foucault argues, emerge within institutional arrangements and are subject to a number of influences. Because of this, there are difficulties in distinguishing forms of knowledge and practice. In the public health field these distinctions are particularly difficult to make as the research and theoretical knowledge base has developed in interaction with health education/promotion practice. Practitioners have probably far outnumbered researchers and academics in the field. Moreover, this practice has been carried out by an extremely wide group of professions. The knowledge base has emerged (and is emerging) from a number of different sites. The emergence of psychopathology in France in Foucault's account shows some similarities with public health development (Foucault 1967).

The construction of objects of psychiatric investigation in eighteenth- and nineteenth-century France was dependent upon a whole number of conditions, including the existence of other discourses. Relationships between attendants of the insane and physicians, families, occupations, entrepreneurs, religious communities, and the local authorities all came to bear on the specific way psychotherapeutic concepts emerged. All these networks influenced the way people became classified as mad or sane. In the eighteenth century this complex of forces allowed certain authorities to designate madness a legitimate object of enquiry. By the end of the nineteenth century, medicine emerged as the dominant authority in delimiting this problem – though it was not the only one. It was primarily this medical authority which, by systems of referral, classification of behaviour and people, was able to build an institutional network that resulted in the development of asylums and attendant caring professions. The development of these institutions led to more clearly differentiated specification of the mad and sub-groups of the mad as well as appropriate treatment regimes.

The body of knowledge known as psychopathology, then, cannot be reduced to a gradually discovered set of objects of study to be conceptualized and classified. This knowledge was produced in mutual interdependence with the behaviour of families, the legal procedures, courts of law, and the mentally ill themselves. This analysis suggests ways of viewing the current development of the body of knowledge or discursive formation of health promotion.

To picture the emergence of health promotion as a body of knowledge, a discipline, or set of disciplines, we must look to: the institutions that practise and teach it; the professions that are involved in furthering its development; the political, social, and policy contexts in which it thrives or struggles; the different health cultures that exist to influence and draw upon it; as well as the bordering disciplines that feed, compete with, and influence its existence. A description of theoretical development within health promotion should take account of all of these features. The development of public health as a system of institutions, government functions, and set of related professions can be viewed in a somewhat similar manner. The complex network of public health and health promotion relationships crosses the public and private realms, involves the state and citizens, corporate actors, professionals and academic researchers as well as a range of field practitioners. The systems of knowledge we know as health promotion and public health are formed in these networks. Attempts to systematize and order these fields of study or disciplines often run up against 'interested parties' and create conflict. The knowledge base represents such interests, including professional processes.

Professional implications

Change in the knowledge base or paradigm of health promotion has been possible only through the efforts of those working within health promotion and public health. Equally, further change will have profound implications for those working in these fields. The structure of bodies of knowledge and the boundaries between different domains of study affect working experience, professional identity, and inter-professional relationships. Disciplines and bodies of knowledge are part of the major socializing mechanisms of the professions. Systems of selection, induction, graduation, and career channelling instil motivational commitments and forms of professional identity. Particular professional careers often possess their own distinctive heroic images and role models. Even within disciplines there may be sub-identities, associated with specific segments – medical sub-specialities being a case in point (Bucher and Stelling 1970).

The form of knowledge will mediate and regulate experience, identity, and working relationships. It follows that changes in this form of knowledge will change and disrupt these experiences, professional identities, and working relationships. Transmission of knowledge has specific effects. Modern concepts of health and disease, which underlie the physician's role, are represented in the medical school curriculum, for example (Armstrong 1977; Atkinson 1981). Certain curricula invite strong professional allegiance by rigidly classifying the different subjects and allowing little cross-over between topics during training. Other curricula encourage the mixing of different disciplines and expect less subject or professional identity until later in careers.

Bernstein (1971) has typified the English and the American education systems, respectively, in this way. Rigid division within a body of knowledge, such as medicine, psychiatry, or general practice, may reflect and perpetuate inter-professional differences.

Recent changes in government policy in the UK may help to break down historical divisions in the training and education of health promotion and public health professionals. The 'Our Healthier Nation' White Paper(1997) and its progeny, including a policy document on workforce developments (DoH 2000) indicated a commitment to multi-disciplinary training and new roles for public health specialists at local and national levels. This will inevitably lead to a new emergent disciplinary base to the training, and one that recognizes the multi-disciplinarity of public health and health promotion.

These changes in conceptual structures within the new public health and health promotion fields will require a realignment of professional loyalties. The reorientation of health services referred to in the Ottawa Charter requires a reorientation in the ways health carers and promoters relate to one another. New working relationships and allegiances will need to develop to work to a new theoretical framework. New cross-disciplinary alliances may be formed to develop particular areas of study. Marketers, for example, may ally with public health medicine to work as social marketers. These new alliances will raise questions of professional identity. Are the doctors, nurses, psychologists, and sociologists working in this field still identified as such or do they call themselves health promoters? Will courses in health promotion and public health stand as a post-qualification training or will they stand as a recognizable training in themselves? Attempts at addressing this are evident in the recent White Papers produced by the UK government but they will clearly bear on the nature of the development of health promotion as a discipline.

The current change and ferment in the health promotion field are suggestive of disciplinary development and formation. Alternatively, this development may be seen as part of a more general tendency towards multi-disciplinarity in the medical and other academic fields, representing a post-modernization of the curriculm (Turner 1990). A feature of the new public health and of health promotion is a much broader focus than either public health or health education. Again this is evident in publications and policy papers produced by academics and governments across the developed world in the last decade or so. A broad conception of the health field was established early (Lalonde 1974; Green and Anderson 1986) and was more recently developed (Kickbusch and de Leeuw 1999; Labonte 1993). With such a breadth of focus – human biology, environment, lifestyle, and health care organization – a broad disciplinary input is highly appropriate.

Social science has played a major, even cathartic role in developing the current range of concepts used, broadening the knowledge and practice base of health promotion. Sociology and psychology in particular have made significant contributions, positing theories of behaviour related to health by reference to social constructs. Social psychological reasons for morbidity and individual health action have been put forward by some (Rosenstock 1974; Fishbein 1967; Festinger 1957; Bandura 1977; Marks *et al.* 2000), whilst explanations referring to social structures and macro-processes as determinants of health have been emphasized by others (Doyal 1979; Hart 1985; Aggleton 1990; O'Neill 1983; Donati 1988; Wilkinson 1996; Marmot and Wilkinson 1999).

These social sciences have drawn the interest of other disciplines in health promotion, most notably education (Campbell 1985), economics (Maynard *et al.* 1989), and communication theory (Green 1980). These, along with sociology, psychology, and epidemiology, may be called primary feeder disciplines in that they have made a major and direct contribution to health promotion theory (and practice) but they are increasingly supported by secondary feeder disciplines whose contribution is at present less obvious. These would include ethics and philosophy, social policy, genetics, and marketing. All these primary and secondary feeder disciplines are given space in this book in an attempt to demonstrate the breadth of health promotion theory. They consolidate what for many has been a growing, even irritating, feeling that the bio-medical model of health promotion no longer offers an adequate explanation of why people think and behave in the way they do.

Adoption of a multi-disciplinary approach to health promotion could avoid such a blinkered approach and may be more appropriate to the health issues of the late twentieth century. Multi-disciplinarity may be, in part, an answer to criticism aimed at bio-medically orientated health promotion. The current development of the knowledge base might be able to draw more fruitfully on feeder disciplines – primary and secondary.

Summary

Health promotion is an important and vital force in the new public health movement. Recent development in health promotion and public health has been rapid, fitting within broader shifts in medicine and health policy in the twentieth and early twenty-first centuries. Within this change, health promotion may be seen to be developing both independently and in inter-action with the public health movement. Such rapid change is characteristic of paradigm shifts within bodies of knowledge and the emergence of new disciplinary alliances or even new disciplines. Given this, we might predict significant development of health promotion knowledge and practice along the lines of disciplinary formation. It is, however, still too early to predict the outcome of this development. Disciplinary development is a complex and often subtle process and dependent on a large number of social, political, and inter-disciplinary factors. Moreover, paradigm shifts are not usually definitive or conclusive. More typically they occur along a continuum of change.

Much is at stake during periods of change. Professional power and identities are profoundly influenced by changes in their knowledge base. The appropriateness of a medical role in health promotion and public health may continue to be debated. Issues of professional co-ordination and leadership may be, indeed are being, discussed.

Adding to the complexity of current ferment within the health promotion field is the contribution to be made from a wide variety of disciplines. This is particularly important within the current concern for efficiency, effective use of resources, and the construction of an appropriate evidence base for health promotion practice. Whilst social science has played an important part in these recent developments, other disciplines also have a contribution to make. Another road for development is increased inter-disciplinarity within health promotion and public health; in which case the contributions from the variety of contributors to this volume will be especially relevant. If multi-disciplinarity is to be a feature of health promotion of the future, there is a need to consider the health promotion disciplines together in one volume.

References

Aggleton, P. (1990) *Health*, London: Routledge.

Anderson, R. (1984) 'Health promotion: an overview', *European Monographs in Health Education Research* 6: 1–126.

Armstrong, D. (1977) 'The structure of medical education', *Medical Education* 11: 244–8.

—— (1988) 'Historical origins of health behaviour', in R. Anderson, J. Davies, I. Kickbusch, D. McQueen, and R. Turner (eds) *Health Behaviour Research and Health Promotion*, Oxford and New York: Oxford University Press.

Arney, W. A. and Bergman, B. J. (1984) *Medicine and the Management of Living*, Chicago: Chicago University Press.

Atkinson, P. (1981) *The Clinical Experience: The Construction and Reconstruction of Medical Reality*, Farnborough: Gower.

Bandura, A. (1977) *Social Learning Theory*, Englewood Cliffs, NJ: Prentice-Hall.

Basaglia, F. O. (1986) 'The changing culture of health and the difficulties of public health to cope with it', in *Vienna Dialogue on Health Policy and Health Promotion – Towards a New Conception of Public Health*, Eurosocial Research and Discussion Papers, European Social Development Programme.

Bernstein, B. (1971) 'On the classification and training of educational knowledge', in M. F. D. Young (ed.) *Knowledge and Control*, London: Collier Macmillan.

Bracht, N. (ed.) (1999) *Health Promotion at the Community Level*, Thousand Oaks, CA: Sage.

Bucher, R. and Stelling, J. (1970) 'Professions in process', in J. A. Jackson (ed.) *Professions and Professionalization*, London: Cambridge University Press.

Bunton, R. and Petersen, A. (2002) 'Genetics, governance and ethics', *Critical Public Health*, special issue.

Bunton, R., Nettleton, S., and Burrows, R. (eds) (1995) *The Sociology of Health Promotion: Critical Analyses of Consumption, Lifestyle and Risk*, London: Routledge.

Burrows, R. and Pleace, N. (2000) (eds) *Wired Welfare. Discussion Document*, York: University of York, Centre for Housing Studies.

Campbell, G. (ed.) (1985) *New Directions in Health Education*, London: Palmer.

Chave, S. P. (1986) 'The origins and development of public health', *Oxford Textbook of Public Health*, Vol. 1, Milton Keynes: Open University Press.

Davies, J. K. and Macdonald, G. (1998) *Quality, Evidence and Effectiveness in Health Promotion: Striving for Certainties*, London: Routledge.

Department of Health (1997) *Our Healthier Nation*, London: HMSO.

—— (2000) *A Health Service for all Talents; Developing the NHS Workforce*, London: DoH.

Donati, P. (1988) 'The need for new social policy perspectives in health behaviour research', in R. Anderson, J. Davies, I. Kickbusch, D. McQueen, and D. Turner (eds) *Health Behaviour Research and Health Promotion*, Oxford and New York: Oxford University Press.

Downie, R. S., Tannahill, C., and Tannahill, A. (1996) *Health Promotion: Models and Values*, Oxford: Oxford University Press.

Doyal, L. (1979) *The Political Economy of Health*, London: Pluto.

Draper, P. (1991) *Health through Public Policy: The Greening of Public Health*, London: Greenprint.

Dubos, R. J. (1959) *Mirage of Health*, New York: Harper & Bros.

Festinger, L. (1957) *A Theory of Cognitive Dissonance*, Stanford, CA: Stanford University Press.

Fishbein, M. (1967) 'Attitude and the prediction of behaviour', in M. Fishbein (ed.) *Readings in Attitude Theory and Measurement*, New York: Wiley.

Fleck, L. (1979) *Genesis and Development of Scientific Fact*, Chicago: University of Chicago Press.

Foucault, M. (1967) *Madness and Civilization*, London: Allen Lane.

—— (1970) *The Archaeology of Knowledge*, London: Tavistock.

—— (1973) *The Birth of the Clinic*, London: Tavistock.

Freidson, E. (1970) *Profession of Medicine: A Study of the Sociology of Applied Knowledge*, New York: Dodd, Mead.

Frenk, J. (1993) 'The New Public Health,' *Annual Review of Public Health* 14: 459–90.

Green, L. W. (1980) *Health Education Planning: A Diagnostic Approach*, Palo Alto, CA: Mayfield.

—— and Anderson, C. L. (1986) *Community Health*, 5th edition, St Louis, MO: Times Mirror/Mosby.

Griffiths, S. and Hunter, D. (eds) (1999) *Perspectives in Public Health*, Abingdon: Radcliffe Medical Press.

Hart, N. (1985) *The Sociology of Health and Medicine*, Ormskirk: Causeway Press.

Holton, G. (ed.) (1973) *Modern Sciences and the Intellectual Tradition: Thematic Origins of Scientific Thought*, Cambridge, MA: Harvard University Press.

Holzner, B. and Marx, J. H. (1979) *Knowledge Application*, Boston, MA: Allyn & Bacon.

Judge, K. and Bauld, L. (2001) 'Strong Theory Flexible Methods: evaluating complex community initiatives' *Critical Public Health* Vol II, No 1, 2001.

Keble, L. and Loader, B. D. (eds) (2001) '*Community Informatics*, London: Routledge.

Kerr, A., Cunningham-Burley, S., and Amos, A. (1997) 'The new genetics: professionals' discursive boundaries', *Sociological Review* 45: 279–303.

Kickbusch, I. (1997) 'Think health; what makes the difference?' *Health Promotion International* 12(4): 265–72.

Kickbusch, I. and de Leeuw, E. (1999) 'Global public health: revisiting healthy public policy at the global level', *Health Promotion International* 14(4): 285–88.

Kuhn, T. S. (1962) *The Structure of Scientific Revolutions*, Chicago: University of Chicago Press.

—— (1970) *The Structure of Scientific Revolutions*, revised edition, Chicago: University of Chicago Press.

Labonte, R. (1993) 'A holosphere of healthy and sustainable communities', *Australian Journal of Public Health* 17: 4–12.

Lalonde, M. (1974) *A New Perspective on the Health of Canadians*, Ottawa: Information Canada.

Latour, B. (1987) *Science in Action*, Milton Keynes: Open University Press.

—— (1993) *We Have Never Been Modern*, Hemel Hempstead: Harvester Wheatsheaf.

Latour, B. and Woolar, S. (1986) *Laboratory Life* 2nd edition, Princeton, NJ: Princeton University Press.

Macdonald, G. (2000) 'A new evidence framework for health promotion practice', *Health Education Journal* 59: 3–11.

MacDonald, T. (1998) Rethinking Health Promotion: a Global Approach, London: Routledge.

McQueen, D. V. (1988) 'Thoughts on the ideological origins of health promotion', *Health Promotion*, Oxford: Oxford University Press.

—— (2000) 'Perspectives on health promotion: theory evidence, practice and the emergence of complexity', *Health Promotion International* 15: 95–7.

Marks, D., Murray, M., Evans, B., and Willig, C. (2000) *Health Psychology; Theory Research and Practice*, London: Sage.

Marmot, M. and Wilkinson, R. (1999) *Social Determinants of Health*, Oxford: OUP.

Maynard, A., Godfrey, C., and Hardman, G. (1989) *Priorities for Health Promotion – An Economic Approach*, York: Centre for Health Economies, University of York.

Morley, D., Rohde, J., and Williams, G. (1986) *Practising Health for All*, Oxford: Oxford University Press.

Mumford, L. (1934) *Technics and Civilization*, New York: Harcourt Brace.

Nielson, L. (1999) 'The Icelandic health sector data base: legal and ethical considerations', in T. A. Caulfield and B. Williams-Jones (eds) *The Commercialization of Genetic Research: Ethical, Legal, and Policy Issues*, New York, Boston, Dordrecht, London, Moscow: Kluwer/Plenum Publishers.

Nutbeam, D. (1999) 'The challenge to provide "evidence" in health promotion', *Health Promotion International* 14: 99–101.

O'Neill, P. (1983) *Health Crisis 2000*, London: Heinemann.

Perkins, E., Simnett, I., and Wright, L. (eds) (1999) *Evidence Based Health Promotion*, Chichester: John Wiley.

Peterson, A. and Bunton, R. (2002) *The New Genetics and the Public's Health* London: Routledge.

Poland, B., Green, L., and Rootman, I. (eds) (2000) *Settings for Health Promotion: Linking Theory to Practice*, Thousand Oaks, CA: Sage.

Porter, D. (1998) 'Public health', in W. F. Brynum and R. Porter (eds) *Companion Encyclopedia of the History of Medicine*, vol. 2, London: Routledge.

Raeburn, J. and Rootman, I. (1998) *People Centred Health Promotion*, Chichester: John Wiley.

Ritzle, G. (1975) *Sociology: A Multiparadigm Science*, Boston, MA: Allyn & Bacon.

Rootman, I. (1985) 'Using health promotion to reduce alcohol problems,' in M. Grant (ed.) *Alcohol Policies*, Copenhagen: WHO.

Rosen, G. (1958) *A History of Public Health*, New York: MD Publications.

Rosenstock, I. M. (1974) 'Historial origins of the health belief model', *Health Education Monographs* 2: 409–19.

Scottish Office Department of Health (1997) *The Scottish Health Service. Ready for the Future*, Edinburgh: Stationery Office.

—— (1998) *Working Together for a Healthier Scotland*, Edinburgh: Stationery Office.

Simpson, R. and Issaak, S. (1982) *On Selecting a Definition of Health Promotion. A Guide for Local Planning Bodies*, Toronto: Addiction Research Foundation.

Speller, V., Learmonth, A., and Harrison, D. (1997) 'The search for evidence of effective health promotion', *British Medical Journal*, 315, 361–63.

Sutherland, I. (ed.) (1979) *Health Education Perspectives and Choices*, London: Allen & Unwin.

Tannahill, A. (1985) 'What is health promotion?', *Health Education Journal* 44(4): 167–8.

Tones, B. K. (1983) *Education and Health Promotion: New Directions*, Institute for Health Education, Vol. 21: 121–31.

Turner, B. S. (1992) *Regulating Bodies*, London: Routledge.

—— (1995) *Medical Knowledge and Social Power*. 2nd edition, London: Sage.

Turner, B. (1990) 'The interdisciplinary curriculum: from social medicine to postmodernism', *Sociology of Health and Illness* 12(1): 241–8.

Wilkinson, R. (1996) *Unhealthy Societies: the Afflictions of Inequalities*, London: Routledge.

WHO (World Health Organization) (1984) *Health Promotion: European Monographs in Health and Health Education*, 6, Copenhagen: WHO.

—— (1985) *Health Promotion: A Discussion Document on the Concept and Principles*, Copenhagen: WHO.

—— (1988) *The Adelaide Recommendations: Healthy Public Policy*, Copenhagen: WHO/EURO.

—— (1991) *To Create Supportive Environments for Health. The Sundsvall Handbook*, Geneva: WHO.

Winslow, C. E. (1920) 'The untilled fields of public health', 51, *Science* 23: 30.

Zimmern, R. (1999) 'Genetics', in S. Griffiths and D. J. Hunter (eds) *Perspectives in Public Health*, Oxon: Radcliffe Medical Press.

Part I
Primary disciplines

2 Psychology and health promotion

Simon Murphy and Paul Bennett

Introduction

Health promotion has historically drawn on many disciplines and knowledge bases to inform its practice, but it has generally been acknowledged that psychology has been the most important contributor discipline and one which helps to operationalize strategies (Bennett and Murphy 1997; Bennett *et al.* 1995). This is illustrated by models of health promotion that have clearly drawn on psychological theory. Green *et al.* (1980), for example, propose the PRECEDE model of behaviour. The model suggests three factors that effect behaviour change: predisposing, enabling, and reinforcing. The first of these influences an individual's motivation and includes attitudes, beliefs, and values. The second either encourages or discourages behaviour and includes external cues or barriers. The third refers to the reinforcement or rewards that the individual receives from the behaviour change. As such it explicitly draws on psychological theories that include the health belief model and social learning theory. In fact, the primacy accorded psychological theory has provided a strong theoretical basis to the development and implementation of some of the most important evaluative programmes that have been conducted (e.g. Maccoby 1988; Puska *et al.* 1985).

Psychology can therefore play an important role in identifying relevant aims and objectives for health promotion and suggesting effective approaches. Despite this, health promotion interventions have frequently been criticized for being atheoretical or for using inappropriate psychological theory (Bunton *et al.* 1991; Bennett and Murphy 1997). This has led to calls for a more rigorous application of psychological theories within health promotion evaluation designs (Schaalma *et al.* 1996) and for an increased role for psychology in informing approaches that focus on physical and social environments and psycho-social aspects of health (Bennett and Murphy 1997).

It could be argued that psychology has traditionally been viewed as a discipline that has guided health education approaches that target individuals and which increases our understanding of how to influence them effectively in regard to behaviour change. We would argue that a more sophisticated view of psychological theory is needed in the light of strategies that aim to create supportive environments, develop healthy public policy, increase personal resources, and strengthen community action (WHO 1991) – one that acknowledges social exchange, community involvement, and a holistic view of health. This chapter therefore provides both a historical overview of the main psychological theories that have been utilized within health promotion initiatives and suggests potential future developments for the application of theory to practice.

Communication theories

The earliest health promotion initiatives adopted a 'hypodermic' model of behavioural change (Bennett and Murphy 1997), the roots of which can be found in theories of mass communication developed in the 1950s and 1960s, at Yale University in particular. These approaches assumed a relatively stable link between knowledge, attitudes, and behaviours. Therefore if information could be provided in a sufficiently persuasive manner and from appropriate sources, this would engender attitudinal change, which would in turn directly result in behavioural change. The assumption of a strong knowledge–attitude–behaviour link has been challenged by research and the relative ineffectiveness of programmes based on this premise. The limits of mass media campaigns are illustrated by Wimbush *et al.* (1998), who assessed the effect of a mass media campaign in Scotland designed to promote walking. Although awareness of the campaign was high (70 per cent), it had no impact on behaviour and of only 16 per cent who were aware of a telephone helpline, only 5 per cent utilized it. Researchers have however, continued to develop theories of mass communication whilst moderating the objectives of such approaches. Winett (1995), for example, argues for a change of goal, from that of behaviour to knowledge, whilst McGuire (1985) has argued for outcome effectiveness to be examined within a five step response: attention, comprehension, yielding, retention, and behaviour.

Providing a more sophisticated account of how messages are received and responded to has often resulted in more positive outcomes. McGuire emphasizes the need to understand target audiences beliefs, an analysis of competing information, and perceived barriers to change before launching any campaign. This approach is supported by Leathar (1981), who found that the key factors to influence young men's drinking in Glasgow were the time spent and social costs of drinking. These factors, not health warnings related to units drunk per week (the intended campaign), became the focus of the message. The need for research that informs message content is supported by Kreuter *et al.* (1999), who found that overweight adults who received tailored information booklets had greater positive thoughts about the material and behavioural change intentions compared to those that received untailored materials. Similarly, initiatives that supplement information campaigns with environmental components, that address barriers to change, may prove to be more successful. Boots and Midford (1999) report positive outcomes, especially for females, associated with a mass media campaign that aimed to promote the use of designated drivers to reduce drink driving in Australia. Significantly, television advertising was supplemented by a nightclub campaign that provided free soft drinks for drivers of two or more passengers.

A further development in the field of communication research is provided by the Elaboration Likelihood Model (Petty and Cacioppo 1986). This suggests that the influence of media output is the result of an interaction between message factors and the cognitive state of the recipient, namely their pre-existing beliefs and interests. Individuals are more likely to 'centrally process' messages if they are 'motivated to receive an argument', because either it is congruent with their pre-existing beliefs, or has personal relevance to them, or they have the intellectual capacity to understand the message. Such processing involves evaluation of arguments, assessment of conclusions, and their integration within existing belief structures. Any resulting attitude change is likely to be enduring and predictive of behaviour. In contrast, 'peripheral processing' is likely to occur when individuals are unmotivated to receive an argument, have low issue involvement, or incongruent beliefs. Such processing involves a response to the credibility and attractiveness of the source, but is likely to be transient and not predictive of behaviour. Indeed, the attractiveness of the source has been shown to be most important to those with low comprehension of message content (Ratneshwar and Chaiken 1991). As such, this theory again stresses the need to understand existing beliefs and tailor messages accordingly, but also suggests that those who are unmotivated may be influenced by the careful selection of who delivers the message or the type of emotional appeal chosen. For example, Scollay *et al.* (1992) reported that a message source known to be HIV positive or to have AIDS resulted in greater increases in knowledge, less risky attitudes, and safer behavioural intentions than a neutral source.

Protection motivation theory (PMT)

One approach to communication that has proved particularly popular with health promoters is the use of fear messages. Early studies of the impact of fear arousing communications focused on the manipulation of levels of fear. A classic study by Janis and Feshbach (1953) exemplifies this type of research. It involved three conditions in which high school students sat through a 15 minute lecture and slide presentation on dental hygiene. Level of threat was manipulated by varying the degree of personally threatening slides in each presentation. Immediately after the presentations, students in the high arousal group reported higher levels of motivation to care for their teeth than the other groups. One week later, however, they had retained less information and their behaviour did not differ from that of any other group.

An explanation of this effect may be found in Protection Motivation Theory (PMT) (Rogers 1983), which was developed to explain the underlying processes that influence individuals' responses to such fear-arousing communication. It posits that individuals will respond to information either in an adaptive or maladaptive manner, dependent on their appraisal of threat and their own ability to respond to that threat. Threat appraisal is a function of both perceived susceptibility to illness and its severity, while coping appraisal is a function of both outcome and self-efficacy beliefs. An individual is most likely to behave in adaptive manner in response to a fear-arousing health message if they believe they are: susceptible to disease; that the disease will have severe consequences; they perceive a link between protective behaviours and reduced risk; and consider themselves capable of engaging in them. These combine to produce protection motivation, measured as an intention to behave in either an adaptive or maladaptive manner.

Rogers argues that the most persuasive messages are those that arouse fear, increase the sense of severity, and importantly emphasize the efficacy of response. This view is supported by Solomon and DeJong (1986), who found that video instruction based on fear techniques was ineffective in changing behaviour and concluded that fear needs to be balanced with constructive information. Without such information, fear can produce resistance to the message (Franzkowiak 1987), denial that it applies to the individual (Soames-Job 1988), and encourage the targeted risk behaviours. For example, Louira (1988) found fear messages increased drug usage and Malfetti (1985) found that it was counter-productive to drink driving. This is because coping appraisal can also result in what health promoters may see as maladaptive responses, such as denial or blunting (information avoidance). For the individual concerned, such responses serve a protective purpose as they represent an emotional coping plan in the face of a health threat.

Blunting and monitoring (information seeking) represent distinct cognitive coping styles. Individuals with a monitoring style would seek out information about AIDS while those with a blunting style would ignore or distract themselves from it. Studies of monitoring and blunting behaviour have found a modest yet significant relationship between monitoring and health-promoting behaviours (van Zuuren and Dooper 1999). Such styles of coping have also been conceptualized as repression / sensitization (Byrne 1961), with repressors dealing with threatening information through avoidance and sensitizers seeking out information about threat. These concepts are also similar to degree of information receptivity (Atkin 1973), which is defined as the amount of attention individuals pay to random encounters of information, for example when they come across items in a newspaper. This effect of such coping behaviour is illustrated by Keller and Block (1999), who found that when individuals' prior intentions are incompatible with fear messages, that denial of relevance and shallow message processing were effective methods of reducing negative emotional responses.

Unfortunately, health messages frequently emphasize vulnerability and severity whilst neglecting efficacy. This is illustrated by a recent content analysis of breast self-examination leaflets which found that they contained an unbalanced proportion of threat to efficacy arguments (Kline and Mattson 2000). Neglecting the dimension of efficacy can result in only those least at risk responding to fear messages. Indeed, fear messages have been shown to motivate change under conditions of low levels of perceived vulnerability (Higbee 1969), high self-esteem (Rosen *et al.* 1982) and high self-efficacy (Strecher *et al.* 1986; Maddux and Rogers 1983). Given the heterogeneous nature of population beliefs and self-efficacy, it could be argued that the use of fear within 'mass' media campaigns is inappropriate as it runs the risk of reinforcing risk behaviours and encouraging denial amongst some of its audience.

More effective may be approaches that tailor fear messages based on an understanding of the diversity of the potential audiences. Block and Keller (1998), for example, examined the utility of PMT in the light of stages of change theory (see below). They measured student responses to safe-sex brochures that manipulated levels of vulnerability and severity in the message. Results suggested that people at different stages of change were affected by different aspects of PMT, with those at precontemplation motivated by vulnerability messages, those at contemplation by severity messages, and those at the action stage by efficacy messages. It may also be advantageous to re-orientate the traditional focus on threat and coping appraisal within health promotion fear messages. Keller (1999) found that whilst high fear appeals followed by avoidance recommendations was persuasive for those already following the recommendations, those most at risk were more responsive when the recommendations were followed by a fear appeal, rather than the other way round. They argue that those at risk perceived themselves as more susceptible, consequences as more severe, recommendations more efficacious and to have higher self-efficacy due to lower levels of message discounting.

The theory of planned behaviour (TPB)

Previous criticisms of attitude-behaviour theories also resulted in the development of the theory of planned behaviour (TPB) (Ajzen and Madden 1986). This was a modification of an earlier model, the theory of reasoned action (Ajzen and Fishbein 1980). It suggests that the closest predictor of behaviour is one's intention to engage in it. This, in turn, is derived from a summation of the individual's attitudes towards that behaviour (including behavioural outcome beliefs) and their perceived social norms relating to that behaviour (including motivation to conform to that norm). Intentions were also influenced by an individual's perceived behavioural control, which derived from external and internal factors. Support for this theory is demonstrated by the fact that young people's perception of their peers' attitude and behaviour is an important predictor of sexual activity (Billy and Udry 1985). Perception of such norms can support preventive health behaviour or inhibit them, as changes in the gay community in relation to safe sex have illustrated (Fisher 1988). Approaches to education using such a model would therefore need to focus on changing or supporting existing norms and values at the group level so that preventive behaviour became a norm. Kristal *et al.* (2000), in an evaluation of a successful worksite nutrition intervention, identify the importance of what they term 'predisposing factors', such as dietary norms and environmental factors that support the development of knowledge and skills within initiatives. Norms are particularly influential when they reflect values that are central to a group's identity and when they are communicated by trustworthy or high-status sources within the group. They are less influential when groups are smaller and less cohesive, with norms that are heterogeneous or changing (Fisher 1988).

Norms can exert an influence in one of two ways: via normative or informational social influence. Informational social influence operates via the communication of information and the modelling of behaviour through social networks. This can affect such things as perceived vulnerability, knowledge, and attitudes to prevention. These informational influences can be varied and interact; for example, individuals may be exposed to conflicting information on vulnerability from a non-mediated channel (such as a friend) and a mediated channel (such as television). As we have outlined, an individual's receptivity to and the persuasiveness of such conflicting messages may depend on their perceptions of the source of that information (Walster and Festinger 1962) or how information from mediated channels (such as newspapers and television) is communicated via non-mediated channels (such as friends and family). Reardon and Rogers (1988) have argued that much of the information received from the mass media is disseminated through inter-personal communication networks. This of course recognizes a complex process of social change, much like the one proposed by the diffusion of innovation theory. Kraft and Rise (1988) argue that such interpersonal communication is the key to attitude change and information uptake and Flay (1986) maintains that it increases the likelihood that it will influence behaviour. This is supported by Pinfold (1999) who reports on an intervention study that sought to reduce diarrhoea in rural north-eastern Thailand by promoting hand washing via a variety of media such as posters, stickers, leaflets, comics, and badges. Examination of reduced fingertip contamination was found for those reporting a secondary non-mediated source of information, namely schoolchildren.

Normative social influence may influence individuals because of fear of sanctions for non-conformity or because they serve a social comparison function; for example, risk is often viewed as a value, judged against peers (Levinger and Schneider 1964). This can affect such things as the levels of acceptable risk taking, as well as the perceived effect of protective behaviour on normative status. Hillier *et al.* (1998) in a qualitative study found that young people's knowledge of safe sex was high but ambivalence about using condoms focused on difficulties in negotiation and, in particular, normative concern regarding a sullied sexual reputation. It could be argued that influencing such norms is a long-term activity, although in some cases social norms can be seen to change in a relatively short space of time. Poesoenen and Kontula (1999), for example, report an increase in positive attitudes to purchasing and carrying condoms amongst sexually active Finnish female adolescents between 1990 and 1994 so that they resembled sexually active males.

Understanding how norms are interpreted and negotiated in relation to risk behaviours is essential for health promotion. For example, Plumridge and Chetwynd (1998), utilizing a discourse analytic approach, examined how young injecting drug users accounted for sharing injecting equipment. Results suggested that whilst individuals saw themselves as morally responsible, they nevertheless shared equipment with others who were seen to be in need, desperate and powerless. The responsibility for sharing was seen to lie with the borrower. This led the authors to suggest the need to encourage a community that takes equal responsibility for protective norms.

Diffusion of innovation theory

Diffusion of innovation theory was proposed by Rogers (1983) as a way of explaining the spread of new ideas and behaviours within society. Like the TPB, it emphasizes the importance of normative beliefs and behaviour. Rogers focuses on three main areas to explain how innovations are successfully diffused. They are the characteristics of the innovation, the classification of individuals within communities, and interpersonal communication. The first of these provides guidance for how initiatives are presented, as successful innovations typically involve minimal costs or commitment, are simple to understand or implement, result in observable benefits, and are perceived to be part of an existing social norm. If these conditions are met, the entry and legitimization of an innovation typically follow an S-shaped curve, with what are termed 'early innovators' accepting the innovation. They are usually from high socio-economic groups who seek information and so can be reached by mass media campaigns. Their adoption brings the innovation to the attention of a minority of 'early adopters' – opinion leaders within the community who are more typical, have good communication networks and status. They bring the innovation to the attention of those in their community via interpersonal communication channels and modelled behaviour. If the innovation is perceived to possess benefits that outweigh its costs, the next group – the 'early majority' – decide to adopt it. These in turn influence the 'late majority', who have lower social status, gain information from those around them, and begin to conform to the emerging social norm. There is a final slowing of the diffusion process as a minority with more traditional views, termed 'laggards', resist acceptance but are influenced by compliance to the majority.

Viewing communities as heterogeneous suggests that health promotion should progress through stages with different communication channels and messages for each group. Unlike the traditional communication theories discussed earlier, the theory recognizes that health promotion messages are interpreted and exchanged via social networks. Rogers suggests a process where change agencies develop innovations and change agents communicate information about and promote the innovation to recipients of the innovation. Havelock (1974) argues that rapid diffusion is more likely to occur if the decision is imposed from above by such a change agency, rather than from below and collectively. However, it can be seen that change can occur without such top-down processes in the area of media advocacy and the rise of health coalition groups such as ASH and the Terrence Higgins Trust.

The formal testing of diffusion of innovation theory has proved difficult. The diffusion process can be spread over a long period of time, requiring longitudinal studies and detailed process research. The costs involved in conducting such research have meant that the majority of studies have depended on respondent recall of environmental and behavioural changes within cross-sectional designs, with little objective verification of self-reports (Macdonald 1992). A recent review of 1210 published health promotion articles conducted by Oldenburg *et al.* (1999) found that only 1 per cent could be categorized as diffusion research. This led the authors to call for an increase in systematic empirical studies in this area. Accordingly, while diffusion of innovation theory has high face validity, its empirical status has yet to be fully understood.

Social learning theory (SLT)

Social learning theory (SLT) (Bandura 1977) states that behaviour is the outcome of an interaction between cognitive processes and environmental events. One of its basic tenets is that behaviour is guided by expected consequences. The more positive these are the greater the reinforcement, hence one is more likely to engage in that behaviour. When the expected consequences are negative, they act as a form of punishment which reduces the frequency of the behaviour or causes it to cease. When individuals avoid such punishments by engaging in an alternative form of behaviour, it is termed negative reinforcement. These processes are important mediators of the uptake and maintenance of many health-related behaviours. New smokers frequently gain social reinforcement from their peers smoking, and from disapproval or punishment from their parents. If they persist, they are rewarded for smoking cigarettes through the changes in mood and attention within seconds of inhalation (Ashton and Stepney 1982). When many individuals quit smoking, they experience withdrawal effects which are alleviated by smoking a further cigarette (negative reinforcement). The importance of understanding the idiosyncratic nature of perceived rewards and punishments and the need to emphasize the rewards associated with protective behaviours within initiatives are illustrated by a study conducted by Detweiler *et al.* (1999). They examined the relative effectiveness of factual information that either emphasized the positive outcomes of using or the negative consequences of not using sunscreen. Pre and post measures of attitudes and intentions were collected and behaviour was assessed via a redeemable voucher for sunscreen. Results showed that compared to messages that emphasized the losses in not using sunscreen, those that emphasized the gains were associated with significantly higher requests for sunscreen and greater intentions to reapply sunscreen at the beach and to use higher factor sunscreen.

This is not to say that individuals are motivated by immediate behaviour-consequence contingencies. Instead they can actively plan and work towards both short- and long-term reinforcers. Such a perspective helps to explain why behaviours persist in the light of negative consequences. Short-term rewards, like the physiological reward associated with smoking, are more influential than potential long-term negative consequences, which may not be actively imagined and in some cases can be actively denied. One of the main aims of health promotion is to bring such long-term consequences to mind, a process called self-regulation. Two aspects of SLT appear to be particularly important to health promotion activities which seek to encourage and support self-regulation. These are the role of expectancies and the process of vicarious learning.

It is argued that behaviours are influenced by two sets of expectancies. The first, action-outcome expectancies, reflect the degree to which individuals believe that an action will lead to a particular outcome, for example that smoking causes cancer. This outcome is then considered in terms of its value to the individual. Second, self-efficacy expectations reflect the extent to which individuals believe themselves capable of the behaviour being considered, for example: I can give up smoking. In other words, the smoker will only attempt to quit smoking if they believe that smoking cessation will reduce their risk for disease, place a high value on this behavioural outcome, and believe they are capable of doing so. Outcome and efficacy beliefs have been shown to be important moderators of a number of health-related behaviours, including resisting peer pressure to smoke or use drugs (Stacy *et al.* 1992), weight loss (Bagozzi and Warshaw 1990), engaging in safer sex practices (O'Leary *et al.* 1992), and breast self-examination (Rippetoe and Rogers 1987). The most powerful determinants of behaviours appear to be domain-specific efficacy beliefs, examples of which are provided by Marlatt *et al.* (1994) in relation to different stages of drug and alcohol misuse. These include resistance self-efficacy beliefs in avoiding first use, harm-reduction self-efficacy beliefs, action self-efficacy beliefs in attaining abstinence or controlled consumption, coping self-efficacy beliefs to avoid relapse, and recovery self-efficacy beliefs to recover from any relapse. Such cognitive variables provide a clear structure for health promotion initiatives and in some cases have been utilized as measures of outcome effectiveness. Hallam and Petosa (1998), for example, in an evaluation of a worksite programme seeking to increase exercise adherence, found significant increases in self-regulation and outcome expectancy compared to a control.

Vicarious learning has proved particularly important to health promotion, being the notion that one can learn behaviours and their outcomes and establish efficacy expectancies through observation of others. For example, whilst smoking initiation may be associated with aversive physical consequences, observation of smoking in others suggests a pleasurable and rewarding behaviour, so individuals persevere in the expectation of future enjoyment. Such modelling of behaviour can come directly from families and peers: those who smoke, for example, are more likely to have family and friends who do so (Ashton and Stepney 1982), whilst indirect modelling can come from the mass media. Hence the concerns that have been raised about the depiction of smoking in the media and the over-representiveness of televisual depictions of alcohol consumption with few negative consequences (Smith *et al.* 1988). Of course, there are individual differences in the degree to which people are influenced by modelling experiences and not all models are equally influential. In general, people are more likely to perform the behaviour they observe if the model is similar to themselves; that is, of the same sex, age, or race (Ratneshwar and Chaiken 1991). In addition, high-status persons, either from within the social sphere of the individual, or from wider spheres such as sports or the media, exert a stronger influence on behaviour than low-status individuals (Winett *et al.* 1989). Modelling can therefore be utilized within health promotion as a way of promoting normative health behaviours and as a way to teach the efficacy skills necessary to achieve behavioural change.

The health belief model (HBM)

The health belief model (HBM) was originally developed in an attempt to understand low compliance rates to screening and prevention recommendations. The model consists of five dimensions: perceived susceptibility (subjective perceptions of risk in relation to the health threat), perceived severity (evaluations of the consequences of the threat), perceived benefits (assessments of the efficacy of preventive actions), barriers (assessment of difficulties and negative consequences of preventive behaviour), and cues to action (triggers for the decision making process). More recently health motivation – that is, an individual's readiness to be concerned about their health – was added to the model. Each factor is viewed as impacting on decision making, although no clear operalization of how they combine to influence such decisions has been forthcoming. Reviews of the efficacy of the model (Harrison *et al.* 1992) have found only a modest correlation between HBM variables and behaviours, typically −0.21 for barriers, 0.15 for susceptibility, 0.13 for benefits, with severity (0.08) least important. Despite this, the HBM provides a strong framework for health promotion programmes, stressing the need to identify a link between an individual's risk behaviour and disease, to highlight the severity of the disease and to make it relatively easy to engage in behaviour likely to lead to a reduction in risk for that disease.

Influencing risk perception has traditionally proved to be difficult. A number of studies have shown that health care and information-seeking behaviour is associated with perceived threat/vulnerability to illness (Crawford 1974; Lenz 1984). However, numerous researchers have found evidence that individuals, whilst acknowledging a general social risk, downplay personal risk. This has been defined variously as an unrealistic optimism (Weinstein 1989), unique invulnerability (Perloff and Fetzer 1986), illusion of uniqueness (Snyder 1978), and self-serving bias (Larwood 1978), all of which act as a form of coping. Young people in particular are said to be more involved in such coping behaviour, as they explore new roles without a full sense of the potential risks involved (Bennett *et al.* 1995; Chapman and Fitzgerald 1982; Flay 1986; and Franzkowiak 1987). Risk taking is also used as an attempt to raise self-esteem and as a response to peer groups pressure (Simons and Miller 1987). Failing to acknowledge the effect of risk perceptions and coping cognitions can result in initiatives failing those most in need. A study by Hanlon *et al.* (1998) found that only certain groups responded positively to a workplace screening programme. An examination of the effect of respondent characteristics showed that reductions in risk behaviours were found in those with lower levels of perceived risk for CHD and higher perceived health status. Those with greater perceived risk and lower perceived health were more likely to see the health check as threatening.

Reducing environmental barriers to healthy behaviours may be one of the most effective approaches to health promotion, their importance demonstrated by Damron *et al.* (1999), who report lack of transportation and child care as common barriers for attendance at a nutritional education programme increasing fruit and vegetable consumption amongst women. Large-scale disease prevention programmes that have focused on whole communities, such as the North Karelia Project (Puska *et al.* 1985) and Heartbeat Wales (Nutbeam *et al.* 1993), have emphasized the reduction of environmental barriers to behaviours. This approach has resulted in the development of healthy eating choices in restaurants and food retailers and the provision of exercise facilities in communities. Evaluation of such programmes has proved difficult, not least because of problems in maintaining non-intervention reference communities and the fact that environmental manipulations are traditionally supplemented by mass media campaigns and skills training, making it difficult to isolate the effect of barrier reduction. However, initiatives conducted in more controllable environments, such as schools and the workplace, suggest that increasing the availability and the promotion of health food choices can improve healthy eating (Glanz *et al.* 1995) and that increasing exercise facilities and providing time off for exercise can increase levels of exercise (Linegar *et al.* 1991).

More common are approaches that increase the barriers to unhealthy behaviours. It could be argued that social policy approaches to health promotion are implicitly based on assumptions common to the health belief model, in that legislation and taxation can act as effective barriers to unhealthy behaviours and facilitators of healthy behaviours. Economic measures related to health promotion have been largely confined to taxation on tobacco and alcohol. The price of alcohol impacts on levels of consumption (Central Statistics Office 1980), particularly for wines and spirits: beer consumption may be less sensitive to price (Godfrey 1990). It has been argued that these effects may hold not just for 'sensible' drinkers, but also those who are manifesting alcohol-related problems (Sales *et al.* 1989). Increases in tobacco taxation may also be the most effective measure in reducing consumption rates, with an estimated reduction in consumption of 4 per cent for every 10 per cent price rise (Brownson *et al.* 1995). The use of taxation seems to be a particularly effective deterrent amongst the young, who are three times more likely to be affected by price rises than older adults (Lewit *et al.* 1981). These findings, however, must now be interpreted against an increasing trade in bootleg alcohol and tobacco from the continent. Legislating the availability of unhealthy products and behaviours has also proved problematic. In theory, laws that prevent young people's access to such things as tobacco represent a significant barrier, but as Brownson *et al.* (1995) have highlighted, enforcing such laws without a licensing scheme such as that applied to alcohol has been difficult. Prohibition approaches to the availability of alcohol and other drugs meanwhile have proved controversial and politically sensitive, with many questioning its effectiveness. Whilst prohibition may be seen as a necessary barrier by some, others have called for more modest barriers to availability. Godfrey (1990), for example, has suggested restricting outlets for drugs such as alcohol, thereby increasing transaction costs and reducing cues.

Cues to action can prompt existing behaviour, but can also trigger any intended behaviour change. Such cues can occur in the social environment (for example a family member falling ill or the onset of physical symptoms) and within the physical environment. Examples of the latter include product labelling such as health warnings on cigarettes and nutritional information on food, although evidence suggests that they reinforce existing behaviour rather than prompting the consideration of behaviour change. For example, Levy *et al.* (2000) found that consumers did not necessarily understand dietary fat information on food labels and that label comprehension was not associated with fat intake. Similarly, Glanz *et al.* (1995) found the public rarely understood nutritional information on food packaging especially amongst those with low incomes. Similarly, health warnings on cigarettes have been found to be ineffective in changing existing smokers' behaviour, although they may serve to prevent smoking initiation (Richards *et al.* 1989). However, Russell *et al.* (1999) report on the effectiveness of a relatively simple environmental cue on physical activity. They examined whether a sign limiting lift use to physically challenged individuals and staff would increase stair use amongst university students. Behavioural observations showed an increase in stair use from 39.7 per cent to 41.9 per cent, with greater stair use amongst males, those under 30, and between Monday and Thursday (but for some reason not Friday!).

Cues to action can act not only as prompts for healthy behaviours, but also as reminders to behave in unhealthy ways. Consequently it has been argued that health promotion should strive to limit and legislate against such things as tobacco and alcohol advertising and the depiction of unhealthy behaviours in the media. Support for restrictions on advertising can be found in longitudinal studies that have examined attitudes to advertising and smoking behaviour. Chapman and Fitzgerald (1982) found a preference for the most heavily advertised brands amongst under-age smokers, whilst Aitken *et al.* (1991) found that positive attitudes to tobacco advertising was associated with intention to smoke amongst 11 to 14 year olds, a relationship which increased in strength over time. It could be argued that media depictions of unhealthy behaviours can influence perceptions of appropriate social norms via modelled behaviour and cue prompts to behaviour. Calls for reforms in the way that such things as alcohol consumption is portrayed in the media is supported by Smith *et al.* (1988), who found 80 per cent of popular programmes making verbal or visual references to alcohol and its depiction as an acceptable personal coping strategy. Similarly, Pechmann and Shih (1999) examined the effect of smoking scenes in movies on non-smoking schoolchildren compared to the same scenes with the smoking behaviour edited out. Results showed that the smoking scenes enhanced pupils' perceptions of smoking status and intention to smoke.

Stages of change theory

One of the first 'stages of change' models was proposed by Prochaska and DiClemente (1984). Unlike previously described models, it suggests that individuals pass through different stages of cognitive processing when undertaking decision making. Prochaska and DiClemente analysed motivation to change across a wide range of areas and identified five major stages that individuals can pass through: precontemplation, contemplation, preparation, action, and maintenance or relapse.

In the precontemplation stage, change is not being considered, whether through ignorance, denial, or demoralization. In the contemplation stage, the individual is considering change at some remote level but is not yet committed to change, and has not thought through how this may be achieved. Health promotion initiatives for individuals at these stages would therefore aim to raise awareness, highlight risk, and suggest effective changes. As the individual moves to the preparation stage, they begin actively considering and planning change. As its name implies, the action stage is when behavioural change actually occurs. For these individuals it is important to address the development of skills and goal setting. After about two months any behavioural change is considered significantly established for the individual to be considered in the maintenance stage. However, individuals who reach the action stage may fail to maintain any changes made, and relapse back to any one of the previous stages. Interventions such as that described by Marlatt and Gordon (1980) in relation to smoking cessation explicitly address issues of relapse by developing methods to resist high-risk social situations and negative attributions for failure. As such, the model is cyclic and bi-directional: individuals involved in behavioural change may start at any point in the process, and progress or move back to an earlier stage at any time.

A criticism of the theory is that the processes that facilitate these transitions are less considered. Other models that have utilized the concept of stages, such as the Health Action Process (Schwarzer 1992), provide more detail regarding movement between stages, particularly the important role of action-outcome expectancies, self-efficacy, and the role of the social and physical environment. It has been argued that the popularity of such stage models within health promotion is because they provide both order and direction for initiatives (Laitakari 1998). Research utilizing stages of change has shown that individuals classified within different stages have demonstrated different needs. For example, Jaffe *et al.* (1999) in an examination of incentives and barriers to physical activity for working women found that while precontemplators had few positive expectations regarding exercise, contemplators had positive expectations but reported the higher number of perceived barriers. While evaluations have suggested that in certain circumstances, tailoring initiatives to stages can result in positive outcomes. For example, in an evaluation of a worksite exercise programme, Peterson and Aldana (1999) examined the effectiveness of written messages tailored to individuals' reported stage of change compared to non-tailored messages for a comparison group. Six weeks after the material was received, they reported greater movement from lower to higher stages amongst those who had received the stage-based materials.

Social environments and holistic health

From a brief review of existing research it can be seen that psychological theories have traditionally provided a strong structure and direction to health promotion initiatives seeking to influence health risk behaviours. We end this chapter by highlighting potential developments in the contribution of psychology and the role of psychology in supporting efforts to improve psychological and social health.

The expectancy-valued theories that have been outlined assume that behaviour is an outcome of formal decision making. However, this may not always be the case – indeed, much of our behaviour appears to be habitual and relatively 'thoughtless' (Hunt and Martin 1988). This may be most apparent in relation to dietary habits, with individuals citing habit and taste for their choice of food, even when considering original decision making. When rationality does influence decision making, it is not always governed by a desire to preserve health, an assumption of many of the theories so far discussed. For example, Ingham and van Zessen (1997) found 36 per cent of their sample of young people reporting consideration of the risks associated with unsafe sex only after the event. While Jacobson (1981) found working-class smokers made rational choices to smoke as a way of coping with stress and adverse material circumstances. Such issues highlight the need to examine how habitual behaviours are maintained and negotiated within people's social environments and to understand how meaning is achieved. In such interactions, participants bring their own understandings and expectations of appropriate behaviours. Behaviour is then shaped by the mutual responses of the participants. Existing patterns of behaviour are therefore open to modification and change is dependent upon the individuals involved and the circumstances in which they find themselves. As Winett (1995) states:

> Psychologists have traditionally focused on cognition and behaviour as the figure, with environment often the distant amorphous ground (or context). A reversal of figure and ground is not suggested; rather, cognitions and behaviour and the environment must receive equal and specific attention.
>
> (Winett 1995: 348)

An example of such an approach is provided by De-Bourdeaudhhuij and Van-Oost (1998), who examined 92 families to assess reciprocal influences on eating behaviours. Results highlighted the influence of children on chosen products and in particular the influence of adolescents on the consumption of unhealthy products by all the family. Similarly, Backett (1990) found that women within families were less likely to exercise regularly than their male partners. These differences frequently did not correspond with desired levels of exercise. Rather, they reflected women's negotiated role within their family, and their affording higher priority to other family commitments than to their own participation in regular exercise. Similarly, although a majority of women were the main providers of food within the households, they may actually exert little control over the choice of foodstuffs. Instead, they frequently found themselves having to negotiate with a variety of differing food choices of family members. One of the few health promotion initiatives to utilize such an approach is reported by Johnson and Nicklas (1995). Their 'Heart Smart Family' was targeted at families with children identified as at high risk for CHD. It involved a 12–16 week programme which focused on increasing awareness of health issues, skills development, and problem solving skills. Following the programme, parents evidenced lowered blood pressures, increased exercise levels, and decreased intake of total fat, saturated fat, and sodium. A clinically significant reduction in children's blood pressure was also observed. In a similar vein, Burke *et al.* (1999) report positive increases in a range of health behaviours, self-efficacy, and reductions in perceived barriers to health following a 16 week randomized control programme aimed at newly married couples. They suggest that such initiatives can usefully focus on points in the lifespan when attitudes are re-evaluated.

The importance of other social environments, such as school, has been highlighted by recent analysis, which found that positive perceptions of the school environment and perceptions of teachers as supportive were associated with higher levels of health-promoting behaviours. Similarly, social environments associated with gender roles (Dorn 1983) and with socio-economic status (SES) have been shown to have a similar influence. This is illustrated by work conducted by Chamberlin and O'Neill (1998), which shows that smokers in lower SES groups have more limited expectations of health, lower perceived effectiveness regarding health-promoting behaviours, and greater situational pressure to engage in health-damaging behaviours compared to their higher SES counterparts.

Finally it must be stated that our discussion has focused predominately on the role of psychology in understanding the influences on health risk and protective behaviour. Psychology, however, has an important role in guiding and suggesting potential outcomes for initiatives that adopt a more holistic approach to health (Repucci *et al.* 1999). This reflects definitions of health promotion provided by WHO (1986) who state that it is

> the process of enabling people to increase control over, and to improve, their health. To reach a state of complete physical, mental and social well-being, an individual or group must be able to identify and to realize aspirations, to satisfy needs, and to change or cope with the environment . . . Therefore, health promotion is not just the responsibility of the health sector, but goes beyond healthy lifestyles to well-being.

Here such concepts as intra- and inter- group processes, participation, empowerment, self-esteem and self-efficacy, which have been traditionally viewed as process measures, become important outcomes.

This type of approach, which places the emphasis on personal growth, development, and empowerment, shares many of the assumptions of the psychological perspective of humanism (e.g. Rogers 1951; Maslow 1970). Most relevant for health promotion is its emphasis on human growth and development and its assumption that individuals are motivated by a desire to develop and self-actualize, a tendency toward fulfilment of all capabilities. Although having a significant influence on therapeutic techniques (Rogers 1967), humanism has largely been neglected within the design and evaluation of health promotion initiative. Taylor (1990), however, identified two possible approaches to health promotion using this perspective. The first, a humanistic approach, takes a client-centred approach, and involves the individual determining their health needs and developing the resources and skills to meet them. The second, a more radical humanist approach, again focused on client-centred participatory learning, but also recognizes that such learning occurs within a social context of relationships. According to this model, health promotion should encourage the development of social, organizational, and economic networks to support individual change. This, he argued, should lead to the development of community groups and collective and individual empowerment. This obviously mirrors work undertaken within community development initiatives where 'a community identifies its needs or objectives, orders (or ranks) these needs or objectives, develops the confidence and will to work at these needs or objectives, finds the resources (internal and/or external) to deal with these needs and objectives (and) takes action' (Ross and Lappin 1967). This area may represent the greatest potential for health promoters and psychologists to work together to achieve true population health.

References

Aitken, P. P., Eadie, D. R., Hastings, G. B., and Haywood, A. J. (1991) 'Predisposing effects of cigarette advertising on children's intentions to smoke when older', *British Journal of Addiction* 86: 383–90.

Ajzen, I. and Fishbein, M. (1980) *Understanding Attitudes and Predicting Social Behavior*, Englewood Cliffs, NJ: Prentice Hall.

Ajzen, I. and Madden, T. (1986) 'Prediction of goal-directed behaviour: Attitudes, intentions and perceived behavioral control', *Journal of Experimental Social Psychology* 22: 453–74.

Ashton, H. and Stepney, R. (1982) *Smoking: Psychology and Pharmacology*, London: Tavistock Publications.

Atkin, C. K. (1973) 'Instrumental utilities and information seeking', in P. Clarke (ed.) *New Models for Communication Research*, Beverly Hills, CA: Sage, pp. 205–39.

Backett, K. (1990) 'Studying health in families: a qualitative approach', in A. Cunningham, S. Burly, and N. McKeganey (eds) *Readings in Medical Sociology*, London: Routledge.

Bagozzi, R. P. and Warshaw, P. R. (1990) 'Trying to consume', *Journal of Consumer Research* 17: 127–40.

Bandura, A. (1977) 'Self-efficacy: Toward a unifying theory of behavioural change', *Psychological Review* 84: 191–215.

Beck, A. T. (1976) *Cognitive Therapy and the Emotional Disorders*, New York: International Universities Press.

Bennett, P. and Murphy, S. (1997) *Psychology and Health Promotion*, Buckingham: Open University Press.

Bennett, P., Murphy, S., and Carroll, D. (1995) 'Psychology, health promotion and aesthemiology', *Health Care Analysis* 3: 15–26.

Billy, J. and Udry, J. (1985) 'The influence of male and female best friends on sexual behaviour', *Adolescence* 20: 21–32.

Block, L. G. and Keller, P. A. (1998) 'Beyond protection motivation: An integrative theory of health appeals', *Journal of Applied Social Psychology* 28 (17): 1584–608.

Boots, K. and Midford, R. (1999) '"Pick a skipper": An evaluation of a designated driver programme to prevent alcohol-related injury in a regional Australian city', *Health Promotion International* 14 (4): 337–45.

Brownson, R., Koffman, D., Novotny, T., Hughes, R., and Eriksen, M. (1995) 'Environmental and policy interventions to control tobacco use and prevent cardiovascular disease', *Health Education Quarterly*, 22 (4): 478–98.

Bunton, R., Murphy, S., and Bennett, P. (1991) 'Theories of behaviour change and their use in health promotion: some neglected areas', *Health Education Research* 6 (2): 153–62.

Burke, V., Giangiulio, N., Gilliam, H. F., Beilin, L. J., Houghton, S., and Milligan, R. A. (1999) 'Health promotion in couples adapting to a shared lifstyle', *Health Education Research*, 14 (2): 269–88.

Byrne, D. (1961) 'The repression-sensitization scale: rationale, reliability and validity', *Journal of Personality*, 29: 344–49.

Central Statistics Office (1980) 'A change in revenue from an indirect tax change', *Economic Trends*, March: 97–107.

Chamberlin, K. and O'Neill, D. (1998) 'Understanding social class differences in health: a qualitative analysis of smokers' health beliefs', *Psychology and Health* 13 (6): 1105–19.

Chapman, S. and Fitzgerald, B. (1982) 'Brand preferences and and advertising recall in adolescent smokers: some implications for health promotion', *American Journal of Public Health*, 72: 491–4.

Crawford, J. (1974) 'Task uncertainty, decision importance and group reinforcement as determinants of communication processes in groups', *Journal of Personality and Social Psychology* 29: 619–27.

Damron, D., Langenberg, P., Anliker, J., Ballesteros, M., Feldman, R., and Havas, S. (1999) 'Factors associated with attendance in a voluntary nutrition education program', *American Journal of Health Promotion* 13 (5): 268–75.

De-Bourdeaudhuij, I. and Van-Oost, P. (1998) 'Family members' influence on decision making about food: Differences in perception and relationship with healthy eating', *American Journal of Health Promotion* 13 (2): 73–81.

Detweiler, J. B., Bedell, B. T., Salovey, P., Pronin, E., and Rothman, A. J. (1999) 'Message framing and sunscreen use: Gain framed messages motivate beach-goers', *Health Psychology* 18 (2): 189–96.

Dorn, N. (1983) *Alcohol, Youth and the State*, London: Croom Helm.

Fisher, J. (1988) 'Possible effects of reference group-based social influence on AIDS risk behaviour and AIDS prevention', *American Psychologist*, November: 914–20.

Flay, B. (1986) 'Mass media linkages with school based programs for drug abuse prevention', *Journal of School Health* 56 (9): 402–6.

Franzkowiak, P. (1987) 'Risk taking and adolescent development', *Health Promotion* 2: 51–60.

Glanz, K., Lankenau, B., Foerster, S., Temple, S., Mullis, R., and Schmid, T. (1995) 'Environmental and policy approaches to cardiovascular disease prevention through nutrition: opportunities for state and local action', *Health Education Quarterly* 22: 512–27.

Godfrey, C. (1990) 'Modelling demand', in A. Maynard and P. Tether (eds) *Preventing Alcohol and Tobacco Problems. 1*, Avebury: ESRC.

Green, L., Kreuter, M., Deeds, S., and Partridge, K. (1980) *Health Education Planning: A Diagnostic Approach*, Palo Alto, CA: Mayfield.

Hallam, J. and Petosa, R. (1998) 'A worksite intervention to enhance social cognitive theory constructs to promote exercise adherence', *American Journal of Health Promotion* 13 (1): 4–7.

Hamburg, D., Nightingale, E., and Takanishi, D. (1987) 'Facilitating the transitions of adolescence', *Journal of the American Medical Association* 257: 3405–6.

Hanlon, P., Carey, L., Tannahill, C., Kelly, M., Gilmour, H., Tannahill, A., and McEwen, J. (1998) 'Behaviour change following a workplace health check. How much change occurs and who changes?', *Health Promotion International* 13 (2): 131–9.

Harrison, J. A., Mullen, P. D., and Green, L. W. (1992) 'A meta-analysis of studies of the health belief model with adults', *Health Education Research, Theory and Practice* 7: 107–16.

Havelock, R. (1974) *Educational Innovation in the United States*, volume 1. Michigan: University of Michigan.

Higbee, K. (1969) 'Fifteen years of fear arousal. Research on threat appeals 1953–1968', *Psychological Bulletin* 72: 426–44.

Hillier, L., Harrison, L., and Warr, D. (1998) ' "When you carry condoms all the boys think you want it". Negotiating competing discourses about safe sex', *Journal of Adolescence* 21 (1): 15–29.

Hunt, S. M. and Martin, C. J. (1988) 'Health related behaviour change – a test of a new model', *Psychology and Health* 2: 209–30.

Ingham, R. and Van Zessen, G. (1997) 'Towards an alternative model of sexual behaviour: from individual properties to interactional processes', in L. van Camphoudt, M. Cohen, G. Guizzardi, and D. Hausser (eds) *Sexual Interactions and HIV Risk: New Conceptual Perspectives in European Research*, London: Taylor & Francis.

Jacobson, B. (1981) *The Lady killers: Why Smoking Is a Feminist Issue*, London: Pluto Press.

Jaffe, L., Lutter, J. M., Rex, J., Hawkes, C., and Bucaccio, P. (1999) 'Incentives and barriers to physical activity for working women', *American Journal of Health Promotion* 13 (4): 215–18.

Janis, I. L. and Feshbach S. (1953) 'Effects of fear-arousing communications', *Journal of Abnormal and Social Psychology* 48: 78–92.

Johnson, C. C. and Nicklas, T. A. (1995) 'Health ahead – the Heart Smart family approach to prevention of cardiovascular disease', *The American Journal of the Medical Sciences* 310: 127–32.

Keller, P. A. (1999) 'Converting the unconverted. The effect of inclination and opportunity to discount health related fear appeals', *Journal of Applied Psychology* 84 (3): 403–15.

—— and Block, L. G. (1999) 'The effect of affect-based dissonance versus cognitive-based dissonance on motivated reasoning and health related persuasion', *Journal of Experimental Psychology*, 5 (3): 302–13.

Kline, K. N. and Mattson, M. (2000) 'Breast self-examination pamphlets. A content analysis grounded in fear appeals research', *Health Communication* 12 (1): 1–21.

Kraft, P. and Rise, J. (1988) 'Public awareness and acceptance of an HIV/AIDS information campaign in Norway', *Health Education Research* 3 (2): 31–40.

Kreuter, M. W., Bull, F. C., Clark, E. M., and Oswald, D. L. (1999) 'Understanding how people process health information. A comparison of tailored and non-tailored weight-loss materials', *Health Psychology* 18 (5): 487–94.

Kristal, A. R., Glanz, K., Tilley, B. C., and Li, S. (2000) 'Mediating factors in dietary change. Understanding the impact of a worksite nutrition intervention', *Health Education and Behaviour* 27 (1): 112–25.

Laitakari, J. (1998) 'On the practicable applicability of stage models to health promotion and health education', *American Journal of Health Behaviour* 22 (1): 28–38.

Larwood, L. (1978) 'Swine flu: A field study of self-serving bias', *Journal of Applied Social Psychology* 18: 283–89.

Leathar, D. S. (1981) 'Lack of response to health guidance amongst heavy drinkers', in M. R. Turner (ed.) *Preventive Nutrition and Society*, London: Academic Press.

Lenz, E. (1984) 'Information seeking – a component of client decisions and health behaviour', *Advances in Nursing Science* 6: 59–72.

Levinger, G. and Schneider, D. (1969) 'The test of the risk as a value hypothesis', *Journal of Personality and Social Psychology* 11: 165–9.

Levy, L., Patterson, R. E., Kristal, A. R., and Li, S. S. (2000) 'How well do consumers understand percentage daily value of food labels?' *American Journal of Health Promotion* 14 (3): 157–60.

Lewit, E., Coates, D., and Grossman, M. (1981) 'The effects of governmental regulation on teenage smoking', *Journal of Law and Economics* 24: 545–69.

Linegar J., Chesson, C., and Nice, D. (1991) 'Physical fitness gains following simple environmental change', *American Journal of Preventive Medicine* 7: 298–310.

Louria, D. (1988) 'Some concerns about educational approaches in AIDS prevention', in R. Schinazi and A. Nahmias (eds) *AIDS Children, Adolescents and Heterosexual Adults*, New York: Elsevier Science Publications.

Maccoby, N. (1988) 'The community as a focus for health promotion', in S. Spacapan and S. Oskamp (eds) *The Social Psychology of Health*, Newbury Park, CA: Sage.

Macdonald, G. (1992) 'Communication theory and health promotion', in R. Bunton and G. Macdonald (eds) *Health Promotion*, London: Routledge.

McGuire, W. (1985) 'Attitudes and attitude change', in G. Lindzey and E. Aronson (eds) *Handbook of Social Psychology*, volume 2, New York: Random House.

Maddux, J. and Rogers, R. (1983) 'Protection motivation and self-efficacy. A revised theory of fear appeals and attitude change', *Journal of Experimental Social Psychology* 19: 464–79.

Malfetti, J. (1985) 'Public information and education sections of the report of the Presidential Commission on Drunk Driving: A critique and a discussion of research implication', *Accident Analysis and Prevention* 17: 347–53.

Marlatt, G. A. and Gordon, J. R. (1980) 'Determinants of relapse: Implications for the maintenance of behavioural change', in P. O. Davidson and S. M. Davidson (eds) *Behavioral Medicine: Changing Health Lifestyles*, New York: Brunner/Mazel.

Marlatt, G. A., Baer, J. S., and Quigley, L. A. (1994) 'Self-efficacy and addictive behaviour', in A. Bandura (ed.) *Self-efficacy in Changing Societies*, Marbach: Johann Jacobs Foundation.

Maslow, A. H. (1970) *Motivation and Personality*, New York: Harper & Row.

Nutbeam, D., Smith, C., Murphy, S., and Catford J. (1993) 'Maintaining evaluation designs in a long-term community based health promotion programme: Heartbeat Wales case study', *Journal of Epidemiology and Community Health* 47: 127–33.

Oldenburg, B. F., Sallis, J. F., French, M. L., and Owen, N. (1999) 'Health promotion research and the diffusion and institutionalization of interventions', *Health Education Research* 14 (1): 121–30.

O'Leary, A., Goodhart, F., Jemmott, L. S., and Boccher-Lattimore, D. (1992) 'Predictors of safer sex on the college campus: A social cognitive theory analysis', *Journal of American College Health*, 40: 254–63.

Pechmann, C. and Shih, C. F. (1999) 'Smoking scenes in movies and anti-smoking advertisements before movies. Effects on youth', *Journal of Marketing* 63 (3): 1–13.

Perloff, L. and Fetzer, B. (1986) 'Self–other judgements and perceived vulnerability to victimization', *Journal of Personality and Social Psychology* 50: 502–10.

Peterson, T. R. and Aldana, S. G. (1999) 'Improving exercise behaviour: An application of the stages of change model in a worksite setting', *American Journal of Health Promotion* 13 (4): 229–32.

Petty, R. and Cacioppo, J. (1986) 'The elaboration likelihood model of persuasion', in L. Berkowitz (ed.) *Advances in Experimental Social Psychology*, volume 19. Orlando: Academic Press.

Pinfold, J. V. (1999) 'Analysis of different communication channels for promoting hygiene behaviour', *Health Education Research* 14 (5): 629–39.

Plumridge, E. W. and Chetwynd, J. (1998) 'The moral universe of injecting drug users in the era of AIDS: Sharing injecting equipment and the protection of moral standing', *AIDS-Care* 10 (6): 723–33.

Poesoenen, R. and Kontula, O. (1999) 'How are attitudes to condoms related to gender and sexual experiences among adolescents in Finland?', *Health Promotion International* 14 (3): 211–19.

Prochaska, J. O. and DiClemente, C. C. (1984) *The Transtheoretical Approach: Crossing Traditional Boundaries of Change*, Homewood, IL: Irwin.

Puska, P., Nissinen, A., Tuomilehto, J., Salonen, J. T., Koskela, K., McAlister, A., Kottke, T. E., Maccoby, N. and Fraquhar, J. W. (1985) 'The community-based strategy to prevent coronary heart disease: Conclusions from the ten years of the North Karelia Project', *Annual Review of Public Health* 6: 147–93.

Ratneshwar, S. and Chaiken, S. (1991) 'Comprehension's role in persuasion: the case of its moderating effect on the persuasive impact of source cues', *Journal of Consumer Research* 18: 52–62.

Reardon, K. and Rogers, E. (1988) 'Interpersonal versus mass communication: A false dichotomy', *Human Communication Research* 15: 284–303.

Reppucci, N. D., Woolard, J. L., and Fried, C. S. (1999) 'Social, community, and preventive interventions', *Annual Review of Psychology* 50: 387–418.

Richards, J., Fisher, P., and Conner, F. (1989) 'The warnings on cigarette packages are ineffective', *Journal of the American Medical Association* 261: 45.

Rippetoe, P. A. and Rogers, R. W. (1987) 'Effects on components of protection motivation theory on adaptive and maladaptive copings with a health threat', *Journal of Personality and Social Psychology*, 52: 596–604.

Rogers, C. R. (1951) *Client Centered Therapy*, Boston: Houghton Mifflin.

—— (1967) *The Therapeutic Relationship and Its Impact*, Madison: University of Wisconsin Press.

Rogers, E. (1983) *Diffusion of Innovations*, New York: Free Press.

Rosen, T. M., Terry, N., and Leventhal, H. (1982) 'The role of self-esteem and coping in response to a threat communication', *Journal of Research in Personality* 16: 90–107.

Ross, M. G. and Lappin, B. W. (1967) *Community Organisation: Theory, Principles and Practice*, New York: Harper Row.

Russell, W. D., Dzewaltowski, D., and Ryan, G. J. (1999) 'The effectiveness of a point of decision prompt in deterring sedentary behaviour', *American Journal of Health Promotion* 13 (5): 257–9.

Sales J., Duffy, J., Plant, M., and Peck, D. (1989) 'Alcohol consumption, cigarette sales and mortality in the United Kingdom: an analysis of the period 1970–1985', *Drug and Alcohol Dependence* 24: 155–60.

Schaalma, H., Kok, G., Bosker, R., Paercel, G., Peters, L., and Poelman, J. (1996) 'Planned development and evaluation of AIDS education for secondary school students in the Netherlands', *Health Education Quarterly* 23 (4): 469–87.

Schwarzer, R. (1992) 'Self-efficacy in the adoption and maintenance of health behaviors: theoretical approaches and a new model', in R. Schwarzer (ed.) *Self-efficacy: Thought Control of Action*, Washington, DC: Hemisphere.

Scollay, P., Doucett, M., Perry, M., and Winterbottom, B. (1992) 'AIDS education of college students: The effect of an HIV-positive lecturer', *AIDS Education and Prevention* 4: 160–71.

Simons, R. and Miller, M. (1987) 'Adolescent depression: Assessing the impact of negative cognitions and socio-environmental problems', *Social Work* July: 326–30.

Smith, C., Roberts, J. L. and Pendelton, L. L. (1988) 'Booze on the box. The portrayal of alcohol on British television: a content analysis', *Health Education Research* 3: 267–72.

Snyder, C. (1978) 'The illusion of uniqueness', *Humanistic Psychology* 18: 33–41.

Soames-Job, R. F. (1988) 'Effective and ineffective use of fear in health promotion campaigns', *American Journal of Public Health* 78: 163–7.

Solomon, M. Z. and DeJong, W. (1986) 'Recent STD prevention efforts and their implications for AIDS health education', *Health Education Quarterly* 13: 301–16.

Stacy, A. W., Sussman, S., Dent, C. W., Burton, D., and Flay, B. R. (1992) 'Moderators of peer social influence in adolescent smoking', *Personality and Social Psychology Bulletin* 18: 163–72.

Strecher, V., Deveillis, B., Becker, M., and Rosenstock, I. (1986) 'The role of self-efficacy in achieving health behaviour change', *Health Education Quarterly* 13: 301–16.

Taylor, V. (1990) 'Health education: a theoretical mapping', *Health Education Journal* 49: 13–14.

van-Zuuren, F. J. and Dooper, R. (1999) 'Coping style and self reported health promotion and disease detection behaviour', *British Journal of Health Psychology* 4 (1): 81–9.

Walster, E. and Festinger, L. (1962) 'The effectiveness of overheard persuasive communications', *Journal of Abnormal and Social Psychology* 65: 415–26.

Weinstein, N. D. (1989) 'Unrealistic optimism about future life events', *Journal of Personality and Social Psychology* 39: 806–20.

Wimbush, E., MacGregor, A., and Fraser, E. (1998) 'Impact of a national mass media campaign on walking in Scotland', *Health Promotion International* 13 (1): 45–53.

Winett, R. A. (1995) 'A framework for health promotion and disease prevention programs', *American Psychologist*, May: 341–51.

Winett, R. A., King, A. C., and Altman, D. G. (1989) *Health Psychology and Public Health. An Integrative Approach*, New York: Pergamon.

World Health Organization (1986) *Ottawa Charter for Health Promotion*, Canada: WHO.

—— (1991) *Supportive Environments for Health. The Sundsvall Statement*, Geneva: WHO.

3 What is the relevance of sociology for health promotion?

Nicki Thorogood

Introduction

This chapter will be considering how sociology can contribute to both the theory and the practice of health promotion. It is my contention that many sociological categories are implicit in the work of health promotion and that articulating them can only improve our knowledge and how we use it. The chapter falls into four main sectors. The first, 'What is sociology?', offers a short introduction to the main theoretical approaches of the discipline and to its key concepts. Clearly, space here is limited and I would recommend any interested students to refer to more comprehensive introductory texts. The second section, 'Sociology of health and illness', briefly considers the role of the discipline in the field of health and illness. This charts its development from being in the service of medicine, to analysing the professional organization of medicine, to incorporating the perspectives of 'ordinary' people, to its present position of providing a critique of medical knowledge and practice.

The third and fourth sections address themselves in more depth to the project of health promotion. The first of these, 'Sociology as applied to health promotion', considers the ways in which a sociological perspective can aid the work of health promotion. It takes some of the accepted categories of sociology – lay beliefs, social stratification, gender, age, and race – and shows how sociological analysis in these areas can be very useful for the practice of health promotion. The last section, 'A sociology of health promotion', takes a somewhat different tack. In this section the sociological method is applied to health promotion itself. This enables a critical analysis to be made of such aspects of health promotion as its norms and values, its ideological underpinning, as well as its exhortations to making healthy choices. Finally, this section addresses the question of whether health promotion acts as a form of social regulation.

Sociology is a discipline based on critical analysis. By taking a sociological perspective we are able to contribute to an examination of both the role and efficacy of health promotion. Sociology is able to ask not only, 'What is health promotion?' but also, 'Why does it take the form that it does?' 'Is this the most effective form in its own terms?' and, 'How have we come to define what effective is?'

What is sociology?

Sociology attempts to analyse the world through the processes that constitute it, whether this is on a macro or a micro level. The former, which might loosely be called structural sociology, looks at such areas of social organization as the economy, education, religion, and work, and their role in the organization of everyday life. This level of sociology would also examine the workings of the institutions and organizations in which this everyday life takes place: government, industry, schools, families, etc. Sociology would want to know who were considered to be the important people involved. Who benefits from its existence and how? How is it funded? What are its stated aims and objectives? What are its values and assumptions? In short, sociology is asking how society works, at the level of institutions and organizations, and what beliefs and attitudes (ideologies) support or challenge this.

There is another level on which sociology works however, viz. the level of individual behaviour. What do people actually do, and why? How do people make sense of their social world, their family, their schooling, their job? How does this micro level of social behaviour interact with the macro level? The key question is how to integrate the two levels of analysis. What is the relationship between the actions and beliefs of individual people in their daily lives and the structural forces and organizations in which they take place? This is perhaps the heart of sociological enquiry: what is the relationship between individual behaviour (social action) and social structure? Commonly, and too simplistically outlined here, there have been two schools of thought: one that the aggregated actions of individuals are what form the structures and the other that the structures determine the actions of individuals. More useful, I would suggest, is the notion of a dynamic interaction between individual and social structure with influences and changes moving in both directions. This has clear relevance for health promotion, which is, after all, in the business of facilitating change at the level both of the individual and of the organization or structure.

Once again, sociology's key concepts can be of use. Not only is sociology in the business of analysing social processes, but it is also interested in the ways in which society is structured, that is, in describing and analysing the different groups that constitute society. These analyses might include social class, gender, age, and race. Of course, they are not mutually exclusive categories and the relationships between them are also of interest to sociologists: for example, the interaction between the effects of gender and of age. Finally, how groups and categories come to be defined is of interest to sociologists. What does it tell us about a society where people are conceived of in categories such as age, or class, or gender and not, for example, by eye colour or astrological sign?

Overall then, sociology is concerned with understanding how society is organized and by what processes it is maintained or changed. Historically, sociologists have adopted a framework that stresses either conflict or consensus. The conflict theorists roughly follow Marxist or Weberian analyses or some development or integration of the two. These interpretations have in common an analysis of competition between social groups to achieve their own interests; fundamental to them is the inequality between the groups, although this is not necessarily thought to be bad. The consensus view acknowledges the plurality of interest groups in society but stresses the harmonious nature of the whole, with each group having its purpose and its place and all functioning in the best interests of society as a whole. This functionalist view is derived from Durkheim's perspective on social organization and one of its notable contemporary exponents has been Talcott Parsons. Interestingly for this discussion, Parsons took health and illness as examples of key factors in the maintenance of social equilibrium. From this, he developed the concept of 'the sick role' (Parsons 1951). In this view, 'illness and illness behaviour' must follow prescribed forms, with the patient, physician, and any others involved having the shared goal of recovery. This functionalist approach to social analysis sees illness at best as dysfunctional and at worst deviant (and thus subject to sanctions).

Concepts of *power* are therefore also crucial to a sociological interpretation of the world. More recently, macro level theories have been subject to a general critique. Interactionist and ethnomethodological perspectives (Goffman 1959; Garfinkel 1967) draw attention to the importance of the particularity of place. The micro social context in which events take place is integral to their meaning and therefore also to their effect or consequences at both micro and macro levels. Thus, nothing is free of the social context in which it takes place. This kind of theorizing exposed the subjective nature of social life and forced the wider discipline to reconsider its claims to 'scientific objectivity'. The notion of a 'value-free' sociological analysis was revealed as problematic and it became apparent that all theories are generated from within social, political, and economic perspectives. Thus, this theoretical standpoint demands that rigorous analysis acknowledge and articulate these interests and contexts, and not proceed as if they do not exist.

It may be more useful to have an analysis that conceptualizes power as a medium rather than an object. In this sense, individuals or groups cannot 'have power' or indeed be rendered powerless. Power can only be exercised, not possessed; it is the medium which exists between social actors, the vehicle through which social relations are expressed.

This more fluid notion of power enables an interpretation of the world that can account for both structural and individual levels of action and the relationship between them (Foucault 1979; Giddens 1979).

These sociological concepts of power, social process, and organization can contribute very usefully to the project of health promotion. I suggest this might take two forms. First, sociological analysis can provide information and understanding, which would make health promotion more effective. Second, sociology can offer a critical analysis of health promotion, its theory, and its practice. These approaches might be referred to as sociology as applied to health promotion and the sociology of health promotion. The latter parts of this chapter will address these approaches in more depth. First, however, it seems appropriate to consider the relationship between sociology and health.

Sociology of health and illness

Medical dominance

Initially sociology was recruited into the field of health and illness in the service of medicine. Medical education saw the need for its students to understand the relationship between health care and the society in which it takes place. Of prime interest were the concerns of the clinicians. Why, for example, did people consult so often with apparently trivial conditions? What was the relationship between the experience of illness and the decision to seek help? How could doctors ensure compliance on the part of their patients? Indeed, what sort of relationship should a doctor and patient have?

In addition to this, medicine, particularly public health medicine (at that stage in its interim guise as community medicine), needed to know how or indeed *which* social factors contributed to the epidemiology of disease. Data were called for on housing, clients, income, employment, etc.

Thus it is apparent that sociology could assist medicine in its task, both in improving the provision of health care to the individual and in analysing the social origins of disease. In its early days, this was sociology as applied to medicine, with sociology's agenda very much set by the interests of medicine. This approach fits well into the consensus model outlined in this chapter, and indeed Parsons was the main exponent of medical sociology during the 1950s.

Medicine as a profession

Early medical sociology developed a related interest in the sociology of the medical profession. Who were doctors? How did they operate as a group? What were the sociological characteristics of the medical profession and how did they maintain their position? This approach did therefore shift the balance from sociology as applied to medicine to the sociology of medicine, even if this was confined to an analysis of the profession (Freidson 1970; Herzlich 1973). Thus sociology was contributing to medical education and practice, and now was forming a critique of the profession of medicine and the implications of this for the delivery of health care.

Incorporating lay perspectives

The group most obviously missing from medical sociological enquiry were patients. What was their experience of illness, of medicine? How was health maintained and illness dealt with in the lay sphere? What kinds of doctoring did people want? How did they go about getting it?

A cursory foray into this kind of approach immediately calls into question the definitions of health and illness that were in use. Are medical definitions of health and illness those used by a lay population? How might they differ? Indeed, is medicine the sole, even the most important way in which ordinary people deal with their illness? Armstrong points out that, until 1954, it was assumed that the experience of symptoms led to a medical consultation:

> The study [Koos 1954] reported that people seemed to experience symptoms much more frequently than their rate of medical consultations would indicate. The researchers were surprised at this because they had assumed, as had medicine for a century and a half, that symptoms as indicators of disease almost invariably led to help seeking behaviour.
>
> (Armstrong 1989: 3)

The significance of this shift in emphasis within medical sociology, from a medical to a lay perspective, was to prompt an intra-disciplinary debate about terminology. 'Medical sociology' evolved into sociology as applied to medicine, and ultimately became the sociology of health and illness (which is now the journal title), which is intended to include all the foregoing aspects whilst not limiting the discipline to a medical agenda (see, for example, Dingwall 1976). This allowed for the discipline to address the relationship between health and other major sociological categories, for example, gender, race, class, age (see examples in Black *et al.* 1984). This has clear parallels with the disciplinary development of health education and health promotion and their relation to medicine (Rodmell and Watt 1986).

A critique of the medical model

Perhaps most importantly for health promotion, this expansion of sociology's remit has allowed it to produce a critique of the medical model and to undertake the project of understanding how health and illness fit into the experience of everyday life. At a structural level, sociology has criticized medicine as a tool to support capitalist development and exploitation (Navarro 1974; Doyal 1979). Medical dominance in the social world has led to a moral critique (Illich 1976), which charges medicine with creating a dependent 'lay' population that is increasingly reliant on the medical profession. Related to this 'de-skilling' thesis is Illich's charge of iatrogenesis; that is, that, far from healing, the practice of biomedicine actually creates illness, as for example may result from the risks of surgery, anaesthesia, immunization, or adverse drug reactions. There is also a large critical literature on the role of medicine in mental health (Szasz 1961; Foucault 1967; Sedgwick 1982; Laing and Esterson 1973).

This structural level of critique would also address ways of improving health that take into account the influence of factors traditionally beyond the scope of medicine. These might include employment, family structure, housing, and at a policy level might suggest possible sites of intervention (McKeown 1979; Kennedy 1983; Townsend and Davidson 1982). Understanding how health and illness fit into the experience of everyday life would address lay concepts of health and illness and draw from these lay models of health behaviour which may run counter to or in conjunction with those of scientific medicine. These might include those models/belief systems that are based on class, race, age, or gender experience (Cornwell 1984; Blaxter and Patterson 1982; Dingwall 1976; Thorogood 1990) or which consider systems of health care that exist outside the bio-medical model, that is, alternative or complementary therapies.

Finally, perhaps the field of sociology of health and illness allows a critical perspective on the social role of medicine. This would examine aspects of social life that may be subject to medical regulation. Clearly, any claim to sickness ultimately requires medical sanction, e.g. for work or school. But we also see the 'medicalization' of many other areas of life, e.g. pregnancy and birth, alcohol abuse, immigration laws (TB), crime and deviance. There are few areas of social life on which medicine doesn't have an 'expert' opinion, and sociology can offer insights into how and why these processes take place. Health promotion can therefore clearly benefit from sociology's interest in these areas. What is it that a sociological perspective can add to the theory and practice of health promotion?

Sociology as applied to health promotion

Health promotion makes claims to know not only what constitutes healthy behaviour, but also the best way to go about encouraging people to achieve it. For this, health promotion needs an analysis of the different groups that constitute society: men and women; young and old; rich and poor; black and white. It relies on knowledge of these groups' varying beliefs and attitudes, interests, and concerns. Health promotion, then, implicitly depends on sociological categories when pursuing its ends.

If health promotion's project is to address change at an individual or a structural level, it needs to know the 'raw material' it is working with. It needs to know what people mean by health, how they believe it affects their lives, and what they feel they could or should be doing about it, in order to facilitate any effective behaviour change. Sociology's analysis of power is crucial if health promotion is to acknowledge the constraints on, and the potential for, social change. Sociology, then, is vital for providing the theoretical insights into the nature and practice of health promotion.

The contribution that a sociological perspective can make to the discipline of health education and health promotion largely depends on what the aims and goals of health promotion and education are thought to be. Clearly, views on this will vary both within and without the field. However, let us assume here the broad-based, loose definition that health promotion is about increasing people's control over their own health, and that this goal is to be attained by addressing the twin supporting themes or pillars of lifestyle and structuralist approaches (WHO 1984). This definition raises a number of questions, some of which will be addressed in this chapter. I hope it will serve, however, as a description of the discipline broadly acceptable to most interested parties.

Lay beliefs

Beginning from this point, it is clear that sociology can provide insights at a number of levels. First, let us consider the role of lay beliefs. There is much sociological evidence that the non-professional community does not uncritically adopt 'the medical model' of disease causation and illness. Blaxter and Patterson (1982), for example, undertook a three-generational study of health attitudes and behaviours amongst a group of working-class Scottish women. They found a whole range of explanations was employed as to the cause of a disease, including individual susceptibility, infection and environment, familial tendencies, stress, poverty, and others. These explanations were clearly influenced by the social context of these women's lives: their own relative poverty; their often damp housing; their role as daughter, mother, or grandmother; their age; their own interpretations of illness or scientific medical explanations.

Indeed, for this group, the authors conclude, *cause* is the most important aspect. Diagnosis alone is insufficient, what these women wanted to know was *why* they had got it. This is not uncommon: social and medical anthropologists (Helman 1978; Cornwell 1984; Herzlich 1973; Pill and Stott 1982) all point to the need for people to explain illness and disease in terms of their own experiences – Why me? Why now? (Tuckett 1976). They also acknowledge that these explanations will imply certain actions, whether these be the traditionally prescribed 'doing the month' (Pillsbury 1984) of Chinese post-partum rituals or the commonplace English aphorism 'feed a cold and starve a fever' (Helman 1978). These authors also alert us to the different layers of belief and explanation. What a person may find acceptable as a general explanation of why people get certain forms of disease, may not necessarily be employed as sufficient explanation as to why *they* have got it. Cornwell (1984) distinguishes two levels of account – the public and the private – that characterize this. Thus, other people may have brought it on themselves by neglecting some aspect of approved behaviour, e.g. inadequate hygiene, food, sleep, or excessive smoking, drinking, 'stress', etc.; whereas personally it may be attributed to family disposition, 'bad luck', or environmental influence. Pill and Stott (1982) found a high degree of fatalism about the aetiology of illness amongst their sample of isolated, less well-educated, young, working-class mothers in South Wales. As Stacey explains:

> Ordinary people, in other words, develop explanatory theories to account for their material, social and bodily circumstances. These they apply to

themselves as individuals, but in developing them they draw on all sorts of knowledge and wisdom, some of it derived from their own experiences, some of it handed on by word of mouth, other parts of it derived from highly trained practitioners. These explanations go beyond common sense in that explanations beyond the immediately obvious are included.

(Stacey 1988: 142)

Obviously these findings have a number of implications for health promotion's strategies. For example, understanding the complexity of lay beliefs could be important for making health promotion initiatives relevant in their approach to the language and concepts that are used by those they wish to reach. Indeed, health promotion might consider it essential to incorporate the knowledge of these 'lay' attitudes and behaviours into its programme designs and strategies. This would certainly be in keeping with developing a more sophisticated 'lifestyles approach' and would contribute to four of the Ottawa Charter's five principal areas of health promotion action: namely, creating supportive environments, strengthening community action, developing personal skills, and reorienting health services. Of course, 'lay beliefs' do not exist in a vacuum, totally separated from 'professional' explanations. Medical theories and diagnoses are incorporated into everyday explanations of ill health; commonly, for example, germs, bugs, and viruses. Neither is this traffic only in one direction. Doctors are just as likely to employ lay explanations in their diagnoses, perhaps particularly in their dealings with the general public, but also because doctors, too, are 'ordinary people' in some aspects of their lives. As Stacey points out, 'As well as lay concepts being socially situated, so is professional practice socially contextualized such that it is itself influenced by lay modes of conceptualization' (1988: 152). Helman's paper 'Feed a cold, starve a fever' (1978) illustrates this process in a North London general practice.

The study of lay beliefs takes us further than this however. Not only must we recognize the 'cross-over' in concepts and language between the lay theories and the bio-medical ones, but we must also acknowledge a more general acceptance by professional and lay people of the relevance of socio-economic factors. 'Ordinary people' themselves recognize the effect of social structure in defining their scope for action. This leads us to a consideration of the ways in which sociology's analysis of social stratification can contribute to the health promotion project.

Social stratification

A society can be divided up in many ways. The categories chosen, however, will reflect social norms and values. In the contemporary world the most commonly used aspects of social division are class and/or wealth, age, gender, and race or ethnicity. These categories themselves reflect differences in power relations between the groups. It follows therefore that these categories will be relevant to the kinds of health and illness experienced. Much sociology of health and illness has focused on these variables, analysing the multivariate ways socio-economic factors have a bearing on health. It is my intention here to take each category in turn, considering some examples of the way these aspects of social structure have a bearing on health and illness and therefore indicate the use of this analysis for health promotion.

In the UK the best-known and most comprehensive work on the relationship between social class and health is the report of the Black Committee (DHSS 1980). This report noted that, despite a general improvement over the last century in the population's health, the disparities between classes remained. The Black Report took mortality as the indicator of health and the Registrar General's classification of occupational classes as an indicator of social class. Whilst these are both less than perfect measures in themselves, they work surprisingly well at predicting levels of health. Thus we see continuing inequalities in health between the social classes which show remarkable consistency whether one takes infant mortality, accidental death, incidence of heart disease, or whatever.

Whilst the database and framework for this report are largely epidemiological, the Committee produced four socially based explanations for these differences. These explanations were:

- *Artefact:* this explanation proposed that the results were no more than a reflection of the statistical categories chosen.
- *Natural selection:* this would explain the preponderance of ill health in the lower social classes by suggesting that people with a tendency to ill health will be unable to compete favourably in the occupational market and thus naturally 'drift down' into the lower social classes.
- *Materialist or structuralist:* this proposes that the correlation between social class and health is a consequence of the unequal distribution of socio-economic factors, such as housing, unemployment, and wealth.
- *Cultural/behavioural:* this model attributes health inequalities to the 'lifestyle' differences between the classes.

The Committee themselves favoured a complex interaction between the latter two explanations. The far-reaching political implications of these findings initially caused the report to be suppressed.

There have been many subsequent commentaries on the Black Report, which both summarize and provide a critique of its findings (Hart 1985; Strong 1990). More recently the work has been updated (Whitehead 1987; Davey-Smith *et al.* 1990) to show that these inequalities persist. Indeed, Davey-Smith *et al.* (1990) maintain that what might have been an effect of unsophisticated measures of class in the first instance is not only upheld but accentuated by the use of more complex indicators of social class and health in their own research ten years later.

Other qualitative studies of health and illness also demonstrate a strong relationship between material/structural circumstances and the experience of health and illness. These fieldwork-based sociological studies describe and analyse this relationship as it occurs in daily life. Some also attempt to articulate the relationship between socio-economic circumstances and the products of 'culture', 'lifestyles', or health behaviour (Cornwell 1984; Blaxter and Patterson 1982).

Social capital and relative deprivation

More recently there has been a focus on *relative* inequalities, stemming from the work of Richard Wilkinson. Wilkinson's (1996) thesis, briefly summarized, is that ill health derives from *relative*, rather than absolute inequality. This then would explain the persistence of dramatic (and widening) health inequalities in societies where the overall levels of health and standards of living have increased. This thesis is supported by evidence that suggests those societies with the most egalitarian distribution of wealth (even if the level of wealth is very low) have lower rates of ill health. Perhaps arising from Wilkinson's work, we have seen, in the last five years, a resurgence of the notion of 'social capital'.

'Social capital' is a much-debated concept (see Morrow 1999 for a very good summary and critical appraisal of the main schools of thought on social capital). It has been subject to a range of interpretations, from a highly individualized model to a model that closely resembles the community development movement of the 1960s and 1970s and could, depending on the political will, be used to facilitate that nebulous concept of 'empowerment'. Whilst it does not resolve the problems of the underpinning norms and values in health promotion, in my view, it is – in theory at least – potentially open to facilitating a range of norms and values, not simply those of the health promotion community. The extent to which this position reflects my continued idealism (which I thought long dead and buried) or indicates real change will only be apparent in time – for the next update of this volume!

To some extent, the hope for 'building social capital' as the 'new' approach for health promotion is founded on the change in political culture signalled by the election of a Labour government in 1997. Whatever the reality of its political constraints, that government is at least rhetorically committed to reducing health and other social inequalities and has allowed for the development of some more radical 'integrated' approaches to 'health development' (as it is now called), e.g. the Sure Start and Healthy Living Centres programmes.

It is apparent that sociological analysis has highlighted a key dilemma for health promotion: the tension between either focusing on facilitating structural change or concentrating on an individual behavioural approach is raised again. Clearly, the evidence for also taking a structural level approach for intervention was incontrovertible (Tuckett 1976; Townsend and Davidson 1982; Davey-Smith *et al.* 1990). This is what lay behind the transition of health education into health promotion (Rodmell and Watt 1986), community medicine into the new public health (Ashton and Seymour

1988), and the Alma Ata declaration (WHO 1978) into healthy public policy (amongst other things, see this volume, Chapter 1). This does not by any means imply that the 'lifestyles' approach had been abandoned but rather that it was recognized that to be effective in increasing individuals' or communities' potential for health, the two must be addressed together. Indeed, it is recognized that the two may be theoretically distinct but are in fact practically inseparable. The nagging question raised here is why it appears that, despite the evidence and the theory, the 'lifestyle' approach still predominates. Ten years on we see this has transmuted into (some) notions of social capital and in the persistence of the 'stages of change' model in health promotion (Bunton *et al.* 2000).

It is here that any 'gut feeling' that this is bound to be the case can be given some intellectual credence through sociological analysis. Using the earlier discussion of concepts of power, it can be seen that resistance to policies that imply widespread social, political, and economic change is most likely to come from those social groups who have least to gain. Thus, for example, in relation to the debate about the health effects of alcohol, we see the relationship between government and breweries militating in favour of changes in the types of beverage produced and the point or level of advertising, but not towards massive increases in taxation or constraints on outlets for purchase or consumption. There are, of course, many reasons underlying the way policy decisions are made (see Chapter 7 this volume) and, to refer again to the earlier analysis of forms of power, these will be subject to local variation. Thus policy will vary between nations, within them, and of course over time, as the balance of power and resistance shifts between the interested parties. It is, of course, a matter of political perspective as to whether you see this shifting balance as one of consensus or conflict; as between interest groups that are inherently equal or inherently unequal.

This discussion is also equally applicable to the other variables in social stratification mentioned earlier. I shall now briefly consider the specific relationship between health and illness and gender.

Gender

There have been many sociological studies that demonstrate the effect of gender. Inequality in almost all areas of social life is structured along gender lines, whether this be in employment, education, wealth, family life, or even linguistic use (see, for example, Rowbotham 1974; Stanworth 1983; Barker and Allen 1976; Brannen and Wilson 1986; Spender 1980, amongst many others). This is no less true for health. In the UK the main gender division in relation to health is the difference in morbidity and morality rates. Overall, men have a higher rate of mortality, women a higher rate of morbidity. As Armstrong put it: 'In summary, women get ill but men die' (1989:46). Sociology's role is to unravel why this should be so. What are the social processes that led to this difference in experience? Or indeed is there a purely biological explanation? Whilst there are *some* diseases that are biologically sex specific (gynaecological ones for instance), it is also true that most diseases affect both sexes. Indeed, as Armstrong (1989) goes on to point out, in other social systems the mortality/morbidity patterns are reversed, so it seems that the explanations are social rather than biological.

Drawing on the literature that documents gender inequalities, sociologists of health have formulated links between the general experience of inequality and the unequal experience of health. Thus again we see class – in terms of employment, housing, poverty, and education – having a bearing, not just on health but differentially on women's and men's health.

Perhaps the single most important factor that distinguishes women's experiences from men's is women's role in the (heterosexual) family. This has, of course, been a central tenet of feminist theory (see, for example, Zaretsky 1976; Mitchell and Oakley 1976; Barrett 1980; Delphy 1977; Eisenstein 1979; Millett 1971; Kuhn and Wolpe 1978).

How then does this plethora of research aid the effectiveness of health promotion? It should be clear that understanding and knowledge of differences in gender experiences of health will lead to more specifically focused campaigns. An understanding of the inequalities in gender relations will also lead to a more subtle and effective approach to the structural changes needed to promote health. For example, knowledge of the unequal distribution of resources within families (Brannen and Wilson 1986) would lead healthy public policy initiatives to address levels of child benefit (as it is paid directly to women) rather than family income support (which is not). Initiatives on healthy diet would address (as they have) women's almost total responsibility for the purchase and preparation of the household's food. Indeed, should health promotion, for the benefit of women's health, challenge these accepted social roles?

Given the breadth of the topic, here it is only possible to cast a cursory glance at issues of gender and health. I have concentrated mainly on differences in the experience of health and in the responsibility for health within the family. This neglects one large area of health in which gender is highlighted; that is, the provision of health care. Women are the main providers of health care in both the public and the private spheres, as both paid and unpaid carers (Stacey 1988). This too should feature in the setting of health promotion's aims and strategies at both the individual and collective level.

Age

Age is yet another variable that can determine health status and behaviour. It is clearly a target area for health promotion too, since different age groups have specific health characteristics. Obviously, the growing proportion of people in society who are over the age of 60 is of particular pertinence to the makers of health and social policy. How this work is done may be influenced by sociological analysis.

Should policy makers, for example, be addressing the more general inequality in the distribution of resources for this age group? Should they be using sociological analysis to examine how this might be an effect of their low status as a social group, or whether their low social status is an effect of their lack of resources? Does health promotion have a role in campaigning not just for policy and lifestyle changes but in the whole social and cultural construction of 'the elderly person'?

The same might be said about other socially constructed 'age groups', such as 'middle-aged men', 'fertile women', 'children', or 'youth'. Indeed, each group does have socially specific characteristics, which are related to their experience of health and their health behaviour. It follows too that health education/promotion has long since directed its gaze towards influencing the health and behaviours of these groups. What has perhaps not been explicit is the role of sociology in identifying these people as 'social groups' and in analysing their particular relationships to power. This will of course have a strong bearing on their capacity for social action and resistance as both individual actors and as collectivities. See, for example, Oakley (1984) on women and childbearing; Dorn (1983) on youth subcultures as a 'buffer' to alcohol education; Phillipson (1982) on the construction of old age.

Race, religion, culture, and ethnicity

This category is somewhat harder to define, for the categories themselves are far from fixed or even subject to a general consensus. Nevertheless, one powerful way in which contemporary social inequalities are structured is along lines of 'race'. This is best understood as a political rather than a biological category (IRR 1982a, 1982b, 1985, 1986; Sivanandan 1983; CCCS 1982) in which it is the common experience of racism (as structured oppression) which unites the group. This definition includes aspects of religion, culture, and ethnicity. For example, in the UK currently religious groups such as 'Muslims' and 'Jews' would be appropriate, but not the Church of England (and note it is not to do with the size of the group in question, but its ideological dominance, or lack of it). Cultural groups such as 'the working class' or 'Northerners' might be considered relatively powerless, but not others such as 'Chelsea fans' or 'claret drinkers'. Ethnicity as a concept also depends on an uncritical acceptance of 'common sense'. This renders 'Asian', but not 'American' an 'ethnic group', 'Irish' but not 'English'.

Since, once again, these categories represent inequalities in power, they also represent inequalities in health. Although there may be diseases that are more prevalent amongst some race/ethnic/cultural groups than others (e.g. sickle-cell anaemia, tuberculosis, heart disease; see Bhat *et al.* 1988), these differences, as with gender, may not be fundamentally biological. The higher incidence of tuberculosis amongst 'Asians' in the UK may have more to do with their social conditions as an effect of racism than a biological predisposition. These sociologically defined inequalities can also help explain why some groups have been targeted for health education and promotion intervention rather than others. The consequences of this have, however, not always been straightforwardly beneficial. These 'unintended consequences' of health promotion (itself a debatable phrase) are examined further in the next section.

The emergence of new social-structural categories of sexuality and disability

The contribution of sociology to health promotion in terms of social stratification might now also include disability and sexuality – categories that have become ascendant in the health field, and for sexuality, not just in the arena of HIV/AIDS. Indeed, in the wake of the HIV/AIDS health promotion campaigns (the pinnacle of health promotion in terms of political importance and visibility?), more general health issues for both lesbians and gay men have been highlighted (see, for example, Fish and Wilkinson, 2000; Farquhar *et al.* 2001).

The rise of 'disability' as a category of sociological enquiry has produced a great deal of debate on the relationship between 'health and 'disability' (particularly 'chronic illness'; see Barnes *et al.* 1999, for example). There are not, however, specific health promotion campaigns that target people with disabilities; rather health promotion campaigns seem to use the notion of 'disability' to warn of what might become of you should you ignore the message (for example to not drink and drive; see Nettleton and Burrows 1995).

In summary

This section has addressed the way in which sociological analysis can be used to further the health promotion project. This might be done by 'addressing' aspects of social stratification such as class, gender, age, race, sexuality, and disability, by taking account of the differential nature of power relations between groups, or by explicating the exchange of concepts between 'lay' and 'expert' belief systems. Sociology can make explicit the taken for granted and thereby facilitate more effective targeting of policies and campaigns.

It remains to be asked whether sociology *should* be facilitating this kind of increased effectiveness, this depth of penetration. In whose interests is it? How were these interests defined? How does it fit with the previous analysis of power? The next section moves to a critique of health education promotion.

A sociology of health promotion

This approach asks not what sociology can contribute to the increased effectiveness of health promotion, but *what* is the role of health promotion and can it be uncritically regarded as 'good'? Sociological enquiry can reveal the norms and values that underpin health promotion; it might also ask questions about the nature of health promotion as a discourse.

Norms and values

Previously, Tuckett (1976) addressed the choices for health education from a sociological perspective. He distinguished the three main reasons for health education as being (i) to act as a branch of preventive medicine, (ii) to facilitate effective use of health care resources, and (iii) to provide general education for health. These reasons, he continued, involve health education in choices about ethics and politics and questions of value judgement. They raise questions about what 'healthy' and what 'normal' are.

At this point in the recent history of health education, the debate was focused on whether health education could be effective by encouraging individual change without demanding any wider social or political change. Tuckett (1976) presented the well-documented and now widely accepted evidence (see this chapter) that health education intervention at a *social* level is likely to be much more effective than simply targeting individual lifestyles and behaviour. Tuckett's argument turned on the point that all health education is political (i.e. not to demand a change in the status quo is itself a political act). If it is accepted that this is the case, then arguing against health education taking a political role is invalid.

Here were the signs of the first stirrings of the shift to health promotion, to the goals of Health For All 2000 and healthy public policy, which were so readily adopted. All intervention for health, must, according to Tuckett: 'Consider and influence relevant social norms and values . . . and health norms and values do not exist independently of other norms and values in society' (1976: 60).

Application of this kind of sociological theorizing has led to some very trenchant critiques of the practice of health education (e.g. Rodmell and Watt 1986; Farrant and Russell 1986). Take, for example, Pearson's (1986) excellent exposure of the racist ideologies underpinning many health education campaigns directed at ethnic minorities. She takes as case studies the campaigns about surma, rickets, antenatal care, and general dietary education. These, she reveals, concentrate on 'lifestyle' aspects of 'Asian' behaviour whilst failing to acknowledge those social structural factors which might be contributing to the overall health outcomes. For example, the campaign about lead in eye cosmetics (surma) ignored factors such as the amount of lead acquired in the blood stream from water pipes in the old housing available to this group, or indeed from paint. It also ignored the effect of being constantly in an inner-city, traffic-filled environment. Similarly, rickets has been eradicated in the white British population by national level policy to fortify commonly used food items with the necessary vitamin D. In contrast, the Asian rickets campaign suggested more 'lifestyle' changes: eating more cornflakes and more margarine and exposing themselves to more sunlight. The case is similar with the Asian mother and baby campaign, where late antenatal booking was implicitly assumed to be the problem of the 'client', not a consequence of the way the service was delivered.

Ideological underpinnings

Application of the sociological method of critical analysis, however, takes us further than the individual vs. social structure debate. We reject the 'victim blaming' approach so admirably revealed by a close examination of the effects of concentrating on 'lifestyles' health education. But the level of analysis employed by Pearson (1986) allows us to see the *ideologies* that underpin such strategies. It is not, she says, simply that 'victim blaming' is wrong; that the 'lifestyles' approach is ineffective; it is that these policies are racist, depending as they do on a particular socially constructed view of 'Asian'. This view constructs 'Asians' as a homogeneous group, subject to a single but all-embracing 'culture'. This undifferentiated group is also constructed as particularly prone to certain diseases as a consequence of their ethnic origins (which may of course be highly varied). Action to improve this 'disease proneness' is assumed to be best undertaken by individuals (by changing their lifestyles) but this is regarded as impossible due to the rigid nature of their all-embracing, but now constructed as conservative, culture. This ideology therefore constructs the notion of an 'Asian culture' which is pathological, and indeed a pathological Asian population. Most revealing of all, however, is that the discourse that underpins this ideology is that of scientific medicine. To be Asian is bad for your health; it is no accident that 'pathological' is the term employed.

This kind of critical analysis shows how important it is, not only to 'consider and influence relevant social norms and values' (Tuckett 1976: 60) with regard to the 'target group' for health education and promotion, but also to examine the social norms and values and the underlying ideologies of those doing the targeting. See also the incisive critique by Ahmad (1993), which demonstrates the implicit racism of much social research in the field of 'ethnicity and health'. There is also a useful critical discussion of the concept of 'culture' in the sociology of race and health by both Ahmad and Kelleher in Kelleher and Hillier (1996).

This critical approach is apparent in a number of other areas. Hilary Graham, for example, in her work on smoking in pregnancy and amongst mothers of young children (1987), shows how health-promoting strategies recommended by health educators and promoters do not take into account the material realities of these women's lives. It is not simply that they cannot afford the recommendations; indeed, in the case of smoking, they may well stand to gain financially. Instead, it is that it simply does not make sense, in the context of their daily routines, to adopt these strategies. As Graham shows, when trapped at home all day with young children and little disposable income, smoking makes sense. You cannot have a physical break from this full-time caring responsibility; you cannot even shut yourself away for half an hour or take a lunch break as another worker would. You must be constantly physically present, alert, and available. Sitting down for ten minutes with a cup of coffee and a cigarette can provide a much-needed break to this routine. In addition to which, the costs are low and the calories few.

Making healthy choices

The implication for health education and promotion of this kind of sociological study is that the picture may not be as straightforward as it seems. Definitions of 'healthy' and 'normal' are not fixed. 'Choice' is not equally available to all people and choices are themselves circumscribed by material conditions. As Graham concludes in her earlier work on women's roles as carers:

> From the picture of family health, which emerges in this book, routine and not choice is the concept which policy makers and professionals need to confront: for choice occurs within, and is contoured by, the routines of everyday life.
>
> (Graham 1984: 188)

'Choice' is a key concept in health education and one that bears closer examination. As the example above demonstrates, 'choice' is constructed and constrained by many factors. Kerr and Charles's (1983) work on food and diet within households similarly shows that factors that are equally important for promoting and maintaining family health can sometimes be in opposition to the healthy behaviour promoted by professionals. For example, the key to many 'white British' families' dietary pattern is contained in the socially significant notion of 'a proper dinner'. 'A proper dinner', as Murcott (1983) has shown, is central to women's role of caring for the family. As Graham goes on to summarize:

> A cooked dinner is seen to constitute a proper meal. Correctly served, it consists of 'proper' meat and 'real' vegetables. Sausages and baked beans do not qualify on either score, whilst chops and peas do. The Sunday dinner epitomises proper eating, for both children and adults; in many families it may be the only occasion on which they eat fresh vegetables (Kerr and Charles, 1983: 11). Kerr and Charles noted in their survey of mothers in York that, in eating properly on Sunday, some families found themselves forced to eat badly (in their terms) throughout the week. The cost of meat, in particular, can force families to make cuts in their consumption of other foods, in fruit and fresh vegetables for instance.
>
> (Graham 1984: 132)

The important point here for health promotion is that 'healthy behaviour' is not uncomplicatedly related to material circumstances. It has a symbolic element, which can be of overriding importance when determining 'choice'. Sociology's role is to draw attention to this.

A critique of health promotion's strategies

This suggests some attention must be paid to the methods employed by health education/promotion. The simple knowledge-action-behaviour change implicit in many health education campaigns is shown to have, at best, limited success (Tones 1986; Bunton *et al.* 2000). Developments in health promotion have suggested that this information-giving approach is a necessary but not a sufficient condition for change. Alongside it should be an 'empowerment' model which emphasizes both 'rationality and free choice' (Tones 1986: 7). This is to be achieved through facilitating decision-making skills and clarification of values and will promote collective social and political action by acknowledging the structural constraints on free choice. A more sophisticated approach to this is the community development model. This acknowledges that 'the community' in question will have pre-existing knowledge and values which will influence the way in which information is received and acted on, choices and decisions made. It recognizes too that these communities might also have something to offer. This then might form part of a strategy to 'build social capital'.

The remaining strategy for health promotion /education is the mass-market campaign, which is closely related to the first, preventive, information-giving approach. There is no space here for in-depth critique of this model, but suffice to say that in its own terms it can never be more than superficial. From a critical perspective it might be asked if advertising can ever be a suitable medium for promoting 'health', which is neither product nor commodity, or for 'selling' a negative message (see, for example, Rhodes and Shaughnessy 1989a).

Thus, health education has been criticized for too narrow an approach, focusing on individual behavioural change in a socio-economic vacuum. Health promotion has acknowledged that good health is not achieved by a series of individually located changes but by situating them in a wider context that both actively promotes and facilitates these choices. What health promotion has perhaps failed to recognize is that 'the healthy choice' is not a unitary concept and that there are many social, cultural, and symbolic meanings, which need also to be taken into account.

An example of a health promotion campaign that failed on these grounds was the Health Education Authority response to HIV/AIDS during the 1980s and 90s. Many critical works levied attacks at the 'norms and values' that were attributed to targeted groups, but also, and perhaps most importantly, to the ideologies and values that underpinned the campaign but that were not articulated (Watney 1988a).

Sociologists highlighted the dilemma facing government-sponsored health education bodies between, on the one hand, the clear need for information on a vital public health issue and, on the other, a political and social reluctance to raise the profile of sex (Wellings 1988; Watney 1988b). The reason for this tension was revealed as a resistance to undertaking any public education campaign which addressed forms of sexual relationship that might be perceived as undermining 'traditional family values' (Jessopp and Thorogood 1990). What emerged was a campaign that gave out muddled messages and we must turn to sociological analyses to suggest some reasons for this.

Critiques drew attention to the racism, homophobia, and erotophobia (e.g. Watney 1988b) that underpinned national HIV/AIDS health education and promotion strategies. The consequences of this, however, was not simply to increase prejudice but to reduce the effectiveness of these measures. The targeting of 'high-risk groups' drew attention away from the fact that it was the behaviour, not the group membership, which carried the risk, thereby engendering complacency amongst those whose sexual behaviour was 'risky', but whose group membership identity was not. It also fails to make the information relevant to the lives of the target group.

As Holland *et al.* (1900a, 1990b) make very clear in their work, national health/education campaigns directed at young people have neglected to take gender relations into account. This is crucial since the 'prevailing definition of sexuality can also render girls relatively powerless to define what happens in an individual sexual encounter' (1990a: 8). Young women were encouraged to take responsibility for protected sex whilst no consideration was given to the context of power relations in which their relationships take place. As Holland *et al.* say elsewhere in this paper:

> Government health education policy on the risks facing young women is currently totally uninformed on the social constructions of female sexuality . . . Knowledge of young women's sexuality needs to be analysed if health education is to be effective in helping to contain the AIDS epidemic.
>
> (Holland *et al.* 1990a: 3)

Sociological analyses of power and the relationships between individual agency and social structure are therefore vital for making health education and promotion campaigns relevant to the target groups' lived experiences. Sociology is necessary for articulating the framework within which 'choice' can be exercised, and for understanding how adjustments to this framework might be made. In the example of young women's supposed responsibility for safer sex we see not only how socially constructed gender relations act to make girls both responsible and blameworthy, but also how the dominant values of male sexuality and patriarchal ideology have underpinned health education and promotion strategies so far. This may render them less effective in achieving behavioural changes but it does serve to reinforce the social, political, and ideological status quo.

Organizational change: the rise (and fall) of public health

The statutory and organizational framework within which health promotion practice takes place was not discussed in the first edition of this chapter. To some extent the national or even international context of health promotion practice lies beyond the remit of a discussion of the relevance of *sociology* for health promotion. Nevertheless, a sociology *of* health promotion might well address the regulatory framework in which the discursive practices of 'health promotion' are constructed (for example, Lupton 1995; Bunton *et al.* 1995; Petersen and Lupton 1996; Thorogood 2000). These accounts provide a sociological critique of the organization and practices of public health and offer insights into the 'social role' of health promotion as practice. This might include a discussion of the shifting organizational forms of health education, promotion and now development, and its relationship to the wider discourse of public health.

Thus, since the original publication of this chapter, government-sponsored health promotion in England has undergone yet another re-organization, and is now the responsibility of the Health Development Agency, presumably to reflect a more integrated approach to the task, or to mark a reduction in dedicated funding. A more unexpected change since that time was the rise in fortune of public health as Departments of Public Health became responsible for advising on local Health Authority commissioning. The boom is over however as Primary Care Trusts take over from Health Authorities and there is no formal role for public health within them. This means that health promotion (or development) may too find itself subsumed into 'primary care'. This constant shifting might be an indication, from a 'sociology *for*' perspective, of a 'lack of focus' or a constant drive to better, more effective practice, or, from a 'sociology *of*' perspective, its shifting position as a regulatory technology.

Evidence-based everything

A change at a conceptual level that has occurred since 1992 has been the rise of the 'evidence-based' movement. Whilst this has undergone lengthy critique, not least in the arena of the sociology of health and illness, it is still a powerful tenet of Department of Health thinking and impacts upon both policy development and the research agenda. Nevertheless, despite the old reliance on the k-a-b model of health promotion persists (Bunton *et al.* 2000). This suggests that it derives from a particular conceptual framework of health promotion – that is a 'top down' one where 'health professionals' know what is best (based on evidence of course) and do their level best to impart it to those for whom it would be of benefit (usually 'the deprived' or otherwise marginal groups). Again, from a 'sociology for' perspective, we might suggest that this might finally wither away with a radical social capital/community development approach (although I really never expected to start sounding so passionate!). However, from a 'sociology of' perspective, it is simply another formation to be analysed and accounted for as part of the shifting discourse of public health.

Health education and promotion as regulation

Perhaps sociologists should be asking whether there are consequences of health promotion which lie beyond facilitating healthy behaviour. Does health promotion act as an agent of social regulation? Are 'healthy choices' themselves an expression of prevalent social norms and values?

As we have seen, choice is constructed and constrained by socially organized power relations, which themselves create the routines or 'normal' relations in which 'choice' is exercised. In order to facilitate making the healthy choice, health promotion must take these factors into consideration. We have also seen that there are other discourses – social, cultural, symbolic – which influence decision making.

Health promotion, not surprisingly, supposes making the *healthy* choice to be the most important. It therefore assumes that this is also how any rational person would act. The task for health promotion is then to remove obstacles, both individual and social structural, to this choice. To quote Ashton and Seymour:

> Health promotion works through effective community action. At the heart of this process are communities having their own power and having control of their own initiatives and activities . . . Health promotion supports personal and social development through providing information, education for health and helping develop the skills which they need to make healthy choices.
>
> (Ashton and Seymour 1988: 26)

Although progressive health promotion rhetoric is keen to emphasize the principle of ethical voluntarism (Tones 1986) – that is, the freedom to make any choice – it is clear that some choices are assumed better than others. It is further assumed that once in possession of the information, the clarified norms and values, and the decision-making skills, and with socio-cultural barriers removed, any rational person could not help but make the healthy choice. Thus, healthy behaviour is seen to be synonymous with rational behaviour. This discourse of rationality belongs within the medico-scientific paradigm which itself defines health and disease. This focus therefore privileges the healthy choice and obscures decisions made in other discourses (Thorogood 1995). This may be the maintenance of family values and cohesion though the provision of a 'proper dinner' or smoking as a strategy for coping with bringing up small children, or it may be the regulation of safer sex within heterosexual relationships.

Indeed, we might ask why the discourses of health should be expected to have any prominence in decision making about sex at all. Indeed, it is only in the realm of medicine that 'sex' is considered 'health behaviour' and then it is addressed only in terms of its outcomes, e.g. pregnancy, contraception, abortion, STIs, etc. For most people the role of 'sex' in their everyday lives is not primarily a health concern. More likely to feature are discourses of risk, pleasure, danger, and penetration; and whilst these formulations of experience remain unacknowledged, so the health promotion message will remain ineffective, as the work of Holland *et al.* (1990a, 1990b) and Wilton and Aggleton (1990) in relation to HIV so clearly has shown.

Here then is an inherent tension for health promotion. To acknowledge the possibility of choice within discourses other than health as equally valid would undermine health promotion's claim to scientific rationality. If health promotion were truly to accept all choices as equally valid, the role of *health* promotion would be reduced to promoting access to and decision making about services, and the dominance of the rational, medico-scientific paradigm would be challenged. It would be possible for other social formations to arise, for competing social norms and values to move into ascendance.

At this level, then, health promotion can be conceptualized as a form of social regulation. By allying itself to scientific objectivity, health promotion can continue to promote 'healthy choices' as value free and rational. In doing this it may fail to acknowledge other discourses and simply act to perpetuate existing social relations.

Conclusion

This chapter has aimed to outline the broad basis of the sociological method and to consider the contribution this method has made or might make to health promotion. First, it seems that knowledge generated initially through medical sociology and subsequently through the sociology of health and illness can make a valuable contribution by questioning definitions of 'health' and by examining the social role of medicine. Second, we have seen how sociology can be a useful tool for increasing the effectiveness of health promotion. This might be through analysis of social structure, identification of relevant target groups, consideration of the role of lay beliefs, or in weighing up the relevant merits of individual versus structural approaches. Third, we have seen how a sociological perspective can contribute to a critique of health promotion, both in its methods and in its goals and aims.

What, then, can be concluded about the relevance of sociology for health promotion? I would suggest that a strong case can be made for the inclusion of this disciplinary method in the theory and practice of health promotion for several reasons. The contribution of sociology to the analysis of health and illness has been most notably to challenge medical dominance in defining what health and illness/disease are. It has shown us the narrowness of a medical perspective and the need to recognize other notions of health and illness if we are to understand the experience of everyday life. Obviously, for a practice that seeks to promote 'healthy behaviours' amongst a 'lay' population, these insights are invaluable. As the section on sociology as applied to health promotion demonstrates, the use of sociological categories is implicit in the work of health promotion: acknowledging and articulating this serves to make health promotion more effective in targeting its work. It also serves to alert health promotion's practitioners to the values and assumptions inherent in these categories. This is clearly necessary if the practice is to be responsive to its clients' needs, to be self-aware, self-critical, and accountable.

Finally, because sociology is a discipline based on *critique*, it allows questions to be asked about the nature of health promotion. It can ask questions about the goals and aims of health promotion and examine their consequences in a wider social context. It is not enough for health promoters simply to 'get on with their jobs', they must also be asking themselves those key sociological questions: In whose interests is this? How is power being exercised here? Which values are being prioritized? Use of the sociological method can and should contribute to the theoretical and pragmatic decisions regarding the future of the health promotion project.

Afterword: what has health promotion done for sociology?

With the benefit of ten years' hindsight, one might now comment on the contribution that health promotion has made to sociology. Health promotion has perhaps made its most significant contribution in the explosion of social theorizing about 'risk' and has been the source of many a PhD. Certainly, as a rich field to be mined for critique, case studies, and theoretical development, health promotion has done many of us proud; as well as keeping many sociologists in gainful employment as teachers, researchers, and practitioners – one need only look at the references to this chapter for confirmation!

References

Aggleton, P. and Homans, H. (1988) *Social Aspects of AIDS*, London: Falmer.

Ahmad, W. I. U. (ed.) (1993) *'Race' and Health in Contemporary Britain*, Buckingham: Open University Press.

—— (1996) 'The trouble with culture', in D. Kelleher and S. Hillier (eds) *Researching Cultural Differences in Health*, London: Routledge.

Armstrong, D. (1989) *An Outline of Sociology as Applied to Medicine*, Bristol: J. Wright.

Ashton, J. and Seymour, H. (1988) *The New Public Health*, Milton Keynes: Open University Press.

Barker, D. and Allen, S. (eds) (1976) *Dependence and Exploitation in Work and Marriage*, London: Longman.

Barnes, C., Mercer, G., and Shakespeare, T. (1999) *Exploring Disability: a Sociological Introduction*, Oxford: Polity Press.

Barrett, M. (1980) *Women's Oppression Today*, London: Verso.

Bhat, A., Carr-Hill, R., and Ohn, S. (1988) *Britain's Black Population*, Aldershot: Gower.

Black, N., Boswell, D., Gray, A., Murphy, S., and Popay, J. (eds) (1984) *Health and Disease: A Reader*, Milton Keynes: Open University Press.

Blaxter, M. and Patterson, E. with assistance of Sheila Murray (1982) *Mothers and Daughters: A Three-Generational Study of Health Attitudes and Behaviour*, London: Heinemann Educational Books.

Brannen, J. and Wilson, G. (eds) (1986) *Give and Take in Families: Studies in Resource Distribution*, London: Allen Unwin.

Bunton, R., Nettleton, S., and Burrows, R. (eds) (1995) *The Sociology of Health Promotion: Critical Analyses of Lifestyle Consumption and Risk*, London: Routledge.

Bunton, R., Baldwin, S., Flynn, D., and Whitelaw, S. (2000) 'The "stages of change" model in health promotion: science and ideology', *Critical Public Health*, 10 (1): 55–70.

CCCS (1982) *The Empire Strikes Back*, London: Hutchinson.

Charles, N. and Kerr, M. (1986) 'Just the way it is: gender and age differences in family food consumption', in J. Brannen and G. Wilson (eds) *Give and Take in Families: Studies in Resource Distribution*, London: Allen Unwin.

Cornwell, J. (1984) *Hard Earned Lives*, London: Tavistock.

Davey-Smith, G., Bartley, M., and Blane, D. (1990) 'The Black Report on socio-economic inequalities in health ten years on', *British Medical Journal* 301 (18–25 August): 373–5.

Delphy, C. (1977) *The Main Enemy*, London: Women's Research and Resources Centre.

DHSS (1980) *Inequalities in Health: The Black Report*, London: HMSO.

Dingwall, R. (1976) *Aspects of Illness*, London: Martin Robertson.

Dorn, N. (1983) *Alcohol, Youth and the State*, Bromley: Croom Helm.

Doyal, L. with Pennell, I. (1979) *The Political Economy of Health*, London: Pluto.

Durkheim, E. (1964) *Rules of Sociological Method*, New York: The Free Press.

Eisenstein, Z. (ed.) (1979) *Capitalist Patriarchy and the Case for Socialist Feminism*, New York: Monthly Review Press.

Farrant, W. and Russell, J. (1986) *The Politics of Health Information*, London: Institute of Education, University of London.

Farquhar, C., Bailey, J., and Whittaker, D. (2001) *Are Lesbians Sexually Healthy? A Report of the 'Lesbian Sexual Behaviour and Health Survey'* London: South Bank University Social Science Research Papers No. 11.

Fish, J. and Wilkinson, S. (2000) 'Lesbians and cervical screening', *Psychology of Women Review*, 2 (2): 3–13.

Foucault, M. (1967) *Madness and Civilisation*, London: Tavistock.

—— (1979) *Discipline and Punish: The Birth of the Prison*, Harmondsworth: Peregrine.

Freidson, E. (1961) *Patients' Views of Medical Practice: A Study of Subscribers to a Prepaid Medical Plan in the Bronx*, New York: Russell Sage Foundation.

—— (1970) *Profession of Medicine: A Study of the Sociology of Applied Medicine*, New York: Dodd, Mead.

Garfinkel, H. (1967) *Studies in Ethnomethodology*, Englewood Cliffs, NJ: Prentice-Hall.

Giddens, A. (1979) *Central Problems in Social Theory*, London: Macmillan.

Goffman, E. (1959) *The Presentation of Self in Everyday Life*, Garden City: Doubleday.

Graham, H. (1984) *Women, Health and the Family*, Brighton: Wheatsheaf Falmer.
—— (1987) 'Women's smoking and family health', *Social Science and Medicine* 1: 47–56.
Hart, N. (1985) *The Sociology of Health and Medicine*, Ormskirk: Causeway.
Helman, C. (1978) 'Feed a cold, starve a fever: folk models of infection in an English suburban community, and their relation to medical treatment', *Culture, Medicine and Psychiatry* 2: 107–37.
Herzlich, C. (1973) *Health and Illness: A Social Psychological Analysis*, London: Academic Press.
Holland, J., Ramazanoglu, C., and Scott, S. (1990a) 'Managing risk and experiencing danger: tensions between government AIDS policy and a young women's sexuality', *Gender and Education*, 2 (2): 193–202.
Holland, J., Ramazanoglu, C., Scott, S., Sharp, S., and Thompson, R. (1990b) 'Don't die of ignorance – I nearly died of embarrassment', paper presented to the fourth Social Aspects of AIDS Conference, London.
Illich, I. (1976) *Limits to Medicine*, London: Marion Boyars.
IRR (1982a) *Roots of Racism*, London: Institute of Race Relations.
—— (1982b) *Patterns of Racism*, London: Institute of Race Relations.
—— (1985) *How Racism Came to Britain*, London: Institute of Race Relations.
—— (1986) *The Fight Against Racism*, London: Institute of Race Relations.
Jessopp, L. and Thorogood, N. (1990) 'No sex please, we're British', *Critical Public Health* 2: 10–15.
Kelleher, D. (1996) 'A defence of the use of the terms "ethnicity" and "culture"' in D. Kelleher and S. Hillier (eds) *Researching Cultural Differences in Health*, London: Routledge.
Kennedy, I. (1983) *The Unmasking of Medicine*, London: Paladin.
Kerr, M. and Charles, N. (1983) *Attitudes to the Feeding and Nutrition of Young Children*. Preliminary Report, York: University of York.
Kuhn, A. and Wolpe, A. M. (1978) (eds) *Feminism and Materialism*, London: Routledge & Kegan Paul.
Laing, R. D. and Esterson, A. (1973) *Sanity, Madness and the Family*, Harmondsworth: Penguin.
Lupton, D. (1995) *The Imperative of Health*, London: Sage.
Maclean, M. (1986) 'Households after divorce: the availability of resources and their impact on children', in J. Brannen and G. Wilson (eds) *Give and Take in Families: Studies in Resource Distribution*, London: Allen & Unwin.
McKeown, T. (1979) *The Role of Medicine*, Oxford: Blackwell.
Millett, K. (1971) *Sexual Politics*, London: Sphere.
Mitchell, J. and Oakley, A. (1976) *The Rights and Wrongs of Women*, Harmondsworth: Penguin.
Morrow, V. (1999) 'Conceptualising social capital in relation to health and well-being of children and young people: a critical review' in *The Sociological Review* Vol. 47, No. 4, November: 744–765.
Murcott, A. (ed.) (1983) *The Sociology of Food and Eating*, Aldershot: Gower.
Navarro, V. (1974) *Medicine under Capitalism*, London: Croom Helm.
Nettleton, S. and Burrows, R. (1995) 'Sociological Critiques of Health Promotion' in R. Bunton, S. Nettleton and R. Burrows (eds) *The Sociology of Health Promotion: critical analyses of lifestyle consumption and risk*, London: Routledge.
Oakley, A. (1984) *The Captured Womb*, Oxford and New York: Blackwell.

Parsons, T. (1951) *The Social System*, New York: The Free Press.

Pearson, M. (1986) 'Racist notions of ethnicity and health', in S. Rodmell and A. Watt (eds) *The Politics of Health Education*, London: Routledge & Kegan Paul.

Petersen, A. and Lupton, D. (1996) *The New Public Health: Health and Self in the Age of Risk*, London: Sage.

Phillipson, C. (1982) *Capitalism and the Construction of Old Age*, London: Macmillan.

Pill, R. and Stott, N. C. H. (1982) 'Concepts of illness causation and responsibility: some preliminary data from a sample of working class mothers', *Social Science and Medicine* 16: 43–52.

Pillsbury, B. (1984) 'Doing the month: confinement and convalescence of Chinese women after childbirth', in N. Black *et al.* (eds) *Health and Disease: A Reader*, Milton Keynes: Open University Press.

Rhodes, T. and Shaughnessy, R. (1989a) 'Condom commercial', *New Socialist* June/July 34–5.

—— (1989b) 'Compulsory screening': addressing AIDS in Britain 1986–1989', *Campaign*, 23 January 1989.

Rodmell, S. and Watt, A. (1986) *The Politics of Health Education*, London: Routledge & Kegan Paul.

Rowbotham, S. (1974) *Hidden from History*, London: Pluto.

Sedgwick, P. (1982) *Psychopolitics*, London: Pluto.

Sivanandan, A. (1983) *A Different Hunger*, London: Pluto.

Spender, D. (1980) *Man Made Language*, London: Routledge & Kegan Paul.

Stacey, M. (1988) *The Sociology of Health and Healing*, London: Unwin Hyman.

Stanworth, M. (1983) *Gender and Schooling*, London: Hutchinson.

Strong, P. M. (1990) 'Black on class and mortality: theory, method and history', *Journal of Public Health Medicine* 12 (314): 168–80.

Szasz, T. (1961) *The Myth of Mental Illness*, New York: Harper & Row.

Thorogood, N. (1990) 'Caribbean home remedies and their importance for black women's health care in Britain', in P. Abbott and G. Payne (eds) *New Directions in Sociology of Health*, London: Falmer.

—— (1995) '"London dentist in HIV scare": HIV and dentistry in popular discourse' in R. Bunton, S. Nettleton, and R. Burrow (eds) *The Sociology of Health Promotion: Critical Analyses of Lifestyle Consumption and Risk*, London: Routledge.

—— (2000) 'Sex education as disciplinary technique: policy and practice in England and Wales', *Sexualities* 3 (4), November: 425–38.

Tones, B. K. (1986) 'Health education and the ideology of health promotion: a review of alternative approaches', *Health Education Research* 1: 3–12.

Townsend, P. and Davidson, N. (1982) *Inequalities in Health*, Harmondsworth: Penguin.

Tuckett, D. (1976) *An Introduction to Medical Sociology*, London: Tavistock.

Watney, S. (1988a) 'AIDS, "moral panic" theory and homophobia', in P. Aggleton and H. Homans (eds) *Social Aspects of AIDS*, London: Falmer.

—— (1988b) 'Visual AIDS – advertising ignorance', in P. Aggleton and H. Homans (eds) *Social Aspects of AIDS*, London: Falmer.

Wellings, K. (1988) 'Perceptions of risk – media treatments of AIDS', in P. Aggleton and H. Homans (eds) *Social Aspects of AIDS*, London: Falmer.

Whitehead, M. (1987) *The Health Divide: Inequalities in Health in the 80s*, London: HEA.

WHO (1978) *Alma Ata Declaration*, Copenhagen: WHO/EUR.

—— (1984) *Health Promotion: European Monographs in Health and Health Education*, 6, Copenhagen: WHO/EUR.

Wilkinson, R. (1996) *Unhealthy Societies: the Afflictions of Inequality*, London: Routledge.

Wilton, T. and Aggleton, P. (1990) 'Condoms, coercion and control: heterosexuality and the limits to HIV/AIDS education', paper given at the fourth Social Aspects of AIDS Conference, London.

Zaretsky, E. (1976) *Capitalism, the Family and Personal Life*, London: Pluto.

4 Epidemiology and health promotion

A common understanding

Andrew Tannahill

Introduction

Epidemiology is widely recognized as an important scientific foundation for health promotion. This chapter addresses the important questions 'What has epidemiology contributed to health promotion?' and 'How might health promotion be better served by epidemiology?' Broadly speaking, two interrelated problem areas are encountered: these concern, respectively, the way in which epidemiology is currently brought to bear on health promotion and, more fundamentally, the way in which the term 'epidemiology' is commonly interpreted.

What is epidemiology?

Many definitions of epidemiology exist. Most are along the lines of the following, which is commonly used.

> Epidemiology [is] the study of the distribution and determinants of disease in human populations.
>
> (Barker and Rose 1984: v)

The contributions to health promotion of epidemiology *thus defined* will now be considered. Basic principles of epidemiological investigation will be described, since understanding of the 'whats' of the role of epidemiology in health promotion is best built on knowledge of the 'hows'. Moreover, it is intended that the account will help 'non-epidemiologists' to interpret epidemiological reports and data, and to work profitably with colleagues whose principal expertise (and socialization) lies in epidemiology. Interested readers may wish to supplement the account given here by turning to one or more of the numerous specialist textbooks covering the subject at various levels of complexity (Friedman 1987; Lilienfeld and Lilienfeld 1980; Mausner and Kramer 1985). In so doing, however, they should beware of the existence of considerable variation in the use of common terms and the attendant scope for confusion. This semantic muddle is particularly regrettable in a discipline whose practitioners pride themselves on the 'hardness' of their methodologies and data.

Contributions to health promotion

These may be considered under headings derived from the above definition: distribution of disease and determinants of disease.

Distribution of disease

The study of the distribution of disease – *descriptive* epidemiology – is central to public health. Its relevance to health promotion lies in its being an essential first step in the prevention of ill health. Descriptive epidemiology, as the name suggests, describes aspects of the burden of disease in communities. These aspects are:

1   the *amount* of given diseases, in terms of deaths occurring over a certain period of time (mortality), cases arising in a particular population over a defined time (incidence), or cases existing in a population at a point of time or over a defined time period (point and period prevalence, respectively); and
2   the manner in which particular diseases are distributed according to characteristics of *time, person,* and *place.*

Much of this work may be done using routinely collected data. Mortality data relate to causes of death, and are obtained from death certificates. Morbidity data are concerned with non-fatal disease events, and are obtained from a wide range of sources, including hospital discharge returns, sickness absence certificates, infectious disease notifications, cancer registrations, general practice records, and the national General Household Survey (which collects medical, social, and other information from a random sample of the population of the United Kingdom).

In many instances, however, the information required is unobtainable through routine channels, and special studies are required. These typically take the form of a *cross-sectional study*, in which the situation in a population at or over a given time is studied, usually through investigating a carefully selected representative sample of the population of interest.

Amount of disease

Routine mortality statistics show, for instance, that the major causes of death in Scotland (as in the United Kingdom as a whole) are coronary heart disease (CHD), cancers, and cerebrovascular disease: in 1988, these conditions accounted for 17,963, 14,720, and 8,150 deaths, respectively, representing 29 per cent, 23.8 per cent, and 13.2 per cent of deaths in Scotland in that year

(Registrar General Scotland 1989). Crude figures of this sort are clearly of value to those concerned with the promotion of health, in that they help build up a picture of the burden of serious ill health in a population.

For any given disease, whether we are dealing with mortality, incidence, or prevalence, it is necessary to relate the number of occurrences of interest to the number in the particular population who are at risk of contributing to these occurrences, and to a specified time scale. In other words, we must calculate a *rate* of occurrence. This is done by dividing the number of occurrences of interest in a specified time (or, in the case of point prevalence, at a particular point in time) by the population at risk. A *crude* rate relates to a total population at risk, for example the total population of Scotland in relation to CHD, or the total female population in connection with cancer of the cervix. Thus it can be calculated using appropriate population estimates that in Scotland, in 1988, the crude mortality rate for CHD was 352.6 per 100,000 population and that for cervical cancer was 7.3 per 100,000 women.

As seen below, however, proper comparisons, over time or between populations, require manipulations of such crude figures, to allow for differences in population structure which may make comparison of crude data invalid.

Distribution by time

The scrutiny of routine data, or the repeated or ongoing execution of special studies, over time allows us to identify and describe time trends for particular diseases. Three basic types of time trend are described (Farmer and Miller 1983: 7).

1   *Epidemic* An epidemic is a temporary increase in the incidence of a disease in a population. Influenza is the classic epidemic disease, with a tendency to relatively short-lived upsurges of incidence of various sizes in and around winter. The 'temporary' may, however, refer to a longer time period, hence present-day references to epidemics of coronary heart disease (see below) and the acquired immune deficiency syndrome (AIDS).

2   *Periodic* This refers to the pattern of more or less regular changes in incidence. For example, whooping cough tends to peak every three years or so.

3   *Secular* Secular, or long-term, trends refer to non-periodic changes in disease statistics over a number of years. For example, tuberculosis mortality has declined markedly, and fairly steadily, since the middle of the nineteenth century. On the other hand, mortality from lung cancer in the UK has grown enormously in the twentieth century. So too has coronary heart disease mortality, although this has shown a decline in recent years (albeit less marked than in the United States and Australia) (British Cardiac Society 1987).

Comparison of disease rates over time requires special manipulations of the crude data to make allowance for possible effects of changes in population structure, notably in relation to age and sex. This is, of course, because most diseases show a predilection for particular age groups, and there are many differences in disease experience between the genders. Thus, a comparison of two crude rates at different times, especially many years apart, may be rendered invalid through the later population's containing a larger proportion of old people or women. The process of *standardization* can correct for age and sex differences simultaneously. Alternatively, separate age-standardized rates for males and females can be calculated.

An important method of standardization involves calculation of the standardized mortality ratio (SMR). This permits comparison between a number of populations by the calculation of a single figure for each population, derived using a reference population. A single SMR can be obtained which makes allowance for differences in age and sex structure between populations. Once again, however, separate figures are often calculated for males and females. Suppose we want to compare male mortality from CHD in Scotland with that in the UK as a whole. The UK male population in this instance is the reference population. Taking the Scottish male population, broken down by age group, we multiply the number of individuals in each age band by the mortality rate in the corresponding age band of the whole UK population (*age-specific* rate). Thus we obtain the number of deaths in each age class which would be expected if Scotland had the same mortality experience as the UK as a whole. The total number of expected deaths for the overall male population of Scotland is then derived simply by adding up the calculated numbers for all the age bands. The SMR is finally arrived at by dividing the observed male CHD deaths (those which actually occurred in the Scottish male population) by the total expected deaths and multiplying by 100.

A population with an SMR of 100 has the same overall mortality experience as the reference population. An SMR of >100 indicates a surplus of deaths: a value of, say, 120 represents an excess of mortality of 20 per cent over that which would have occurred had the population experienced the same age-specific mortality as the reference population. An SMR of <100 implies a relatively favourable experience: an SMR of 85, for example, indicates a 15 per cent shortfall of deaths in comparison with the expectation based on the reference population.

SMRs can be calculated for a number of populations, allowing comparison not only with a reference population but with each other. International 'league tables' can be constructed, for example. Moreover, sub-national comparisons may be made: mortality in various cities can be compared, as indeed can the experiences of various districts within cities. Thus, taking the whole of Scotland as the reference population, the SMR for lung cancer in the Greater Glasgow area for the years 1975-88 was 136. For districts within that area, again taking the Scottish population as the standard, the all-causes SMR ranged from around 60 to over 120 (Greater Glasgow Health Board 1990).

The calculation and comparison of SMRs are of benefit to health promotion in quantifying and ranking disease problems, and in identifying places with particularly pressing needs for prevention or other forms of action.

Distribution by person

Characteristics of person which affect the likelihood of occurrence of particular diseases include age, sex, ethnicity, occupation, socio-economic status, marital status, and aspects of lifestyle (such as smoking). Disease rates may be calculated for subsets of the population thus distinguished: for example, we may calculate age-specific mortality rates for accidents (or particular types of accidents), this again helping us to identify priorities for preventive action.

Distribution by place

International, regional, and small area (for example postcode sectors) comparisons of disease distribution may be made. Once more, standardization is required to allow for important differences in population structure.

Determinants of disease

Description of the distribution of disease may throw up some clues as to aetiology, that is to say the causal origins of disease. In other words, descriptive studies may *generate* hypotheses of causation. For instance, a cross-sectional study may show that certain types of respiratory disease are commoner in smokers, leading to the hypothesis that smoking causes these diseases.

Cross-sectional studies may also be used for more advanced exploration into the origins of disease. For example, one such study investigated the prevalence of self-reported symptoms of chronic bronchitis in relation to age, smoking status, and place of residence (characterized as having high or low levels of atmospheric pollution) (Lambert and Reid 1970). Independent associations between the disease (chronic bronchitis) and the suspected risk factors (increasing age, smoking, and atmospheric pollution) were found, but it seemed that in the absence of smoking atmospheric pollution had a relatively small impact.

In general, however, the *testing* of a causal hypothesis requires more sophisticated studies. These may be classified, in order of increasing complexity, as *analytic* (*case-control* and *cohort*) studies and *intervention* studies. Cohort studies will be described first.

Cohort studies

In its simplest form, a cohort study involves recruiting a study population (cohort) free of the disease of interest, categorizing the subjects according to the presence/absence or level of exposure to a suspected risk factor (or risk factors), and following them up over a period of time to see if they develop the disease under investigation. The strength of association between a given risk factor and the disease in question may, in the case of a risk factor classed as present or absent, be calculated by the formula:

$$\text{Relative risk} = \frac{\text{incidence rate in exposed}}{\text{incidence rate in non-exposed}}$$

For a graded risk (such as blood pressure or blood cholesterol level), a separate relative risk may be calculated for a number of classes of risk (for example, diastolic blood pressure 90–99 mmHg, 100–109 mmHg, etc., taking <90mmHg to signify 'non-exposure').

A relative risk of 1 implies an absence of association. Statistical tests are applied to indicate the probability or confidence that the relative risk value truly differs from unity. Subject to such testing, the higher the relative risk, the greater the strength of (positive) association, while a relative risk of less than 1 represents a negative association, suggestive of a protective effect.

It should be noted that positive association, even with a statistically significant and high relative risk, does not necessarily indicate causation. Strength of association, as measured by the relative risk, is only one of a number of factors to be considered in assessing the likelihood that an association is causal (Bradford Hill 1977: 288).

Possibly the most famous cohort study of all time is that concerning smoking and mortality among British doctors, carried out by Doll and Hill (1964). The study involved sending a questionnaire on smoking behaviour to all doctors on the British Medical Register, and following the cohort up for subsequent death. Association between smoking and several causes of death were found. Most notable was the marked association with lung cancer, which, in males, showed a virtually linear relationship between age-standardized mortality rate and number of cigarettes smoked per day.

In terms of health promotion 'message', this study provided evidence that, on a number of preventive grounds, it is advisable not to smoke – or at least not to start. What about people who already smoke? Would they be likely to attain preventive benefits from stopping? A follow-up component of Doll and Hill's classic study offered such hope: analysis of questionnaires enquiring into changes in smoking status demonstrated that the likelihood of dying from lung cancer fell with time after smoking cessation.

The above example dealt with a single risk factor. However, a single cohort study can collect information simultaneously on a number of risk factors. Sophisticated methods of multivariate analysis can then be used to estimate the independent associations of the various risk factors with a particular disease from a morass of potentially interacting risk factors.

The teasing out of the roles of multiple, interacting risk factors is of particular relevance in relation to CHD. Cohort studies such as the Framingham

Study (Dawber 1980) have provided much information on risk factors for CHD, their interrelationships, and their relative weights. The most consistently strong independent associations have been found for age, male gender, blood pressure, cigarette smoking, and blood cholesterol level. Combinations of risk factors mark especially high risks.

So far, we have confined our consideration of analysis to relative risk. Cohort studies yield further measures which are of value to health promotion.

1   *Attributable risk* is the incidence of a given disease in the group exposed to a particular risk factor *minus* that in the non-exposed group. This quantifies the hazards, in probability terms, of being exposed to the risk factor and, conversely, the benefits which accrue to an individual from not being exposed (provided, of course, that status as regards that particular risk factor is the only important difference between the groups).

   For example, the attributable risk for cigarette smoking in relation to lung cancer mortality was found in one study to be 169 per 100,000 per year (188 *minus* 19 per 100,000 per year) (Hammond 1966). Provided that the groups of smokers and non-smokers studied did not differ from each other in relation to any other relevant risk factor, this suggests that a person may avoid an excess risk of 169 per 100,000 per year by not smoking (or, more precisely, by never starting to smoke, since the data do not by themselves indicate reversibility of risk).

2   *Population attributable risk per cent* may be calculated in a number of ways, depending on the data available. Broadly speaking, it takes into account, whether directly or indirectly, how commonplace a risk factor is in the population, and is a measure of the percentage of a disease's incidence which may be ascribed to a particular risk factor. It is therefore a guide to the potential benefits to the population of elimination of a particular risk factor. Thus, for instance, it has been estimated that some 30 per cent of all cancers may be attributed to tobacco (Doll and Peto 1981).

Cohort studies are not undertaken lightly. In general they are unsuitable for rare diseases (due to the lack of events of interest), and, even in the case of relatively common diseases, they tend to require a large study population and a long period of follow-up, and accordingly to be expensive. Cohort studies, therefore, should in the main be reserved for the testing of clearly defined hypotheses.

Case-control studies

This type of analytic study often provides evidence which is further explored through cohort studies. On the whole, case-control studies require fewer study subjects and consume less time than cohort studies. Moreover, they are suitable for the study of rare diseases.

A case-control study starts with an identified group of people with the disease of interest – the *cases*, and a suitable comparison group without the disease – the *controls*. The control group has to be 'matched' to the cases in certain important respects (see Barker and Rose 1984: 84).

Cases and controls are then categorized according to the presence/absence (or level) of past exposure to the risk factor(s) of interest. This will often involve enquiry about the past (for example, history of alcohol consumption), giving rise to the possibility of poor or selective recall, which may bias the results. Moreover, the possibility that the factor under study (for example, diet, weight) has been affected by the onset of the disease in question (for example, peptic ulcer, bowel cancer) has to be borne in mind.

Clearly, if there is a positive association between a risk factor and disease, then a higher proportion of cases than controls would be expected to fall into the 'exposed' category.

Unlike cohort studies, case-control studies do not yield incidence rates. Accordingly, relative risks cannot be calculated directly. However, relative risk may generally be estimated with an acceptable degree of precision, by calculating the so-called *odds ratio* from case-control study data.

Just as a number of relative risks may be calculated for a graded risk in a cohort study, so may odds ratios be calculated for various levels of exposure: biological gradients (close response relationships) may thus be identified.

An example of a case-control study of recent relevance to health promotion is that carried out by Winn *et al.* (1981), which showed an association between the practice of snuff-dipping (which involves placing a wad of tobacco, either loose or in a teabag-like sachet, between cheek and gum) and cancer of the mouth. This study has helped secure regulatory action against snuff-dipping products in the United Kingdom and elsewhere.

Experimental studies

Experimental evidence is the benchmark for judging whether an association is causal, and thus for directing preventive efforts. Whereas the types of study described so far involve merely looking at natural phenomena in populations (and are thus collectively known as *observational studies*), experimental studies into causality entail some sort of direct manipulation of the situation by the researchers (and are consequently often referred to as *intervention studies*).

An intervention study involves assessing the effect (in terms of occurrence of the disease in question) of:

1   administering a suspected causal factor (this approach, for obvious reasons, being confined by and large to animal experiments);
2   removing a suspected causal factor (for example, eliminating a suspected industrial hazard from an industrial environment); or

3   employing an agent or device which protects against a suspected causal
     factor (for instance, using protective clothing as a barrier to a suspected
     occupational factor).

The distinction between intervention studies (designed to test causal
hypotheses) and *preventive trials* (aimed at evaluating the efficacy and safety
of particular preventive packages) is blurred in practice. In an ideal world,
descriptive, analytic, and intervention studies would establish causal factors.
Preventive trials would then help decide how best to combat the identified
factors. In reality, however, trials are used not only to assess the impact on
risk factors but also to gauge outcome in terms of disease onset or mortality:
in other words, to judge causality.

It is helpful to explore the contributions of experimental studies to health
promotion using CHD as an illustration. Not only do studies in this area
abound, but the wide variation in interpretations of the resulting data clearly
demonstrates that the contribution of epidemiology to health promotion is
far from straightforward. Also, of course, this disease topic is of particular
relevance to health promotion in the developed world, not only by virtue of
its place at the top of the mortality league table, but also because the risk
factors concerned have been implicated in the aetiology of numerous other
diseases and amount to a substantial proportion of the lifestyle components
on which health promotion focuses.

The identification of CHD risk factors through observational studies was
referred to above. These findings have formed the basis of a broad consensus
on action required to prevent the disease. What have experimental studies
added to the situation? So far, for reasons which will now be explored, the
short answer to this question has to be confusion.

A number of experimental studies in CHD prevention, some centred on
people identified as being at 'high risk' and others involving a more or less
'mass' approach, have been reviewed by various commentators (Anonymous
1982; Oliver 1983; Shaper 1987; McCormick and Skrabanek 1988; Shea and
Basch 1990). Only two examples will be looked at here, to give a flavour of
the polarization of interpretations of major studies.

The World Health Organization (WHO) European Collaborative Trial of
Multifactorial Prevention of Coronary Heart Disease involved 60,881 men
aged between 40 and 59, working in eighty factories in Belgium, Italy, Poland,
and the UK. Half of them received advice on diet, smoking, weight, blood
pressure, and exercise (WHO European Collaborative Group 1986). One
commentary on this study discarded it as showing 'no difference in coronary
heart disease mortality . . . between the control group and the intervention
group' (McCormick and Skrabanek 1988). This judgment overlooks important variations between the trial centres. In the Belgian component of the trial,
there was a significantly lower total incidence of CHD in those given health
education than in the comparison group. Differences of a similar nature, but
not statistically significant, were found in Italy and Poland (where statistical

significance would be more difficult to reach due to the small number of participant factories and the low population incidence of CHD, respectively). The results of the trial as a whole were weakened considerably by the lack of a positive result (in terms of changes in both risk factors and incidence) in the large UK centre. It could well be that the UK intervention was somehow less suitable or satisfactory than that in other centres.

It will have been noted that the above dismissive critique focused only on CHD mortality, whereas, in Belgium at any rate, beneficial effects of education on the total incidence of CHD were found. Clearly health promotion is concerned with morbidity as well as mortality, and in any case benefits in relation to morbidity might reasonably be expected to precede a reduction in mortality.

It is important to recognize also that the success or failure of health promotion in the prevention of CHD cannot be judged entirely on the basis of an intervention of fairly traditional health education confined to middle-aged men. This brings us to a very different kind of study from the above. The North Karelia Project in Finland followed community pressure for action against CHD. It was set up as a comprehensive, community-based programme, involving health education, specific preventive services, and health protection policies: in other words, action was taken in all spheres of health promotion (Tannahill 1985; Downie *et al.* 1990: 57). Trends in CHD risk factors and mortality were compared with a neighbouring province and with the rest of Finland (Puska *et al.* 1983, 1985; Salonen *et al.* 1983; Shea and Basch 1990; Tuomilehto *et al.* 1986).

Again controversy reigns in the interpretation of the study's findings. It has been widely accepted that the project led to reductions in CHD risk factors, arguably beyond North Karelia, due to 'leakage' of interest and action (thus, it is said, 'diluting' the impact in North Karelia specifically). However, the commonly propounded conclusion that the interventions in North Karelia reduced CHD mortality in the province has been disputed (McCormick and Skrabanek 1988). Indeed, one of the principal investigators stated that the project 'should not be considered as evidence either for or against the aetiological role of the three coronary risk factors [serum cholesterol level, blood pressure, and smoking]' (Salonen 1987). Returning to a point made above, the project was not in fact designed to test causal hypotheses (in other words, it was not an intervention study proper but rather a non-randomized trial). Scepticism over such studies often distils into a fundamental questioning of the risk factors identified through observational studies. It should, however, be noted that the European Collaborative Trial showed that benefit in terms of CHD reduction was significantly related to the extent of risk factor change.

At this stage of the discussion, it is helpful to move away from specifics, to draw together some very basic points of central importance in appraising critiques of experimental studies concerned with CHD prevention.

1   The lack of unequivocal evidence that preventive intervention reduces CHD mortality does not warrant the conclusion that such interventions have been shown to be useless.

2   Critiques have centred on mortality among the under-65s (in the interests of validity of death certification), whereas, given the age distribution of death from CHD, most of the impact in absolute terms would be to be found in the older age groups (Gunning-Schepers *et al.* 1989).
3   There is a tendency for commentators to focus on mortality, thus over-looking or ignoring beneficial effects on CHD morbidity.
4   The beneficial effects of risk factor change on other diseases (such as smoking on lung cancer, blood pressure on strokes, and obesity on osteoarthrosis and disability) must be taken into consideration. (This points to the absurdity of treating CHD in isolation from other health problems, a point which is explored further below.)
5   Favourable effects of lifestyle change on *positive health* – for example of taking up exercise on well-being and fitness – tend to be ignored by the nihilist camp.

These and the preceding arguments serve as reminders that we must appraise *all* the available evidence, rather than latching uncritically on to debunking critiques. While it is vital to encourage reflective practice, we must resist the unhelpful temptation to caricature challenges to accepted doctrines and dogmas as a nihilistic battle-cry to be taken up as an alternative to addressing the implications for established practices posed by health promotion. Passive acceptance of negative arguments, or the mere succumbing to the created climate of uncertainty and inconsistency, militates against professional and public action towards health promotion.

In short, it would be wrong to convert the much-publicized criticisms of population-based preventive strategies into paralysis. An adequate consensus as to modifiable risk factors remains: we must continue in our search for the best means of altering risk status in the population, and in so doing, we must set our efforts in the broader context of the prevention of other diseases and the enhancement of positive health. These last two themes are of importance to further discussions in this chapter.

Summary of contributions of epidemiology to health promotion

We have seen that epidemiology, as defined at the beginning of this chapter, has an important role in identifying and quantifying ill health problems in communities, in assessing the means of and scope for prevention, and in evaluating preventive interventions.

As we have begun to see in the preceding section, however, the application of epidemiology to health promotion has not been without its difficulties. The problem areas will now be examined, starting with shortcomings arising from the way in which epidemiology is brought to bear on health promotion.

Problems areas to date

Unsound programme planning

Epidemiology is generally accepted as a primary feeder discipline for health promotion. In fact it is viewed by many as *the* primary discipline. This is manifest in a widespread tendency to have epidemiology 'drive the system'. That is to say, not only does epidemiology set the health promotion agenda – through identifying and quantifying causes of morbidity and mortality and elucidating foci for prevention – but the resultant catalogue of categories of ill health and risk factors is directly translated into 'health promotion' programmes (figure 4.1).

The end-product is a series, indeed a hotch-potch, of disease- and risk factor-based initiatives. For example, a health authority may devise a CHD prevention programme, a smoking programme, a cancer programme, an alcohol programme, a drugs programme, a human immunodeficiency virus/acquired immune deficiency syndrome (HIV/AIDS) programme, and so on. It is obvious that there are overlaps between such programmes. For example, smoking is associated with CHD and cancers, and tobacco is a drug of addiction; HIV infection is related to illicit drug use and, through effects of intoxication on sexual behaviour, to alcohol use; furthermore, there are common links in the origins of most unhealthful aspects of lifestyle – including factors such as socio-economic disadvantage, unhealthful peer pressure, and the power of vested interests.

Despite these overlaps, the individual programmes commonly proceed in relative, or even absolute, isolation. This lack of co-ordination brings the potential – often realized – for duplication and inconsistency of health

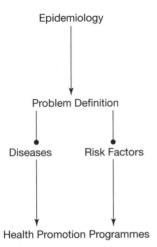

Figure 4.1 Epidemiology driving the health promotion system

education 'messages', which in turn is likely to breed public confusion and rejection.

Furthermore, necessary efforts to secure programmes' permeation of whole communities is thwarted at grass-roots level by the inherent uncoordinated nature of the approach. Important 'gatekeepers' to the community – head-teachers, employers, and so on – are likely to be frustrated and irritated by a disjointed stream of requests to take action on this, that, and the other. Even if programmes *are* established in key parts of the community, they will tend to be piecemeal and (as described above) to involve wasteful, and potentially damaging, duplication. These problems and others are discussed more fully elsewhere (Tannahill 1990).

A *neglect of methodological issues*

The above approach to programme development carries with it important problems regarding methodology. In short, the question of 'how to' is lost in consideration of '*what* to'. Plans become a list of diseases and risk factors to be addressed, often translated into targets for achievement (Tannahill 1987).

Largely implicitly, programmes thus defined rely heavily on outmoded models of health *education*. The assumption is that if people are told what is good – and bad – for them, then healthful attitudes and behaviour will follow in a neat sequence. The consequence of this gross oversimplification (Tannahill and Robertson 1986) is excessive dependence on 'campaigns' and the giving of information and advice, at the expense of notions such as skills development, enabling, and empowerment. This is state of the *ark* practice, not state of the *art*.

An *over-emphasis on individual behaviour*

Epidemiology-driven health promotion places an onus on the individual member of the public to take responsibility for his or her health, without properly addressing ways of 'making healthy choices easier choices'. Health-related behaviour is largely viewed *in vacuo*, isolated from its social context, and there is a tendency to neglect essential regulatory measures which protect health.

These undesirable features are reinforced by narrow approaches to risk appraisal. For example, CHD has been linked to aspects of lifestyle, including diet and smoking. At the same time, despite frequently being referred to as a 'disease of affluence', it has been shown (Townsend *et al.* 1988) to be associated in the developed world with low socio-economic status. The common response to the latter observation is to point to social class differences in the lifestyle factors, and to return the focus to changing individual behaviour – persuading people not to smoke, and so on – as distinct from the more challenging question of how the broad environment might be changed: individuals are expected somehow to shrug off powerful anti-health pressures in their everyday lives and 'do the right things'. A further problem is that the gradient of CHD across employment groups can, in any case, only partly be explained by orthodox risk factors (Marmot *et al.* 1984).

A narrow view of outcomes

An over-reliance on epidemiology in developing health promotion programmes manifests itself also in the definition of desirable outcomes. These tend to relate to disease incidence rates, mortality rates, risk factor prevalences, and uptake rates for specific preventive services. The contribution of other disciplines towards outcome definition is underplayed. Measures of educational outcome, for example, may be viewed (and indeed played down) as *process* measures.

The narrow outcome focus runs the risk of failing to detect human problems in the operation of preventive programmes. For instance, all-out efforts may be made to pass people through health check programmes, with both eyes firmly fixed on considerations such as uptake and pick-up rates, to the neglect of important matters such as necessary support for risk reduction and potential psychological ill effects of screening.

This brings us to the question of how health is envisaged in current epidemiological practice. So far, we have focused on problems relating largely to how epidemiology is used. It is time to look at those which spring directly from how the term 'epidemiology' is interpreted.

An incomplete view of health

It will be recalled that the definition of epidemiology presented at the beginning of the chapter referred exclusively to disease. Epidemiology seen in this light concerns itself with 'objective' measures of diagnosed disease. The inherent view of ill health is incomplete, in that it overlooks important *subjective* aspects. This may be seen in relation to the above brief discussion of health check outcomes: assessment of psychological ill effects requires the investigation of clients' own feelings and experiences.

Moreover, epidemiology as defined so far is deficient in its neglect of the *positive* dimension of health (which embraces well-being and fitness: Downie *et al.* 1990: 23).

A notable consequence of this incomplete view of health has been the almost exclusive concern with *prevention* in the foregoing account. Indeed health promotion in practice is often reduced to a repackaging of preventive medicine. This is well seen, for example, in many examples of 'health promotion' in general medical practice, and of health authority plans for 'health promotion'. Moreover, as indicated above, the ignoring of positive health is a major weakness in nihilist health promotion writings based on the results of experimental studies.

The case for ensuring an emphasis on positive health in health promotion rests on a number of arguments.

1   Most fundamentally, 'health promotion' which is concerned only with a part of health is obviously a misnomer. This begs the question: what *is* health? A whole series of books could be, and indeed have been, written in response to this question (see Seedhouse 1986; Aggleton 1990). Only a brief analysis of some of the critical issues is possible here.

The classic WHO (1946) definition of health – as a state of complete physical, mental, and social well-being, and not merely the absence of disease or infirmity – is a useful starting point for such a discussion. While this definition is open to valid criticism by dint of its Utopian nature, it is surely of value in embracing the sorts of things which people conceptualize as being part of health. It reminds us that health is not merely to do with the physical – there are important mental and social facets – and that it has a positive dimension.

How does the positive dimension (represented by well-being in the WHO definition) relate to the negative dimension (ill health)? This relationship has generally been represented as a single continuum, with positive at one pole and negative at the other. As pointed out by Downie *et al.* (1990: 20), such a portrayal overlooks the fact that ill health and positive health are by no means invariably inversely related to each other: it is quite possible for someone with a serious disease to have a higher level of well-being or fitness than someone who has a 'clean bill of health' from a clinical point of view. Herein lies a vital lesson for health promotion: successful prevention cannot be relied upon to maximize positive health. This is well illustrated by the extreme image of a society which has taken prevention well and truly to heart, and is accordingly remarkably free of ill health, but which is so concerned with risk reduction that its quality of life is seriously impaired.

Health promotion, then, must surely be aimed at achieving a balance between positive health and ill health, as well as between physical, mental, and social aspects of health.

2   A question of ethic arises from the points made above. Surely it is *unethical* for those involved with health promotion to peddle a pale imitation of the real thing?

Personal experience of a teaching session with clinical medical students provides a suitable illustration. On being asked to define health, one of the students suggested 'the absence of clinical signs'. This met with the approval of his colleagues. However, in an ensuing participatory exercise on perceptions of personal health, consideration of matters of illness and disease was conspicuous by its absence: the students were very clearly concerned with issues of mental and social well-being, physical fitness, and self-concept and self-esteem. They were faced, then, with the dilemma of strait-jacketing patients into a narrow 'medical' view of health while couching their own health in much more positive ways. They could offer no defence for this.

3   It is commonly said that a positive focus is more motivational in terms of encouraging the adoption of a healthful way of life. In strictly academic terms the case for accepting this is commonly overstated. However, there are common-sense reasons for giving credence to the argument. Why should people give up pleasurable (if unhealthful) practices or adopt unattractive (albeit healthful) ones *now* for the sake of some possible – but by no means certain – preventive benefit in the future? This question is particularly pressing in relation to disadvantaged people for whom unhealthful practices, such as smoking or misusing alcohol or other drugs, may be the main pleasures in – and only escape from – an other-wise miserable existence; and for whom the future is neither worthy of investment nor amenable to personal influence. It is also especially relevant to young people, insulated by time from pressing awareness of their own mortality.

4   Also of relevance to the question of motivation is the matter of lay perspectives of health, in which the positive dimension figures prominently. It is clearly important for those who seek to promote health to be operating on a basis with which the public may identify.

5   It is widely accepted that a cornerstone of health promotion is *empower-ment*. As well as contributing to this process through informing people and securing environments conducive to health, health promotion can foster attributes which help individuals and communities to become more empowered. These attributes, including a high level of self-esteem and a set of lifeskills, may be seen as components of well-being: nurturing them, therefore, is part of the process of enhancing positive health.

The way ahead

An epidemiology of health

Attention has been drawn to the fact that at present epidemiology is on the whole taken to be concerned with disease, and that this focus is too narrow for effective and ethically acceptable health promotion. Even leaving aside consideration of the impact of epidemiology on health promotion, it is reasonable to suggest that epidemiology should focus on health more fully. After all, although the oldest use of the term appears to have been in connection with epidemics (*Oxford English Dictionary*), the word is derived from the Greek *epi* and *dēmos* and thus means literally 'study on the people', not study of diseases of the people.

The idea of the epidemiology of health was actively endorsed as long ago as the early 1950s, when a book of that title was published in the United States by the New York Academy of Medicine, following a health education conference (Galdston 1953). Galdston referred to the epidemiology of health as 'new', but argued that in actuality it was older than that of disease, and that it was based on an older science – physiology rather than pathology. The book spoke of 'holism', and of an ecological approach, notions which one might have thought of as more modern. A British study of the height, weight, and general condition of two groups of boys was cited as an example of the epidemiology of health, on the grounds that this was a study of the state of health rather than disease. The following definition of the epidemiology of health was presented:

> a discipline, rooted in physiology and trussed by mathematics, whereby essential information on the state of health is to be gained, this information serving to inspire and direct action to maintain and advance the health of the people.
>
> (Galdston 1953: 6)

Galdston warned that the 'new' epidemiology must not be thought of as 'merely the mirror side of the epidemiology of disease', emphasizing, as has been stressed in this chapter, that health is not the same as the absence of disease.

The epidemiology of health must augment a concern with aetiology and pathogenesis by incorporating methods of enquiry into what it is that enables people to attain and maintain good health in the face of all manner of environmental insults. Kelly (1989) highlighted the need for research focused in this way. Referring to the work of Antonovsky (1987), he advocated the application of a 'salutogenic approach', based on the premise that 'misery, pain, illness and pathology is the normal lot of the human being'. The critical question, he argued, is

> how it is that certain individuals and certain groups, certain households and certain societies are better able to withstand the endemic pathological onslaught of lousy social conditions, of noxious environmental hazards, of self-destructive behaviour, or of micro-organisms, while others are not.
>
> (Kelly 1989)

Pulling together key points made in this chapter, there is a need for epidemiology to focus on the distribution and determinants of good health as well as bad. Just as health embraces the subjective as well as the objective, the positive as well as the negative, the physiological as well as the pathological, then so too must the epidemiology of health.

To what extent is such a vision of epidemiology a reality? This question can be answered to a great extent by reference to the prevailing notion of epidemiology which has shaped this chapter. Although some definitions of the term incorporate the word 'health' (Last 1988: 42; Richards and Baker 1988), and despite periodic 'reinventions' of an epidemiology of health (see Brown 1985, for example), in practice the disease model still dominates.

The picture is not, however, wholly bleak. Conventional, 'objective' measures of ill health have come to be supplemented by well-validated indicators such as the Nottingham Health Profile (Hunt *et al.* 1986), which allows for an assessment of health status based on subjective judgements. In addition to standard epidemiological studies, it has become commonplace for researchers and even health authorities to undertake studies of health-related beliefs, attitudes, and behaviours in defined populations, these representing an extension of the cross-sectional study beyond its traditional territories (see, for example, Butler 1987; Health Promotion Research Trust 1987; Dumfries and Galloway Health Board 1990). The expanded health database provided by such innovations is of value in providing further insights into influences on health, and a population profile of health status and health-related knowledge, attitudes and behaviour, through which health promotion challenges may be identified and progress monitored.

Moreover, much work of the sort described in the New York Academy of Medicine book referred to above has been, and is being, conducted in the name of social sciences or even social epidemiology. Somehow such studies appear to be cut off from 'mainstream' – that is, medical – epidemiology. Such longitudinal studies (for example, the West of Scotland Twenty-07 study: Mcintyre *et al.* 1987) are essentially cohort studies in which subjective and objective assessments of positive health and ill health may be made, and through which determinants of good health and poor health may be explored.

There is a pressing need for the various strands identified here to be pulled together into a unified epidemiology of health. This is not a bid for further territorial expansion by 'medical epidemiology': it is a call for, as it were, a broad church of epidemiology presided over by leaders of many different denominations, in which the importance of lay preachers is recognized.

An integrated base for health promotion

Having made a case for adopting a view of epidemiology broader than that which currently dominates, we need to consider how this expanded discipline should be applied to health promotion.

Criticism was made above of the tendency for epidemiology to drive the system, in the sense that problems identified by the epidemiology of disease come to be translated directly into corresponding programmes of action (Figure 4.1). It was pointed out that this is both philosophically and logistically unsound. As the chapter developed, issues of multi-disciplinary teamwork and sensitivity to lay perceptions and perspectives were raised. Health promotion must involve a partnership between various professionals, many agencies, and the community itself. Health promotion planning, implementation, and evaluation need to be based on an epidemiology of health (itself reflecting such partnership) integrated with other sciences which have a bearing on methodology (Figure 4.2). This is consistent with the argument, made in the introduction to this book, that collaboration in practice must be matched by collaboration in theory.

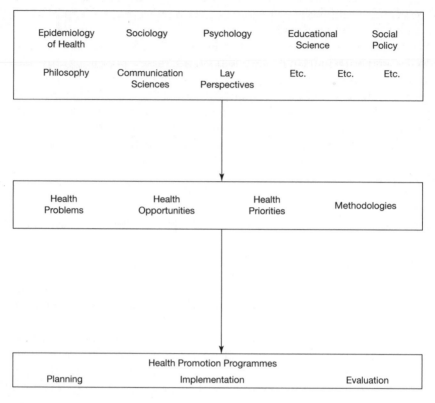

Figure 4.2 An integral base for health promotion

The necessary coalition of disciplines must be firmly founded on an aware-ness of each other's perspectives and expertise, and cemented by the mutual respect which is, eventually, born of proper teamwork. This is a vital challenge in these heady days of the renaissance of public health and advocacy of multi-disciplinary, multi-agency institutes of public health. Not least it is a challenge for epidemiologists.

Summary

Epidemiology, as commonly defined, provides important inputs to health promotion, namely: knowledge of the scale and distribution of important disease; an understanding of causal mechanisms, and thus of the potential for prevention; and methodologies for evaluating preventive initiatives.

Major problems arise from the inappropriate application of epidemiology to health promotion: epidemiological evidence on diseases and risk factors tends to be translated directly into health promotion programmes, to the neglect of methodological issues. This problem is compounded by the narrow

– disease – focus of mainstream epidemiology, and by its emphasis on 'objective' measures.

There is a pressing need for an 'epidemiology of health', which draws on medical and social epidemiology, and on new methods as well as old. This broader-based epidemiology must recognize positive health together with ill health; it must use subjective measures alongside the objective; it must investigate the distribution and determinants of good health as well as bad; it must seek to identify not only health problems, but also health opportunities; it must be concerned not just with pathological mechanisms, but with physiology; and its view of health determinants must be holistic, so that health-related behaviour is properly viewed in its broad environmental context.

This epidemiology of health must then come to form, with other relevant bodies of knowledge, an integrated, multi-disciplinary base on which health promotion may be planned, practised, and evaluated.

References

Aggleton, P. (1990) *Health*, London: Routledge.

Anonymous (1982) 'Trials of coronary heart disease prevention', Editorial, *Lancet* 2: 803–4.

Antonovsky, A. (1987) *Unravelling the Mystery of Health*, San Francisco: Jossey Bass.

Barker, D. J. P. and Rose, G. (1984) *Epidemiology in Medical Practice*, 3rd edition, Edinburgh: Churchill Livingstone.

Bradford Hill, A. (1977) *A Short Textbook of Medical Statistics*, London: Hodder & Stoughton.

British Cardiac Society (1987) *Report of the Working Group on Coronary Disease Prevention*, London: British Cardiac Society.

Brown, V. A. (1985) 'Towards an epidemiology of health: a basis for planning community health programmes', *Health Policy*, 4: 331–40.

Butler, J. R. (1987) *An Apple a Day . . . ? A Study of Lifestyles and Health in Canterbury and Thanet*, Canterbury: University of Kent at Canterbury/Canterbury and Thanet Health Authority.

Dawber, T. R. (1980) *The Framingham Study: The Epidemiology of Atherosclerotic Disease*, Cambridge, MA: Harvard University Press.

Doll, R. and Hill, A. B. (1964) 'Mortality in relation to smoking: ten years' observation of British doctors', *British Medical Journal* i: 1399–410.

Doll, R. and Peto, R. (1981) *The Causes of Cancer*, Oxford: Oxford University Press.

Downie, R. S., Fyfe, C., and Tannahill, A. (1990) *Health Promotion. Models and Values*, Oxford: Oxford University Press.

Dumfries and Galloway Health Board (1990) *Dumfries and Galloway Health and Lifestyle Survey 1990*, Dumfries: Dumfries and Galloway Health Board.

Farmer, R. D. T. and Miller, D. L. (1983) *Lecture Notes on Epidemiology and Community Medicine*, 2nd edition: Oxford: Blackwell.

Friedman, G. D. (1987) *Primer of Epidemiology*, 3rd edition, New York: McGraw-Hill.

Galdston, I. (ed.) (for the New York Academy of Medicine) (1953) *The Epidemiology of Health*, New York: Health Education Council.

Greater Glasgow Health Board (1990) *The Annual Report of the Director of Public Health 1989*, Glasgow: Greater Glasgow Health Board.

Gunning-Schepers, L. J., Barendregt, J. J., and van der Maas, P. J. (1989) 'Population interventions reassessed', *Lancet* i: 479–81.

Hammond, E. C. (1966) 'Smoking in relation to death rates of one million men and women', in W. Haenszel (ed.) *Epidemiological Approaches to the Study of Cancer and Other Chronic Diseases*, National Cancer Institute Monograph 19, US Department of Health, Education and Welfare.

Health Promotion Research Trust (1987) *The Health and Lifestyle Survey*, London: Health Promotion Research Trust.

Hunt, S. M., McEwen, J., and McKenna, S. P. (1986) *Measuring Health Status*, London: Croom Helm.

Kelly, M. (1989) 'Some problems in health promotion research', *Health Promotion* 4: 317–30.

Lambert, P. M. and Reid, D. D. (1970) 'Smoking, air pollution, and bronchitis in Britain', *Lancet* i: 853–7.

Last, J. M. (ed.) (1988) *A Dictionary of Epidemiology*, 2nd edition, New York: Oxford University Press.

Lilienfeld, A. M. and Lilienfeld, D. E. (1980) *Foundations of Epidemiology*, 2nd edition, New York: Oxford University Press.

McCormick, J. and Skrabanek, P. (1988) 'Coronary heart disease is not preventable by population interventions', *Lancet* ii: 839–41.

Mcintyre, S. *et al.* (1989) 'The West of Scotland Twenty-07 study: health in the community', in C. Martin and D. McQueen (eds) *Readings for a New Public Health*, Edinburgh: Edinburgh University Press.

Marmot, M. G., Shipley, M. J., and Rose, G. (1984) 'Inequalities in death – specific explanations of a general pattern?', *Lancet* i: 1003–6.

Mausner, J. S. and Kramer, S. (1985) *Mausner and Bahn. Epidemiology – An Introductory Text*, 2nd edition, Philadelphia: Saunders.

Oliver, M. F. (1983) 'Should we not forget about mass control of coronary risk factors?', *Lancet* ii: 37–8.

Puska, P. *et al.* (1983) 'Change in risk factors for coronary heart disease during 10 years of a community intervention programme (North Karelia project)', *British Medical Journal* 287: 1840–4.

— (1985) 'The community-based strategy to prevent coronary heart disease: conclusions from the ten years of the North Karelia project', *Annual Review of Public Health* 6:147–93.

Registrar General Scotland (1989) *Annual Report 1988*, Edinburgh: HMSO.

Richards, I. D. G. and Baker, M. R. (1988) *The Epidemiology and Prevention of Important Diseases*, Edinburgh: Churchill Livingstone.

Salonen, J. T. (1987) 'Did the North Karelia project reduce coronary mortality?', *Lancet* ii: 269.

— *et al.* (1983) 'Decline in mortality from coronary heart disease in Finland from 1969 to 1979', *British Medical Journal* 286: 1857–60.

Seedhouse, D. (1986) *Health: The Foundations for Achievement*, Chichester: Wiley.

Shaper, A. G. (1987) 'Epidemiology and prevention of ischaemic heart disease', *Current Opinion in Cardiology* 2: 571–85.

Shea, S. and Basch, C. E. (1990) 'A review of five major community-based cardio-vascular disease prevention programmes. Part I: Rationale, design, and theoretical framework', *American Journal of Health Promotion* 4: 203–13.

Tannahill, A. (1985) 'What is health promotion?', *Health Education Journal* 44: 167–8.

—— (1987) 'Regional health promotion planning and monitoring', *Health Education Journal* 46: 125–7.

—— (1990) 'Health education and health promotion: planning for the 1990s', *Health Education Journal* 49: 194–8.

Tannahill, A. and Robertson, G. (1986) 'Health education in medical education: collaboration, not competition', *Medical Teacher* 8: 165–70.

Townsend, P., Davidson, N., and Whitehead, M. (1988) *Inequalities in Health*, Harmondsworth: Penguin.

Tuomilehto, J. *et al.* (1986) 'Decline in cardiovascular mortality in North Karelia and other parts of Finland', *British Medical Journal* 293: 1068–71.

Winn, D. M. *et al.* (1981) 'Snuff dipping and oral cancer amongst women in the Southern United States', *New England Journal of Medicine* 304: 745–9.

WHO (1946) *Constitution*, New York: WHO.

WHO European Collaborative Group (1986) 'European trial of multifactorial prevention of coronary heart disease: final report on the 6-year results', *Lancet* i: 869–72.

5 The contribution of education to health promotion

Katherine Weare

Goals of this chapter

This chapter will explore the contribution of education to health promotion. To do so we need some definition of health promotion. As there is little space to debate the various existing models here, and this topic is discussed in other chapters in this volume, this chapter will make use of the recent definitions and key concepts and principles of the World Health Organization (WHO 1986, 1991, 1997). The vision of health promotion put forward by the WHO is centrally concerned with certain key principles, such as empowerment, democracy, equity, and autonomy, but these are values or goals rather than techniques, and do not tell us how we may achieve them. The chapter suggests that education has a key part to play in the realization of modern health promotion principles and goals. It will put forward a very wide range of educational approaches and strategies that have their uses, as we must not be bedevilled by absolutist thinking, but use whatever works best to achieve our goals.

What do we mean by health promotion?

Empowerment is a central principle

The Ottawa Charter defined health promotion as 'the process of enabling people to increase control over, and to improve, their health' (WHO 1986). The Charter also suggested that health is 'a resource for everyday life, not the objective of living'. The goal of health promotion activity is not therefore to produce behaviour change in a particular direction in order to impose a state of perfect health, but to help people to be as healthy as they wish to be.

It follows that a key principle of health promotion activity is empowerment (Tones and Tilford 1994). The concept of empowerment came originally from community development projects in the late 1970s, and is essentially concerned with the distribution of power, as the name suggests. It is about the active participation of all involved in a process, including, and especially, those who are its intended beneficiaries, using what is now often termed a 'bottom up' rather than a 'top down' approach (Beattie 1991): the activity is undertaken by and with, rather than on behalf of or to, people. Empowerment is predicated on some central principles and values, most notably democracy, equity, and sustainability (WHO 1997).

Empowerment can be for individuals or communities. An empowering community brings together self-empowered individuals, and works with them to build a sense of mutual responsibility to build supportive communities, change personal and social circumstances, challenge political structures, and create healthy environments (Catford and Parish 1989).

Education is central to an empowerment approach to health promotion

Education has a vital role to play in the empowerment process and is thus central to health promotion. It was not always seen this way, however, and in the early 1980s, health education had a rough time of it. Some writers criticized health education for being, as they saw it, a series of individually focused campaigns designed to change lifestyles, and which therefore disempowered people by 'blaming the victim' for their own ill-health (Rodmell and Watt 1986). As a result there was for some time an emphasis on health promotion, which was seen as advocating structural changes to the social, political and public health fabric of society. This polarization lead to the marginalization of health education, and indeed of all educational activity, in favour of socially focused approaches, for some years.

In the mid-1980s there was a fight back on behalf of health education (Tones 1987). It was particularly significant that the Ottawa Charter (WHO 1986) placed education firmly at the heart of health promotion when it suggested five areas for action within health promotion, one of which was predominantly individual and educational: 'the enhancement of the individual with the knowledge, skills and motivation to make competent decisions about their health'.

Health education and health promotion tend now to be seen as 'overlapping spheres' (Green and Kreuter 1991) and the differences between them as about levels of intervention rather than ideology or values. It is now seen as appropriate to include approaches that are aimed predominantly at individuals in the full repertoire of wider health promotion interventions. Tones and Tilford (1994) suggest a helpful way forward which puts the two into a clear, symbiotic, and synergistic relationship:

> Health promotion consists of any combination of education and related legal, fiscal, economic, environmental and organizational interventions designed to facilitate the achievement of health and the prevention of disease.

They summarize it in the much quoted formula: 'Health Promotion = Health Education × Healthy Public Policy'.

Health education in any case is now seen as containing social approaches. Tones and Tilford see it as being concerned with attempts to change knowledge, attitudes, and behaviour through learning in its broadest sense, including the knowledge, attitudes, and behaviour that relate to social issues, and many typologies of health education include social change and radical models (Draper *et al.* 1980).

The settings approach

The 'settings' approach is another 'big idea' in WHO's vision of health promotion (WHO 1991). The settings approach focuses attention on the total context in which health-related activity takes place, where not only the physical environment but the surrounding ethos and relationships can support, or indeed undermine, health. It recognizes that health is the product of a myriad of interconnected and interacting physical, social, and psychological factors.

Starting with the seminal 'healthy cities', the settings approach has given rise to several context-specific initiatives, including those that involve education, such as 'health-promoting schools' (WHO *et al.* 1993; WHO 1997) and, more recently, 'health-promoting universities' (Tsouros *et al.* 1998) and 'health-promoting medical schools' (White 1998). Applying the settings approach to educational institutions has led to a broadening of the traditional focus on the curriculum and the individual student, to one in which the totality of the life of the institution is taken into account. This includes, for example, the institution's organization, management structures, relationships, and physical environment – the total context which shapes the health of all those who learn and work there. Looking even more broadly, the institution is seen as part of its wider community, reaching out to, and supported by, for example the families of students, social work services, health agencies, the police, the media, in fact a whole host of interested and relevant agencies.

Settings are by no means value free. The Thessaloniki Conference, the most recent WHO pronouncement on the health-promoting school, emphasized the extent to which certain key principles need to underpin the activity: they include empowerment, democracy, equity, and sustainability (WHO 1997).

The relationship between education and health promotion

To date there has been something of a stand-off between the practice of education and the goals of health promotion. For example, the efforts that have been made to develop a health-promoting approach in educational settings such as schools, colleges, and universities have been bedevilled by the commonly held view from educational establishments that the promotion of health is not their main goal. Educators have tended to see their task as ensuring the academic success of their students, and see health education and health promotion as irrelevant to this, believing that they do not have the time, the resources, or the responsibility to devote themselves to the promotion of the mental, physical, or social health of students (Abercrombie *et al.* 1998).

However, some recent developments are starting to bring health promotion and education closer together in very heartening ways. Those involved in health promotion are starting to appreciate the need to respect the educational goals of the school, to map health promotion goals onto these, and make links with them that reflect areas of mutual interest, rather than expecting schools simply to adopt 'foreign' health-related goals (St Leger and Nutbeam 2000). At the same time, recent research in mainstream education is uncovering some useful areas of congruence with the concerns of health promotion, as we shall see.

Educational settings – the key elements that make for success

Work on educational environments: four key features

In recent years, work in mainstream education has broadened its focus from a concern solely with the individual learner, to look more widely at the kind of educational environments that are conducive to learning, often called the 'effective' school, university, or college. This new holistic perspective has in itself brought the study of education closer to the 'settings' concept. Furthermore the findings of a wide range of educational studies on effective institutions have been impressively consistent, whether they are related to students' academic performance, their social behaviour, or their attitudes to school, or to teachers' professional performance and morale. They demonstrate clearly that there need not be a conflict between traditional academic goals and the goals of health promotion.

Four key elements have been shown to be crucial to the effectiveness of an educational institution, in both its academic and its health-related dimensions. They are: the encouragement of autonomy in staff and students; clarity about rules, boundaries, and expectations; a high degree of participation by students and staff; and supportive relationships. Each of these four elements demonstrably leads to better academic achievement, greater interest in learning, less drop out, higher levels of self-esteem, and reduced levels of health-damaging behaviour in students. They also lead to better teaching, improved morale, lower stress levels, and lower absenteeism in staff (Fraser and Walberg 1991; Wubbels *et al.* 1991; Tunstall 1994; Thurlow 1995).

The importance of taking a holistic, settings approach has also been amply demonstrated by this research on the effectiveness of educational institutions. Strategies that work on a range of inter-related fronts at once have been shown to be more likely to make long-term changes to students' attitudes and behaviour across a wide range of issues than are limited and uni-dimensional approaches. This applies not only to programmes designed to tackle health issues, such as reducing alcohol, tobacco and drug use, and violence (Durlak

1995; Durlak and Wells 1997), but also and to those that attempt to improve academic outcomes (Fraser and Walberg 1991). Looking specifically at the four elements – autonomy, clarity, participation, and relationships – although they are highly influential separately, they are even more so when they are found together, when they reinforce one another (Hawkins and Catalano 1992; Solomon *et al.* 1992). For example, teachers who feel more supported and involved in the decision making of the institution are more likely to set clear goals for their students (Moos 1991). Students learn more effectively if they are happy in their work, believe in themselves, like their teachers, and feel the place where they study is supporting them (Aspey and Roebuck 1977; Hawkins and Catalano 1992). Some researchers have suggested that the factors cannot be understood in isolation (Marshall and Weinstein 1984) but are all facets of one another.

We will now explore each of the four factors in turn, look briefly at the evidence for their significance in both education and health promotion, and suggest some broad parameters for how they may be achieved.

Autonomy

The centrality of autonomy to empowerment

The empowering vision of health promotion embodied in the Ottawa Charter necessarily implies autonomy. If we accept the WHO definition of health as a resource not a goal, then free choice has to be at the centre of the concept, and the goals of empowerment must be self-determination and independence. So a state of good physical health which a person or community had not freely chosen and over which they did not have control could not be described as good health at all in the sense of 'complete physical, social and mental well-being' (WHO 1946). The person or community could not be said to be socially and mentally 'well' if they were being coerced. So approaches that have as their intended outcome solely a change in behaviour of an individual or population in a healthier direction, and which measure their success entirely on this criterion, cannot be described as truly health-promoting – they are 'healthist', putting health before people and their human and political rights, and subverting the essential health-promoting principle of voluntarism (Green and Kreuter 1991).

The centrality of autonomy to education

Autonomy is not just a central principle of modern health promotion; it is coming to be seen as a vital principle in mainstream education too, as evidence emerges for its centrality to academic learning. Students have been shown to have higher academic attainments, enjoy learning, be more motivated, attend better, and are happier at school if they are encouraged to think for themselves, to work as independently as their age, stage, and personality allows and have high degrees of responsibility and freedom (Wubbels *et al.* 1991). The goal of education then becomes to help learners become reflective and appropriately critical, self-motivated, self-directed and self-disciplined, and responsible for their own behaviour and learning (Elias and Kress 1994).

So, what kind of education do we need to help learners develop autonomy?

Education is much more than the transmission of facts

At first sight it might appear that to achieve autonomy we should just give people the facts and let them make up their own minds. The world of health education in practice – in the school, the clinic, or the doctor's surgery – is still dominated by the commonsense view of 'give the learner the facts (e.g. the helpful and informative leaflet, the lecture on the dangers of drugs by the policeman, or the chat on diet from the health professional) and they will surely then follow the advice and be healthy'. This view is based on what is sometimes called the 'rational educational' model, the fundamental assumption of which is that people are basically rational, and their behaviour driven by logically derived principles (Williams 1984). According to this view, people need to be given factually correct information and then they will probably make a sensible decision. If, after being given the correct information, a person chooses not to take the healthy course of action, that is their right: it is entirely up to them and the educator has no mandate to interfere further (Baelz 1979).

This approach has the benefit of intellectual purity; however in practice it is far too naïve to be of much use to anyone. It does not take into account the constraints that surround us and which prevent most of us, either literally or at least in our minds, from being free to make sensible decisions and healthy choices (Tones 1986). Studies of health education interventions and reviews of health promotion initiatives (Liedekerken 1990; Veen 1995) show time and again that unhealthy behaviour rarely stems from a lack of knowledge or information. Most of us, including the young, know only too well what is good for us, but find it hard to respond to healthy messages. Even the most highly motivated find healthy lifestyles hard to sustain (Miller and Rollnick 1991). We live in a society where we are besieged daily by cleverly crafted but health-damaging messages devised and funded by large corporations, in a society that constantly puts corporate gain before health. If left to ourselves, we would probably bow to the pressure and follow the path so seductively set before us by the advertisers. Simply providing information is of little defence in these circumstances; there is too much else going on all around us that is undermining this information. If information is all we have to protect us, we will almost certainly remain where we are, and be drawn into habits we may know are bad for us but which we feel powerless to change.

The rational educational model does not exist in isolation – it has under-pinnings in mainstream education. It is the health education version of what was, until this century, the 'commonsense' view of education as 'giving people facts'. This unreflective view of education sees learning as a straightforward process whereby, through the examination of the world directly with the sense organs, or being told what other people have already found out, a person adds to their mental store of facts. Again this may, and indeed should, sound hopelessly naïve, but today much educational practice is still predicated on these assumptions.

There are good educational as well as health-related reasons for seeing the 'education as facts' approach as too limited to be of much use. As other chapters in this volume suggest, both psychology and sociology have demonstrated that the world is largely a construct of the human mind: the way we classify objects is shaped, and in some ways actively created, by the ways in which our minds perceive them. Minds are not empty bottles to be filled, or blank pages to be written on: they are complex systems that actively interact with the world, both to transform and be transformed by our lived experience. What we learn from an experience is largely a feature of what we already know (Ausbel *et al.* 1978), and we learn by adding links to our existing mental framework (Gagne 1965), assimilating new information into old patterns as far as possible, and only accommodating our minds when the fit becomes too uncomfortable (Piaget and Inhelder 1958). So a serious study of education emphasizes learning as a process of becoming, not as an accumulation of bits of information (Entwistle and Ramden 1983; Barrows and Tamblyn 1980).

Nor is the ability to memorize facts a particularly useful skill in the twenty-first century. Theories of social change (Tofler 1980) suggest that knowledge is expanding so fast that memorizing enough data for everyday practice is an impossible task, and in any case pointless, as much of what is learnt today will be superseded tomorrow. People no longer train for one career: with the changing job market they may tackle several in a lifetime. Data retrieval systems mean that we can call up the facts we need quickly. In this context the most useful skills are being able to solve problems, think rationally and logically, deduce conclusions, generalize and transfer learning from one context to another (Mayer 1979). Schon (1983) has categorized such learning in the professional context as becoming a 'reflective practitioner', a state of competence that is far more helpful than being able to remember facts. We are now also starting to appreciate the vital importance of emotional and social competences to success in education and in later life (Goleman 1996), an issue that will be explored in some detail later.

Being autonomous is something we achieve, not something we are

We need to see autonomy as an end point, something that educators help people achieve by all the educational forces at their disposal, not an innate feature with which they start out. It is also a relative not an absolute concept, and always a matter of degree: none of us can do exactly what we wish all the time – the knock-on effects on others to whom we have responsibility could be disastrous. Nor is it appropriate to allow young children a high degree of independence before they are ready to cope with it: their early needs are for boundaries and structure, not untrammelled freedom. The growth of autonomy is about gradually internalizing a sense of inner structure, security, and power; and for this one has first to experience this stability in the outside world. From the very beginning the child needs to be encouraged to become increasingly independent, and to internalize a sense of power, but needs to be able to rely on boundaries and rules to which they can return as needed.

People have been shown to learn best where the degree of freedom is suited to their age, stage, and personality (Moos 1991). Less mature and more anxious learners need higher degrees of structure and organization but still benefit from being given as much autonomy as they can handle, while more mature and confident students can cope with higher levels of choice. But this does not mean that education should lapse back to the behaviour change model for the young and then try to retrieve it for older learners. Autonomy must always be the clear goal, and all learners need to be steadily moved towards independence and autonomy, whatever their starting point, a step at a time.

Being effective in real life

Education may sometimes begin in the classroom, but if learners are to be autonomous, it must end by making a difference to how they act in the real world. The concept of 'action competences', developed in health promotion in Northern Europe, particularly Denmark (Bruun Jensen 1994; WHO 1997), is a particularly useful one here. This concept suggests that competences cannot be said to be really learned until they have been put into practice to empower people to change their real-life circumstances, their environments, and with it their personal behaviour and feelings. To become autonomous, empowered, and independent, we need to be able to apply our learning outside of the context in which we learn it, and to new and real-life situations.

In order to be effective in real-life situations, we need to recognize the generic base of what we are learning, not just its specific application. Traditionally, school health education has tended to concentrate on health topics, such as drug misuse, diet, and exercise. However, the empowerment approach to health promotion sees behaviour that relates to physical health, and to specific issues such as smoking or sexual behaviour, as determined by deeper attitudes such as self-esteem and empathy. It therefore teaches generic competences such as communication, assertiveness, and decision making, rather than focusing on specific topics, imparting information, or teaching isolated behaviours (Macdonald 1994). The ability to generalize is a difficult one to acquire, especially when we are young, when our thinking is more concrete than when we are older (Houghton 1991), but it is one of the most vital of competences for achieving autonomy.

Many initiatives fail to have any long-term impact because they do not help students to generalize their learning (Beelmann *et al.* 1994), while approaches that explicitly help students practise in real-life situations have been shown to be highly effective (Durlak *et al.* 1994). 'Coaching', where the teacher works alongside the learner, helping them cope with real-life situations, has similarly become increasingly popular as a teaching method, both for children and adults. Teaching these generic, foundation competences is more likely to help students change their behaviour, for example in preventing and/or reducing violence, aggression, bullying, truancy, school dropout rate, teenage pregnancy and drug abuse, than teaching that concentrates on those specific behaviours (Caplan *et al.* 1992; Durlak 1995). In fact, approaches that teach specific skills to avoid drug misuse, child abuse, suicide prevention, or sexual behaviour have been shown to backfire at times, and exacerbate the very problems they were supposed to tackle (Botvin and Dusenbury 1989).

Clarity

The importance of clarity

The second vital factor in any educational setting is clarity, and it takes many different forms. Clarity means making sure that people know what is expected of them and what they can expect; knowing what their place and role are; and what the rules, structures, and most of all the boundaries are. Such clarity makes it safe for people to take risks, to trust, to take part, to build relationships, and gradually practise the kind of independent action and thought that leads to autonomy. People do not operate effectively in situations that are unclear or uncertain; they tend to become anxious and defensive. The younger and less confident we are, the more we need clarity: studies of child development demonstrate clearly that children need to be raised by trustworthy and consistent carers (Winnicott 1984).

In educational contexts, students have been shown to have higher attainments, be more motivated, and attend better in situations with a high degree of structure and clear rules, where teachers demonstrate strong leadership and direction and have high expectations (Wubbels *et al.* 1991; Haertel *et al.* 1981). Rutter *et al.* (1979) found that pupils performed better in more structured schools in which they received more praise and positive rewards and where staff had high expectations of them. Teachers too are more motivated and effective where goals are clear, where they have clear and positive feedback on their performance, and where there is strong leadership from the top (Little 1982; Moos 1991; Devlin 1998).

Learning skills

A basic element that contributes to clarity is knowing clearly what we have to learn. Approaches to education that focus on behaviour and skills can bring a welcome degree of clarity to the learning process. The 'behaviour change' approach is often dismissed by both health education and mainstream education as ideologically unsound, de-powering, manipulative, coercive, and top-down. However, the teaching of behaviours and skills is not *a priori* ethically unsound, it depends on how it is used and who controls it. Behavioural skills-based approaches can be used in ways that are voluntaristic and learner-centred, so long as the management of them is put in the hands of the students themselves (Besalel-Azrin *et al.* 1977).

With adults the teaching of behavioural skills is always voluntaristic, and the most successful behaviour modification programmes are those which people devise for themselves, with or without the help of professionals, to get their behaviour under their own control and to help them reach their own goals (Watson and Tharp 1985). Some behavioural skills programmes have been specifically concerned with helping young people to set their own goals and manage their own progress, through self-reflection, self-assessment, self-recording, and self-reinforcement (Nelson *et al.* 1991), and such programmes have been shown to be very effective (Niness 1995; Webber *et al.* 1993). So if used within the overall context of an empowerment approach, and with the goal of achieving autonomy, the learning of behavioural and cognitive skills produces a high degree of clarity, and can form a useful part of the overall strategy.

The elements of behaviour change theory are vital in helping us to understand what really helps people to change. The copious experience developed by years of careful experimentation has shown that people learn best when they undergo explicit and extensive learning of skills, through learning problem-solving strategies and routines, and are helped to generalize these skills to new situations. They need to learn the skills in ordered and structured environments, which give them clear cues about what needs to be done, and which reinforce their behaviour consistently and positively. They also need to be taught by teachers who model these behaviours consistently and positively themselves (Elias 1990; Grossman and Hughes 1992).

Studies that have compared skills-based approaches with those that teach only values and attitudes have consistently demonstrated the advantages of a skills approach (Hawkins and Catalano 1992; Fertman and Chubb 1992; Vaughan and Lancelotta 1990). For example, a study that directly compared students taught the 'just say no' approach to drug avoidance with students taught a systematic programme of specific drug refusal techniques, which taught appropriate social skills, and which provided them with a rationale for each response, showed that only the skills group showed significant gains in their ability to refuse drugs in follow-up situations (Jones *et al.* 1990). The importance and relevance of skills training have been shown time and again, across a broad range of cultures (Guttman 1994; Hon and Watkins 1995).

The recognition of the importance of such skills-based work has long been accepted in health education. The WHO's approaches for young people have been heavily based on a systematic and comprehensive 'Life Skills' approach, which has been shown to be effective across a wide range of issues, from mental health to sexuality, and again to be relevant across a range of countries and cultures (Lee 1994; Buczkiewicz and Carnegie 2001).

Understanding clearly where people are starting from

Another way in which clarity can be achieved is by carefully determining the starting point of any educational enterprise before embarking on it. If we are to educate effectively, we need to find out where people are starting from and tailor the learning experience to suit them. One of the most important ways in which people differ in their starting points is age and stage of development. People do not develop in a linear way: every child moves through distinct cognitive stages, each with their own rules and principles of logic and causality (Piaget and Inhelder 1958). 'Stages' are not confined to children: as people age so they change emotionally and attitudinally, and the beliefs, needs, and interests of a person of 16 will be very different to those of the same person at 60.

The idea of 'starting where people are' has a long and eminent history. Rousseau, with his beliefs about the need to 'educate the child according to his nature' inspired the child-centred education movement that shaped the theory and practice of primary school education in a powerful way. The developmentally based theories of Abraham Maslow (1971) have had a major impact on education, including health education. He suggests that human needs exist at various levels. For most people the 'lower' ones must be satisfied before they are able to consider the 'higher' ones. Once a person has the basic necessities to keep alive, such as food and water, she or he can move on to more 'long-term' physical needs, such as safety and shelter. With physical needs under control, emotional needs can then surface. The most fundamental emotional need is to feel loved and wanted. Not until this is satisfied can a person feel good about themselves and acquire self-esteem. They then may feel able to address their higher intellectual needs. These begin with 'self-actualization', which includes personal achievements, creative expression, and self-fulfilment. Ultimately, the most mature people are able to look outside of themselves and their immediate relationships and be concerned with wider issues, but such attributes as altruism and impartial rational understanding are only likely to be achieved if more self-centred needs have already been satisfied.

Techniques for finding out where young people are starting from

Taking into account a person's stage of development has long been a fundamental principle of much modern health education. For example, the concept of a 'health career' underlay several curriculum projects of the 1970s and early 1980s (e.g. Schools Health Education Project, 1982). More recently the principle has been used to underpin some novel research strategies that are being used to illuminate the particular, and sometimes peculiar, ways in which children and young people think about health-related issues. These techniques are loosely based on the kind of 'projective' methods that were used in the 1950s in the US (Oppenheim 1996), and involve asking learners to respond spontaneously, with writing and/or drawing, to an open-ended invitation, which can be completed in a whole range of ways, and has no 'right answer'. The technique most widely used in a health context is 'draw and write' (Wetton and McCoy 1998). Others include 'bubble dialogue', filling in dialogue and/or thoughts in a bubble over the head of a cartoon figure, and/or completing an 'unfinished sentence' (Weare and Gray, 1994). Research using these approaches has been carried out right across Europe on a huge range of health-related issues, and the results used to underpin a variety of educational projects, some on professional development (Weare and Gray, 1994) and some on curriculum development (Wetton and McCoy 1998).

However, the idea that education must start where people are is far from being universally accepted in health promotion practice. There are still many examples of unhelpful 'one size fits all' thinking and, more worryingly, approaches, strategies, and campaigns that have proved counter-productive and even harmful. In particular, there has been a long tradition of 'moral panic' inspired education on drugs, alcohol, and smoking aimed at young people, which has attempted to emphasize to adolescents the need to avoid long-term health problems and minimize risk through avoiding drug and tobacco use, sometimes using 'scare tactics' to attempt to frighten learners into a healthier lifestyle. These approaches are not only ineffective, but are often counter-productive: they should thus be seen as not only pointless but possibly very dangerous for schools to use (de Meyrick 2001). At best, young people will probably block out horrific or gory images, as the mind has a highly useful defence mechanism for forgetting such things quite quickly. It also fails to understand the mindset of the young. Given their age and stage, most adolescents are necessarily motivated by short-term hedonism and self-centred optimism. They think they are tougher than others are and thus see the threat of addiction as a challenge rather than a risk, believing they are strong enough to resist. In any case, they have little concern for their futures and may well find the idea of living beyond 40 more a threat than an inducement!

Building from where people are, in a spiral, co-ordinated way

Piaget (Piaget and Inhelder 1958) has demonstrated that what is engaging to the learner is the 'nearly new', something with which she or he is largely familiar and therefore can understand, but which contains a note of dissonance which makes it intriguing. To be effective, the educational task must be right for the learner. Bruner (1966) has shown that learning is most effective when it is organized into a 'spiral' in which issues are revisited in increasing depth as time goes on, rather than in a linear series of 'one-off' experiences. People also learn best when their experiences are brought

together and reinforce one another. Effective education should not therefore tackle topics in isolation, but use a co-ordinated approach, where the
different learning experiences are organized to complement one another by,
for example, studying the same issue in different contexts during the same
period of time.

The importance of using a clear, step by step, coherent and co-ordinated
approach to the study of health, rather than a series of isolated one-off lessons,
has long been supported by those at the forefront of health education, and
underpins many of the key health education curriculum development projects
in the school context (Metcalfe *et al.* 1993). The European Network of Health
Promoting Schools has always put the need for effective co-ordination
at school, district, and national level at the heart of its guidelines (WHO
et al. 1993).

Positive expectations, climates, and policies

Clarity needs to be present, not just in the overt curriculum, but throughout
the whole life of the institution. All too often the rhetorical messages of a
school or college are undermined by unarticulated but highly influential real-
life attitudes and practices. The effect of the 'hidden curriculum' – the often
unspoken and unwritten expectations and norms of an educational institution
on the attitudes, achievements, and behaviour of those who learn and work
there – has long been recognized in health education school curriculum
projects (Metcalfe *et al.* 1993).

The evidence for the significance of school climate and the hidden
curriculum is indeed very clear from mainstream educational research.
A review on discipline and the prevention of violence and bullying in schools,
carried out by the Elton Committee, concluded that a positive school climate
was the most effective deterrent for such unwanted behaviours (Elton 1989).
Teacher expectations of students have long been known to be a vital determinant of student performance, and often they are conveyed in very subtle
ways, with a look, a word, or a nuance. Hamacheck (1978) reviewed the
literature many years ago, and concluded that the evidence for the impact of
teacher expectations on student performance was immense. School climates
need to be positive and to value all students. Again the behavioural approach
is pragmatically useful here, showing clearly that it is more effective to reward
wanted behaviour and ignore unwanted behaviour than to fix attention on
unwanted behaviour through punishing it (Nelson *et al.* 1991).

One way in which educational institutions can achieve greater clarity and
develop positive climates is by making explicit their values and norms
and determining clear procedures, through the development of sound policies.
In recent years in the UK, schools and institutions of higher education have
been put under a great deal of external scrutiny, which has required them to
have clear policies on a range of issues, including some that relate to health
education, such as personal, social and health education itself, and also sex

education, responses to drugs, and bullying. The need to develop similar policies is beginning to be felt in higher education too (Tsouros *et al.* 1998). Policies need to be developed actively and in partnership with all who learn and work in an educational institution so that all feel a sense of responsibility for them and ownership of them, and not simply have them imposed from above. If so, they are likely to have a beneficial impact.

This brings us on to the third key factor, participation.

Participation

Empowerment necessarily involves engagement and participation – it is very much something that people do together, not something that is done to them. Again the need for participation is supported by sound evidence from mainstream educational research. The degree of participation that the educational institution encourages is a strong determinant of the morale and performance of students and teachers and pupils (Moos 1991). For example, a study by Bryk and Driscoll (1988) found that schools with shared values and a common agenda of activities produced students who were more interested and who had higher levels of achievement than less 'communal' schools. While in 'communal' schools that encouraged participation and engagement, the incidence of bad behaviour, absence, and dropout rates were lower. These results have been replicated elsewhere (Elton 1989). Fantuzzo *et al.* (1988) looked at twenty-six studies that compared student-initiated and managed classroom interventions with those initiated by teachers, and found that the student interventions were more likely to change student behaviour.

Recent developments in education have emphasized the need for a shift in focus from teaching to learning and in power from teacher to the learner (Sotto 1994). The emphasis is no longer on what the teacher is doing, which may or may not be having an impact, but on what the student actually learns. Along with this shift, we have a change in the leadership role of the teacher, from didactic expert to facilitator, involving learners in responsibility for learning, as far as their age and stage allow. This has long been recognized as an appropriate role for those who teach adults, but there is evidence that such a relationship can be highly effective with younger students too. For example, Schaps *et al.* (1996) found that students did better in classrooms where they had more influence over both the content of what they learned and the classrooms in which they learned it. There is copious work in health education which emphasizes the idea of shared responsibility between teacher and student, for example in the democratic approach used to develop action competences in schools in Denmark (Bruun Jensen 1994), and in the developing use of 'circle time' in many different classroom contexts (Mosley 1996).

The need for active engagement

Cognitive psychology has shown us that people are more likely to be influenced by their learning if they have to engage with it actively and make it their own in some way (Bligh 1980). Students need to spend as little time as possible on passive tasks such as reading and listening, and as much as possible in participatory and active learning (Kolb 1984). Although, as we have seen, very young and/or insecure children need the security of a regular classroom routine, most people respond better when varied methods of teaching and learning are used. Approaches to learning that employ a range of methods have been shown to be more effective than those that use a limited range (DuPaul and Eckert 1994). Work on learning styles (Kolb 1984) has shown that people learn in many different ways, so using a range of styles allows for the use of a range of learning experiences to match these different styles, as well as helping learners to develop a wider repertoire than their usually preferred style. It also helps people to generalize their learning, by giving them a range of examples to which they can apply what they have learned, and practise it in a range of contexts which, as we have seen, is a vital part of becoming autonomous.

Health education for children and young people has led the field of education in finding ways to apply this insight, and has developed a wealth of strategies for involving people in their learning in varied and active ways. Teaching and learning in health education make use of a very wide range of methods, such as simulations, games, role plays, discussions, and video, often using small groups and an active 'workshop' style. The principles of active learning have inspired many of the most influential curriculum projects and initiatives through the years (Schools Health Education Project 1982; Metcalfe *et al.* 1993; HEA 1989, 2001).

Equity

A further key principle of health promotion, and one that relates directly to participation, is that of equity. It means that educational institutions need to value diversity and widen opportunity and participation, so that all students from all sectors of the community and with all levels of ability can achieve their potential. In an educational context this often requires a major realignment from the traditional approach of competition and elitism.

The achievement of equity is perhaps the biggest challenge facing educational institutions today. The statistical association of social class and ethnic origin with educational achievement is well known, and has hardly changed since the 1960s: if anything the gap is widening. To take the UK for instance, working-class children and those from certain ethnic backgrounds, especially Afro-Caribbean, do worse on all educational measures, such as tests of attainment, examination results, and entrance to higher education (Foster *et al.* 1996). Work on school exclusions suggests that Afro-Caribbean children are four times as likely to be excluded as white children (Smith 1998).

Although some of the causes of this differential distribution of educational achievement may lie in the home and the neighbourhood, educational institutions play a strong part too, amplifying the differences which pupils bring with them to the classroom (Elton 1989). For some time we have known that many teachers have unhelpfully low expectations of children from working-class backgrounds and certain ethnic groups (Fuchs 1973), which can result in pupils being given very different images of their own abilities, and different educational experiences and challenges (Young 1971). Schools and teachers are by no means immune from overt or institutional racism: a recent UK survey showed that one in ten trainee teachers has racist attitudes (Wilkins 1999). Such differences tend to impact not only on academic achievement but on health-related behaviour too. Willis (1984) points out that many of those students in his study of a secondary school who smoked or abused drugs were underachievers, and argues that their 'unhealthy' habits can be partly seen as their way of getting back at an education that they feel does not meet their needs.

There is now in the UK a major drive towards social inclusion and greater participation in higher education by all groups in society (Ball 1998). If they wish to overcome these problems, educational institutions will need to tackle their own attitudes and practices. This has been shown to be possible; for example Rogers (1994) describes an Australian school programme which explicitly taught teachers not to be fatalistic and determinist, but to start where pupils are and build on their positive attributes.

Relationships and the emotions

The centrality of relationships and emotions to health

In the West at least, with its philosophy rooted in positivism and rationality, there have traditionally been major conceptual divides between the mind, the body, the emotions, and the surrounding context of social relationships. Education has tended to be seen as being all about the mind, while a medicalized view of health has seen it as being all about the body. In both disciplines, the emotions and social relationships have tended to be regarded as either irrelevant, or as 'noise in the system' that need to be managed but are not themselves of central interest.

In contrast to this divisive thinking, modern health education has long based its practice on research that suggests that relationships and emotions have a central part to play in both education and health. Research has shown that we tend to choose to look after our health, according to how we feel about, for example, the level of control we have in the world (Becker 1974), or the extent to which others care about us (Seligman 1991). Similarly, we are more likely to look after the health of others if we feel bonded with them, at a family or community level (Adams and Smithies 1990).

Recently, the extent to which relationships and emotions affect physical health very directly has become strikingly clear. There is strong evidence that those who experience negative emotions and poor relationships for long periods are much more prone to illness. Depression appears to hinder recovery from illness or surgery and makes death more likely (Goleman 1996), and has been linked to suppression of the immune system, and hence to illnesses such as colds and flu (Glaser and Glaser 1987; Seligman 1991). Anger, high levels of hostility, and a sense of having no control have been convincingly linked with heart disease (Williams 1984; Marmot *et al.* 1997). Meanwhile the experience and expression of positive emotion, for example through learning to laugh more often, or to look on the positive side of an experience, has been linked with positive physical health outcomes (Seligman 1991; Holden 1998).

The centrality of relationships and emotion to education

This interest in relationships and emotions in health education is starting to be supported by similar concerns in mainstream education. As we have seen, Maslow's theory has demonstrated that emotional needs such as self-esteem and loving and caring underpin the ability to move onto higher goals such as intellectual understanding. More recently, scientists such as Gardner (Gardner *et al.* 1995) have been highly influential in obtaining recognition for emotional and social competence as valuable in their own right, not just as a stepping stone to intellectual development. Gardner's work on 'multiple intelligences', has brought relationships and emotions into a central position in education. He suggests that limiting the definition of what we mean by 'intelligence' to the cognitive and intellectual is too restrictive and narrow. He has identified seven separate intelligences, some of which are traditional (e.g. logical and spatial) but two of which are concerned with relationships and emotions. 'Interpersonal intelligence' is the ability to understand others, how they work, what motivates them, and how to work co-operatively with them. 'Intra personal intelligence' is the ability to understand oneself, to form an accurate model of oneself, and use it to operate effectively in life. Gardner suggests educators need to treat these emotional and social forms of intelligence as being of equal worth to those more traditionally transmitted by education.

In the mid-1990s, Goleman's seminal book *Emotional Intelligence* (1996) had a major impact on mainstream educational thinking by demonstrating in an accessible and popular way the extent to which emotional and social abilities are fundamental to success in life. He cites many different studies which show that emotional and social competences such as resilience, getting on with others, handling frustrations, and managing emotions, are far better predictors of career success at work than is IQ. He suggests that the various forms of intelligence, both the traditional cognitive ones and the newly identified social and emotional ones, support one another, and are indeed fundamentally inseparable: by directing the attention towards what matters, emotional and social intelligences help people to think clearly, prioritize, decide, anticipate, and plan. Without an emotional value to attach to an activity, all decisions can appear equally good.

The evidence for the educational importance of supportive relationships

The importance of social relationships is supported by work on educational environments. The quality of relationships in an educational setting has been shown to be a crucial factor in producing high levels of staff and student performance and positive attitudes: caring, warm and supportive relationships have been shown to be essential if pupils are to learn, and teachers to teach, more effectively. Major international reviews of the evidence have suggested that students learn more and have higher attainments, enjoy learning, are more motivated, and attend better, if their teachers are 'more understanding, helpful and friendly' (Wubbels *et al.* 1991), if they work in contexts that are characterized by 'higher levels of cohesiveness' and 'less social friction' (Haertel *et al.* 1981) and are emotionally attached to their school or college (Battistich *et al.* 1997; Hawkins and Catalano 1992; Solomon *et al.* 1992). Educational contexts that are unsupportive and have poor relationships have been shown to induce depression and absenteeism in staff and pupils (Moos 1991). Bad relationships is one of the most commonly cited causes of staff stress (Kyriacou 1996), while high levels of support, particularly from the head teacher, have consistently been shown to reduce the likelihood of teacher burnout (Sarros and Sarros 1992).

Relationship skills and emotional literacy can be taught

Not only is the importance of relationships and emotions in education now being accepted, we are coming to understand how these issues can be taught. Those engaged in the caring sector, and in particular counselling and therapy, have long accepted that people can, for example, be encouraged to get in touch with their feelings, to be able to identify them, own them, listen to what they are telling them, and communicate more openly and effectively with others. Emotional and social education is starting to be found in schools, facilitated by organizations that lobby for the introduction of 'emotional literacy' in the UK such as Antidote (Antidote 1998), or 'social and emotional learning' in the US such as CASEL (Elias *et al.* 1997). There has been considerable work in recent years which has demonstrated in detail some of the ways in which schools and other institutions can teach emotional and social intelligence (Elias *et al.* 1997; Salovey and Sluyter 1997).

In realizing the importance of emotional and social education, mainstream education starting to catch up with health education, and supply the scientific evidence for approaches which to health educators have long had intuitive validity. Health education has been in the forefront of educational initiatives that take the learner's emotional state into account, and that recognize that if people are to be empowered, they have to be able to manage, not be disabled by, their own emotions. From the early days in the 1970s, many major school-based developments in health education have been centrally concerned with the development of self-esteem and relationship skills, and with the role of the teacher as pastoral tutor and counsellor. This emphasis continued through the 1990s in some key European curriculum projects on health education in general (Metcalfe *et al.* 1993) and on mental and emotional health in particular. Emotional and social education are now seen as playing a pivotal role in the health-promoting school.

Conclusion

As we have seen, education has a central part to play in the achievement of an empowering health promotion; without it health promotion would, as Green and Kreuter (1991) point out, tend to become coercive. It is clear that a very wide range of educational approaches and strategies have their uses, including those often derided by health promoters and health educators, such as a behavioural skills approach, so long as the basic principles of empowerment and autonomy are respected, and are the goal of the activity. We have also seen that health promotion has a major role to play in the development of mainstream education, often leading the way in, for example, recognizing the importance of emotion, relationships, active approaches to learning, and partnership. Health promotion and education have been, and will always remain, intertwined, and it is essential that practitioners in both fields understand this, can see where their interests come together, and can reinforce and support one another (Weare, 2000).

References

Abercrombie, N., Gatrell, T., and Thomas, C. (1998) 'Universities and health in the twenty first century' in A. Tsouros, G. Dowding, J. Thompson, and M. Dooris (eds) *Health Promoting Universities*, Copenhagen: WHO Regional Office for Europe, pp. 29–34.

Adams, L. and Smithies, J. (1990) *Community Participation and Health Promotion*, London: HEA.

Antidote (1998) *Realizing the Potential: Emotional Education for All*, London: Antidote.

Aspey, D. and Roebuck, F. (1977) *Kids Don't Learn from People They Don't Like*, Massachusetts: Human Resource Development Press.

Ausbel, D. P., Novak, J. S., and Hanesian, H. (1978) *Educational Psychology, a Cognitive View*, 2nd edition, New York: Holt, Rinehart & Winston.

Baelz, P. R. (1979) 'The philosophy of health education', in I. Sutherland (ed.) *Health Education Perspectives and Choices*, London: Allen & Unwin.

Ball, J. (1998) *School Inclusion: The School, the Family and the Community*, London: Joseph Rowntree Foundation.

Barrows, H. S. and Tamblyn, R. M. (1980) *Problem-based Learning*, New York: Springer.

Battistich, V. *et al.* (1997) 'The relationship between students' sense of their school as community and their involvement in problem behaviors', *American Journal of Public Health* 87.

Beattie, A. (1991) 'Knowledge and control in health promotion: a test case for social theory and social policy', in J. Gabe, M. Calnan, and M. Bury (eds) *Sociology of the Health Service*, London: Routledge.

Becker, M. H. (1974) 'The health belief model and personal health behaviour', *Health Education Monographs* 2 (4).

Beelmann, A., Pfingsten, U., and Losel, F. (1994) 'Effects of training social competence in children: A meta-analysis of recent evaluation studies'. *Journal of Clinical Child Psychology*, 23: 260–71.

Besalel-Azrin,V., Azrin, N., and Armstrong, P. (1977) 'The student-oriented class-room: a method of improving student conduct and satisfaction'. *Behavior Therapy*, 8 (2): 193–204.

Bligh, D. (1980) *Methods and Techniques in Post Secondary Education*, Paris: Unesco.

Botvin, G. and Dusenbury, L. (1989) 'Substance abuse prevention and the promotion of competence', in L. Bond and B. Compas (eds) *Primary Prevention and Promotion in the Schools. Primary Prevention of Psychopathology*, Vol. 12, Newbury Park, CA: Sage Publications.

Bruner, J. (1966) *Towards a Theory of Instruction*, Cambridge, MA: Harvard University Press.

Bruun Jensen, B. (1994) 'An action competence approach to health education', in C. Chu and R. Simpson (eds) *Ecological Public Health: From Vision to Practice*, Brisbane: Griffiths University.

Bryk, A. and Driscoll, M. W. (1988) *The High School as Community: Contextual Influences and Consequences for Students and Teachers*, Madison: University of Wisconsin-Madison, National Center on Effective Secondary Schools.

Buczkiewicz, M. and Carnegie, R. (2001) 'The Ugandan life skills initiative', *Health Education* 1: 10–15.

Caplan, M., Weissberg, R., Grober, J., Sivo, P., Grady, K., and Jacoby, C. (1992) 'Social competence promotion with inner-city and suburban young adolescents – effects on social-adjustment and alcohol-use', *Journal of Consulting and Clinical Psychology*, 60 (1): 56–63.

Catford, J. and Parish, R. (1989) '"Heartbeat Wales", new horizons for health promotion in the community – the philosophy and practice of Heartbeat Wales', in D. Seedhouse and A. Cribb (eds) *Changing Ideas In Health Care*, Chichester: John Wiley.

de Meyrick, J. (2001) 'Forget the "blood and gore": An alternative message strategy to help adolescents avoid cigarette smoking', *Health Education* 3: 20–8.

Devlin, T. (1998) *Public Relations and Marketing for Schools*, London: Pitman.

Draper, P., Griffin, J., Dennis, J., and Popay, J. (1980) 'Three types of health education', *British Medical Journal* 281: 493–5.

DuPaul, G. and Eckert, T. (1994) 'The effects of social skills curricula: now you see them, now you don't', *School Psychology Quarterly*, 9 (2): 113–32.

Durlak, C., Rose, E., and Bursuck, W. (1994) 'Preparing high school students with learning disabilities for the transition to postsecondary education: teaching the skills of self-determination', *Journal of Learning Disabilities*, 27 (1): 51–9.

Durlak, J. (1995) *School Based Prevention Programmes for Children and Adolescents*, London: Sage.

Durlak, J., and Wells, A. (1997) 'Primary prevention mental health programs for children and adolescents: a meta-analytic review', *American Journal of Community Psychology*, 25 (2): 115–52.

Elias, M. (1990) 'The role of affect and social relationships in health behaviour and school health curriculum and instruction', *Journal of School Health* 60 (4): 157–63.

Elias, M., and Kress, J. (1994) 'Social decision making and life skills development: a critical thinking approach to health promotion in the middle school', *Journal of School Health*, 64 (2): 62–6.

Elias, M., Zins, J., Weissberg, R., Frey, K., Greenberg, M., Haynes, N., Kessler, R., Schwab-Stone, M., and Shriver, T. (1997) *Promoting Social and Emotional Learning*, Alexandria, VA: ASCD.

Elton, Lord (1989) *Discipline in Schools: Report of the Committee of Enquiry Chaired by Lord Elton*, London: HMSO.

Entwistle, N. J. and Ramsden, P. (1983) *Understanding Students' Learning*, London: Croom Helm.

Fantuzzo, J., Polite, K. C., David, M., and Quinn, Greg (1988) 'An evaluation of the effectiveness of teacher- vs. student-management classroom interventions', *Psychology in the Schools* 25: 154–63.

Fertman, C. and Chubb, N. (1992) 'The effects of a psychoeducational program on adolescents' activity involvement, self-esteem, and locus of control', *Adolescence*, 27 (107): 517–26.

Foster, P., Gomm, R., and Hammersley, M. (1996) *Constructing Educational Inequality*, London: Falmer Press.

Fraser, B. and Walberg, H. (eds) (1991) *Educational Environments*, Oxford: Pergamon.

Fuchs, E. (1973) 'How teachers learn to help pupils fail' in N. Keddie (ed.) *Tinker-Tailor . . . the Myth of Cultural Deprivation*, Harmondsworth: Penguin.

Gagne, R. M. (1965) *The Conditions of Learning*, New York: Holt, Rinehart & Winston.

Gardner, H., Kornhaber, M., and Wake, W. (1995) *Intelligence: Multiple Perspectives*, London: Harcourt Brace College Publishers.

Glaser, R. and Kiecolt-Glaser, J. (1987) 'Stress associated depression in cellular immunity', *Brain, Behaviour and Immunity*, 1.

Goleman, D. (1996) *Emotional Intelligence*, London: Bloomsbury.

Gordon, J. and Grant, G. (1997) *How We Feel*, London: Jessica Kingsley.

Green, L.W. and Kreuter, M.W. (1991) *Health Promotion Planning: an Educational and Environmental Approach*, Toronto: Mayfield.

Grossman, P. and Hughes, J. (1992) 'Self-control interventions with internalizing disorders – a review and analysis', *School Psychology Review*, 21 (2): 229–45.

Guttman, C. (1994) *On the Right Track: Servol's Early Childhood and Adolescent Development Programmes in Trinidad and Tobago. Education for All: Making It Work.* Innovations Series, 5. Paris: UNESCO, Basic Education Division.

Haertel, G., Walberg, H., and Haertel, E. (1981) 'Socio-psychological environments and learning: a quantitative analysis', *British Educational Research Journal*, 7: 27–36.

Hamacheck, D. (1978) *Encounters with the Self*, New York: Holt, Rinehart & Winston.

Hawkins, J., and Catalano, R. (1992) *Communities That Care: Action for Drug Abuse Prevention*, San Francisco: Jossey-Bass.

HEA (1989, 2001) *Health for Life: The HEA Primary School Project*, Walton-on-Thames: Thomas Nelson.

Holden, R. (1998) *Happiness Now*, London: Hodder & Stoughton.

Hon, C., and Watkins, D. (1995) 'Evaluating a social skills training program for Hong Kong students', *Journal of Social Psychology* 135: 527–28.

Houghton, S. (1991) 'Promoting generalization of appropriate behaviour across special and mainstream settings: a case study', *Educational Psychology in Practice*, 7 (1): 49–53.

Jones, R., McDonald, D., Fiore, M., and Arrington,T. (1990) 'A primary preventive approach to children's drug refusal behavior: the impact of rehearsal-plus', *Journal of Pediatric Psychology*, 15: 211–23.

Kolb, D. (1984) *Experiential Learning*, New Jersey: Prentice-Hall.

Kyriacou, C. (1996) 'Teacher stress: a review of some international comparisons'. *Education Section Review*, 20 (1): 17–20.

Lee, J. (1994) 'Prevention, process and product: the role of Life Skills', in D. Trent and C. Reed (eds) *Promotion of Mental Health*, Vol. 3, Aldershot: Avebury.

Liedekerken, P. C. (ed.) (1990) *The Effectiveness of Health Education*, Utrecht, Netherlands: Dutch Health Education Centre.

Little, R. (1982) 'Norms of collegiality and experimentation: workplace conditions of school success'. *American Educational Research* 78: 178–85.

Macdonald, G. (1994) 'Self esteem and the promotion of mental health', in D. Trent and C. Reed (eds) *Promotion of Mental Health*, Vol. 3, Aldershot: Avebury.

Marmot, M., Bosma, H., Hemingway, H., Brunner, E., and Stanfield, S. (1997) 'Contribution of job control and other risk factors to social variations in coronary heart disease incidence', *Lancet* 350: 235–39.

Marshall, H. and Weinstein, R. (1984) 'Classroom factors affecting students' self evaluation: an interactional model', *Review of Educational Research* 54: 301–25.

Maslow, A. (1970) *Motivation and Personality*, 2nd edition, New York: Harper & Row.

Mayer, R. E. (1979) 'Can advance organizers influence meaningful learning?', *Review of Educational Research* 49: 371–83.

Metcalfe, O., Weare, K., Williams, M., and Young, I. (1993) *Promoting the Health of Young People in Europe*, Copenhagen: WHO.

Miller, W. and Rollnick, S. (1991) *Motivational Interviewing: Preparing People for Change*. New York: Guildford Press.

Moos, R. (1991) 'Connections between school, work and family settings', in B. Fraser and H. Walberg (eds) *Educational Environments*, Oxford: Pergamon.

Mosley, J. (1996) *Quality Circle Time*, Cambridge: LDA.

Neilans, T. and Israel, A. (1981) 'Towards maintenance and generalization of behavior change: Teaching children self-regulation and self-instructional skills', *Cognitive Therapy and Research*, 5: 189–95.

Nelson, J., Smith, D., Young, R., and Dodd, J. (1991) 'A review of self-management outcome research conducted with students who exhibit behavioral disorders', *Behavioral Disorders*, 16: 169–79.

Niness, H. (1995) 'The effect of a self management training package on the transfer of aggression control procedures in the absence of supervision', *Behavior Modification*, 19 (4 October): 464–90.

Oppenheim, A. (1996) *Questionnaire Design, Interviewing, and Attitude Measurement*, London: Pinter.

Piaget, J. and Inhelder, B. (1958) *The Growth of Logical Thinking from Childhood to Adolescence*, London: Routledge.

Rodmell, S. and Watt, A. (eds) (1986) *The Politics of Health Education*, London: Routledge.

Rogers, B. (1994) *Behaviour Recovery: A Whole-School Program for Mainstream Schools*, Victoria: Australian Council for Educational Research.

Rutter, M., Maughan, B., Mortimore, P., and Ouston, J. (1979) *Fifteen Thousand Hours: Secondary Schools and their Effects on Children.* Cambridge, MA: Harvard University Press.

Salovey, P. and Sluyter, D. (1997) *Emotional Development and Emotional Intelligence*, New York: Basic Books.

Sarros, J. and Sarros, A. (1992) 'Social support and teacher burnout', *Journal of Educational Administration* 30 (1): 55–69.

Schaps, E., Lewis, C., and Watson, M. (1996) 'Building community in school', *Principal*, November: 29–31.

Schon, D. A. (1983) *The Reflective Practitioner*, New York: Basic Books.

Schools Health Education Project (1982) *Health Education 13–18*, London: Nelson.

Seligman, M. (1991) *Learned Optimism*, Milson's Point, Australia: Random House.

Smith, R. (1998) *No Lessons Learnt*, London: The Children's Society.

Solomon, D., Watson, M., Battistich, V., Schaps, E., and Delucchi, K. (1992) 'Creating a caring community: a school based programme to promote children's prosocial competence', in E. Oser, J. Patty, and A. Dick (eds) *Effective and Responsible Teaching*, San Francisco: Jossey Bass.

Sotto, E. (1994) *When Teaching Becomes Learning*, London: Cassell.

St Leger, L. and Nutbeam, D. (2000) 'A model for mapping linkages between health and education agencies to improve school health', *Journal of School Health* 70 (2): 45–50.

Thurlow, M. (1995) *Staying in School: Strategies for Middle School Students with Learning & Emotional Disabilities. ABC Dropout Prevention and Intervention Series*, Minneapolis: Institute on Community Integration, University of Minnesota.

Tofler, A. (1980) *The Third Wave*, London: Pan.

Tones, K. (1986) 'Health education and the ideology of health promotion: a review of alternative strategies', *Health Education Research: Theory and Practice* 1 (1): 3–12.

—— (1987) 'Promoting health: the contribution of education', *Education for Health in Europe: A Report on a WHO Consultation on Co-ordinated Infrastructure with a Health Promotion Strategy*, Edinburgh: Scottish Health Education Group.

Tones, K. and Tilford, S. (1994) *Health Education, Effectiveness, Efficiency and Equity*, 2nd edition, London: Chapman and Hall.

Tsouros, A., Dowding, G., Thompson, J., and Dooris, M. (eds) (1998) *Health Promoting Universities*, Copenhagen: WHO.

Tunstall, D. (1994) *Social Competence Needs in Young Children: What the Research Says.* Paper presented at the Association for Childhood Education International Study Conference, New Orleans, March 30–April 2.

Vaughan, S., and Lancelotta, G. (1990) 'Teaching interpersonal social skills to poorly accepted students: peer-pairing versus non-peer-pairing', *Journal of School Psychology*, 28: 181–8.

Veen, C. (1995) *Evaluation of the IUHPE Project on the Effectiveness of Health Promotion and Health Education* (12 volumes), Utrecht, Netherlands: Dutch Health Education Centre.

Watson, D. L., and Tharp, R. G. (1985) *Self Directed Behaviour: Self Modification for Personal Adjustment*, 4th edition, Monterey, CA: Brooks/ Cole.

Weare, K. (2000) *Promoting Mental, Emotional and Social Health: A Whole School Approach*, London: Routledge.

Weare, K. and Gray, G. (1994) *Promoting Mental and Emotional Health in the European Network of Health Promoting Schools*, Copenhagen: World Health Organisation.

Webber, J., Scheuermann, B., McCall, C., and Coleman, M. (1993) 'Research on self-monitoring as a behavior management technique in special-education classrooms – a descriptive review', *Remedial and Special Education* 14 (2): 38–56.

Wetton, N. and McCoy, M. (1998) *Confidence to Learn: A Guide to Extending Health Education in the Primary School*, Edinburgh: Health Education Board for Scotland.

White, M. (1998) 'Creating a healthy medical school', in A. Tsouros, G. Dowding, J. Thompson, and M. Dooris (eds) *Health Promoting Universities*, Copenhagen: WHO Regional Office for Europe, pp. 56–65.

WHO (1946) *Constitution*, Geneva: WHO.

—— (1986) *Ottawa Charter For Health Promotion*, Geneva: WHO.

—— (1991) *Sundsvall Statement on Supportive Environments for Health*, Copenhagen: WHO Regional Office for Europe.

—— (1997) *The Health Promoting School: an Investment in Education, Health and Democracy: Conference Report on the First Conference of the European Network of Health Promoting Schools, Thessaloniki, Greece*, Copenhagen: WHO Regional Office for Europe.

WHO, CEC, and CE (1993) *The European Network of Health Promoting Schools: Resource Manual*. Copenhagen: WHO Regional Office for Europe.

Wilkins, C. (1999) *Making 'Good Citizens': the Social and Political Attitudes of PGCE Students*, London: Carfax.

Williams, R. (1984) *The Trusting Heart*, New York: Random House.

Willis, P. (1984) *Learning to Labour*, Aldershot: Gower.

Winnicott, D. (1984) *The Maturational Process and the Facilitating Environment*, London: Hogarth.

Wubbels, T., Brekelmans, M., and Hooymayers, H. (1991) 'Interpersonal teacher behaviour in the classroom', in B. Fraser and H. Walberg (eds) *Educational Environments*, Oxford: Pergamon.

Young, M. (1971) 'An approach to the study of curricula as socially organised knowledge', in M. Young (ed.) *Knowledge and Control*, West Drayton, Middlesex: Collier Macmillan.

Part II
Secondary disciplines

6 Health promotion as social policy

Robin Bunton

Health promotion professes to be centrally concerned with the social policy process and most definitions of health promotion place notions of social structure and policy process at the centre of concerns. Building healthy public policy, for example, was one of the five means of health promotion action to achieve Health For All by the Year 2000 – along with creating supportive environments, strengthening community action, developing personal skills, and reorienting health services. To promote health effectively, we need to be able to understand, analyse, and ultimately influence social and health policy. Social policy should have a substantial input to health promotion, taking health promotion on its own terms. More than this, however, the study of social policy might contribute to our understanding of the emergence of health promotion itself. Health promotion has developed along with and in response to a social and political context particular to the late twentieth century. It has been described as lying at the forefront of social and cultural change (Beattie 1991). Understanding this social and political policy context, and health promotion's place within it, provides important reflection and self-awareness but also allows a better understanding of the limitations on and the possibilities for developing healthy public policy. Health promotion is itself a topic of interest to social policy analysts and is increasingly seen as an area of social policy. There are substantial areas of overlap between the two fields of study.

This chapter examines the contribution which the study of social policy can make to the study of health promotion in both informing the development of healthy public policy and in providing analyses of the possibilities for the governance of health. It outlines the salient features of the academic study of social policy, its focus and perspective, and suggests how these might contribute to health promotion and to healthy public policy in particular. Substance misuse policy is used to illustrate the overlapping interests of health promotion and social policy. Before introducing social policy as a discipline or field of study, we will briefly consider the nature of healthy public policy within health promotion discourse.

Healthy public policy

Defining healthy public policy can be problematic because of variation in the use of the term and inherent conceptual ambiguity (Pederson *et al.* 1988). Though a relatively new term, it is a direct descendant of the 'old' and the 'new' public health movements, and intimately linked to the development of World Health Organization programmes. The conceptual grounding for healthy public policy came from the WHO Assembly's resolution that health be the main social goal of government, including Health For All by the Year 2000. Subsequent conferences and concept statements have given substance to healthy public policy, as did the WHO conference on healthy public policy held in Adelaide (WHO 1988b) which produced the following definition:

> Healthy Public Policy is characterized by an explicit concern for health and equity in all areas of policy and by an accountability for health impact.

The concept anticipates a new culture of public policy that is pluralistic and looks beyond state administrative planning structures to develop and implement policy, calling for multi-sectoral, multi-level, and participative initiatives.

A useful distinction has been made between healthy public policy and public health policy (Hancock 1982). The latter term refers to a narrower set of policies, more usually aimed at the system of caring for ill people. This distinction is a crucial one. Healthy public policy self-consciously aims to go beyond the health care system and its more traditional hospital and physician-based care. Definitions of healthy public policy incorporate very broad visions of health, crossing traditional disciplinary, organizational, and governmental categories. They refer to a concern for manipulating the social policy environment to create a healthy society, implicitly recognizing that the social environment is an important determinant of health. Milio's elegant definition captured this well, describing healthy public policy as 'Ecological in perspective, multi-sectoral in scope and participatory in strategy' (Milio 1987). Being ecological and to some extent holistic, such an approach claims to recognize the complexity of the determinants of health and disease (Milio 1986). Various sectors of society are understood to act in interdependence to regulate, enhance, or endanger health. Governmental sectors outside health are involved in engendering health, such as agriculture, education, transportation, energy, and housing, for example.

The environment has recently received more attention from health promoters and public health practitioners. In 1991 Peter Draper argued for a 'new' approach to public health that was 'green sensitive' and recognized that the human-made environments in rich and poor countries could adversely affect people's health. The 'core' of public health, he claimed, should be environmental in focus taking the physical and the social and economic aspects of existence – the 'total environment' (Draper 1991: 10). Building sustainable environmental policy has been seen as a vital part of healthy public policy generation. The Third International Conference in Sundsvall, Sweden, held in 1991 on 'Supportive Environments for Health', attempted to fuse the focus on health, the environment, and sustainable development (WHO 1992). Analysts such as Draper were drawing upon a broader definition of the environment than health promoters and public health practitioners had been used to. The environment was social as well as physical, produced by humans as well as by nature. Such thinking drew upon thinking from the international study of the environment, such as the World Commission on Environment and Development (Brundtland Report 1987) and the *State of the World* reports coming from the Worldwatch Institute. Since then, environmental issues have climbed higher up the public health policy agenda as well as that of nation states globally. The 1992 Rio Earth Summit focused world attention upon the limits of endless techno-economic development. Sustainable development became a concern as well as a possibility for 'ecological modernization'. This followed on a host of international developments that appeared to embrace environmentalist issues. The call to make health promotion and the 'new' public health more responsible for countering potentially hostile, socio-economic environments at the end of the last century in many ways reflected the preoccupation of nineteenth-century public health activists.

Such approaches to healthy public policy imply new ways of thinking about health and government policy, and they suggest the design of overarching mechanisms linking very different policy sectors. The environment is conceived as a complex web of inter-connected human and non-human systems (Stokols 2000). Governments, it is argued, should view health as a resource and plan to maximize its production by social and economic development. Central government mechanisms have been suggested that vet all policies for their health effect (or gain) in much the same way that treasury departments (Milio 1986) now vet policies. Mobilizing for the development of healthy public policy will require new organizational mechanisms and new means of co-ordination to bring about new alliances. New methods of working will also be necessary.

Though sometimes confused with health promotion policy, healthy public policy takes a broader focus than this neighbouring concept, which tends to refer to the development of specific health promotion programmes such as the development of no-smoking policies or healthy diet policies, or even the establishment of health promotion organizations or structures. Healthy public policy refers to multi-sectoral and collaborative processes involving the participation of all groups and populations affected.

Collaboration and co-ordination are needed to draw upon the wide range of activities required to promote healthy public policy. Participation also features largely. If multi-sectoral collaborative efforts are to be achieved, then different sectors, groups, or communities must be made aware of the health consequences of their actions and be made to commit themselves to change. There has been a call for greater public accountability for health and the development of partnerships in the policy process. Slogans and catchphrases such as 'intersectoral planning', 'community participation', 'putting health on the agenda of policy makers' became synonymous with the Health For All by the Year 2000 movement. Corporate and business interests, non-government bodies, and community organizations were all considered for their potential for preserving and promoting people's health. Mobilizing for healthy public policy is often challenging and involves facilitating, enabling, and empowering sections of the community (Stacey 1988). Such work often appears to lack coherent theoretical or evidence-based backing (Pederson *et al.* 1988) and may be an area in which social policy analysis has much to offer. Understanding how groups and organizations come to act upon and change aspects of their everyday world is central to understanding the healthy public process.

The Adelaide Conference on healthy public policy (WHO 1988b) identified a number of areas for immediate action. It recognized that equity and access to health resources (health care, healthy environments, and other health-enhancing goods and services) are fundamental to promoting and protecting health. Four areas were prioritized: the health of women, food and nutrition, tobacco and alcohol, and the creation of supportive environments. New alliances are recommended as a means of achieving this, such as the joining of public health and ecological movements locally, nationally, and internationally. Commitment to global health is central to these recommendations. There is an inherent refusal to accept the social policy environment unquestionably, along with a call for changes in the social and political environments.

The development of the concept of healthy public policy stresses the need to understand and analyse the policy environment in a very broad sense. It points to the need for analysis of broader beliefs and cultures as well as detailed understanding of the nature of available policy advocates, areas of public support, the nature of key 'stakeholders' and influences of policy, as well as government and organizational structures. Such an area of study could be said to form the *raison d'être* of social policy. The broad focus of concern matches that of the contemporary discipline, though this has not always been the case. There would appear to be a substantial convergence of interest between health promoters and social policy analysts, at least as far as the area of study is concerned. Perspectives may vary considerably within health promotion, as this volume illustrates. Variety also exists within the study of social policy, as the following brief outline of the discipline illustrates.

Social policy

Social policy refers to the sets of arrangements and structures associated with state policies, ranging from broad economic policy to specific areas such as crime control. Social policy is more often used to refer to policies that are 'integrative' in one way or another; that is, they are designed to bind or to bring about harmonization in society in some way (Boulding 1967). Though usually associated with national and local government, social policy may be the result of non-government initiatives or the unintended outcome of a variety of political, social, and organizational imperatives. Social policy also refers to a particular field of academic study, with its own concerns and perspectives. It is the academic study of social policy that is the main concern of this chapter, though these two areas cannot easily be divorced from each other. The study of social policy is in large part influenced by current developments in the social policy environment. In discussing the academic discipline of social policy, it will be useful – necessary even – to refer to recent changes in the social policy environment.

Seen as either a discipline or a field of study incorporating a number of disciplines, social policy is a relatively new development. It emerged very much (along with its allied discipline social administration) in response to unprecedented expansion of the welfare state in the late nineteenth and early twentieth centuries, providing an academic background for the emerging social service occupations (Brown 1983). The subject grew with a distinct institutional focus, studying the nature of a rapidly growing social service provision. In Britain, like many other Western or Northern societies, the end of the Second World War marked a new era of welfare administered by either central or local government, which replaced the piecemeal provision of the nineteenth and early twentieth centuries. General social services became an integral part of state activity attempting to eliminate the so-called 'five great areas of want': poverty, homelessness, ignorance, disease, and idleness (unemployment). In Britain, a number of 'blue-print' documents such as the Beveridge report (Beveridge 1942) appeared, shaping the construction of the welfare state. The introduction of national insurance schemes, family allowances, national assistance, national health services, state education, and children's welfare systems were commonly developed along with local government housing.

The study of social policy reflected these concerns. Marshall, one of the founders of the discipline, defined social policies by their welfare objectives – security, health, and welfare. He contrasts such policies with economic policies, which are less altruistic. Social policies, he has argued, are concerned with collective interventions to promote individual welfare, often using political power to supersede or modify the operations of the economic system (Marshall 1975). Marshall distinguished three aims of social policies: the elimination of poverty, the pursuit of equity, and the maximization of welfare. The study of social policy was intimately linked to reforms on all these fronts and has been dubbed 'the book-keeping of reform' (Rex 1978). Key individuals within the discipline in Britain have been linked to Fabianism and explicitly committed to social reform (Brown 1983).

The focus of social policy is much broader than these concerns, however, and also more critical. Titmuss, another important founder and the first Professor of Social Administration, defined his subject as the study of eight areas:

1   The analysis and description of policy formation and its consequences, intended and unintended.

2   The study of structure, function, organization, planning and administrative processes of institutions and agencies, historical and comparative.
3   The study of social needs and of problems of access to, utilization, and patterns of outcome of services, transactions, and transfers.
4   The analysis of the nature, attributes, and distribution of social costs and diswelfares.
5   The analysis of distributive and allocative patterns in command-over-sources-through-time, and the particular impact of the social services.
6   The study of the roles and functions of selected representatives, professional workers, administrators, and interest groups in the operation of social welfare institutions.
7   The study of the social rights of the citizen as contributor, participant, and user of the social services.
8   The study of the role of government (local and central) as an allocator of values and of rights to social property as expressed through social and administrative law and other rule-making channels.

(Titmuss 1968 quoted in Brown 1983)

This description, demanding though it is, does not exhaust the concerns of the subject. Social policy is not simply concerned with the analysis and critique of administrative institutions and processes and the effects of government welfare policies. It is also interested in the structures and processes of wider society, which create a given distribution of resources, have a bearing on welfare, and, in turn, regulate the institutions that manage that distribution (Walker 1983). All areas of government policy can influence social policy, including 'the social purposes and consequences of agriculture, economic, manpower, fiscal, physical development and social welfare policies' (Rein 1970). Indeed the scope of the discipline or field of study appears to be broadening, as some commentators introduce more areas of concern such as: communications, consumption and shopping, transport and leisure (Cahill 1994). Broader societal structures of kinship, social groups, occupational structures, fiscal structures, and many other organizing principles of society have an influence over welfare and social policy. It is, for example, difficult to conceive of the Western state as existing entirely separately from industry and financial institutions. In most capitalist societies the two are intimately linked. Rather than see social policy as attempting to modify the play of market forces, as Marshall suggested, social policy might be seen to be organized to suit the vested financial interests represented through the political system. The industrial sector has an important influence over social inequalities. The state can respond to this in a number of ways. Low pay, for example, has consistently been responsible for significant levels of poverty. Policies to counter this may be aimed at improving the incomes of those workers by tax incentives or income supplements; governments may also develop minimum wage policies. The state can also attempt to influence the industrial structure itself. Governments are important purchasers of goods and services and can influence industrial development by means such as the regulation of the location of industry.

Social structure may act to limit or undermine social policies to promote equity. Policies to reduce poverty, for example, may conflict with fundamental class interests which not only restrict attempts to introduce a more equitable distribution of resources, but also influence and restrict policies designed to do so. Welfare policies cannot be discussed in isolation from a critique of the social structure (Walker 1983); nor from accounts of the social construction of social policy. There is a need to look at the forces and power relations that underpin the formation of social policies. Such an approach focuses on the functions and outcomes of social policy typical of a number of analysts (Titmuss 1974; Townsend 1975). Social policy examines, then, the rationale and underlying ordering principles that affect the distribution of resources, status, and power between different groups and individuals in society.

Examples of social policy, and its place in broad social structures, can be seen in the analysis of health policy. The place of medical welfare, it has been suggested, promotes particular class interests within capitalist societies (Navarro 1976). Other powerful interests have been dominant in the development of medical and other welfare provision, such as the influence of professional groups (Freidson 1970; Wilding 1982). Recent developments in health policy may be restricting and challenging such interests (Elston 1991). Critiques of such power have influenced the development of health promotion and the new public health (Ashton and Seymour 1988). It has also led to recommendations to develop policies on the professions.

The place of the state as one of the main policy-forming bodies has been the focus of much discussion within social policy. As a potential regulator of social structure, the state has the opportunity to control and regulate as well as to provide security and protection. The fate of particular groups can be influenced in both directions. Feminists, for example, have been ambivalent about the role of the state because of such propensities. On the one hand, the state can assist women to develop new forms of interdependence based in the community and not in more 'repressive' family structures. Community child care initiatives, hostels, employment, and education for women may act in this way, for example, and can strengthen women's interests and counter patriarchal interests. At the same time, however, state provision may have its own repressive functions and serve the needs of capitalism in other ways; it can construct its own version of family life and values which do not suit the needs of women (Fitzgerald 1983; Wilson 1983). State policy has the potential to regulate particular social groups or even to marginalize and 'normalize' them (Small 1988; Pascall 1986; Manning 1985).

State-sponsored social policies, then, have the capacity to proscribe and legitimize particular types of social relationship, or relationships of welfare (Taylor 1996). Social relationships within society are invested with power and conflict, and power struggles exist between different social groups. Critical social policy analysis has described the ways in which social policies can reproduce these unequal relationships by privileging certain group's interests. Power relationships in broader society influence the ways that social and health policies are formed and, consequently, the ways in which services are delivered. Conflicts between different classes, genders, ethnicities, abilities and disabilities, sexualities, ages, and localities may been seen in a number of areas of social policy formation (Williams 1994). The ways that genders, minority ethnic groups or 'races', and people with disabilities are conceived of or constructed, for example, can have profound effects on the ways in which they are included or excluded from society. An example of this is the ways in which policy on institutionalized care for disabled people in the UK has discriminated against disabled people and created inequality between disabled and non-disabled people. Such policy introduces forms of social regulation of disabled people (Barnes 1996). These dangers also exist in areas of health promotion policy. The introduction of new forms of communication, co-ordination, inter-sectoral and inter-agency liaison in healthy public policy, for example, attempts to introduce new types of social relationships – new types of citizenship and governance. There are dangers of manipulation and social control. The regulatory potential of health promotion and public health policy has received some critical attention over the last decade (Baum 1993; Bunton 1992; Bunton *et al.* 1995; Lupton 1995; Petersen 1996, 1997; Petersen and Lupton 1996). Such critical analysis can offer an insight into the unintended consequences of policy development.

Social policy, then, has a very broad range of interests, examining the values, principles, and rationales that govern the distribution of resources and the formation of policies on the one hand, whilst being interested in the impact of such principles on social relationships, behaviours, organizations, professions, and classes, on the other. Such a broad remit requires a broad intellectual base and social policy, as a field of study has developed from and draws upon a range of disciplines including politics, economics, sociology, and history. This eclectic base has also been matched by a strong empirical tradition and programmes of research directed at the analysis of social need: social problems have been a feature of the subject from its inception. A concern for research methodology, fieldwork, and survey analysis has been dominant. Topics such as poverty and ill health, child neglect, and housing have remained common concerns. Indeed we might see the recent resurgence of interest in inequalities in health and health promotion as a reassertion of the place of social policy within the field (Coburn 2000).

Policy process

Social policy is centrally concerned with the processes of policy formation. Questions about how policy development can be brought about more efficiently have concerned the discipline, as they do health promotion. Policy studies is an allied field of study that is drawn upon in this area. Policy itself has been well defined by Blum (1981):

> Policy is a long-term, continuously used standing decision by which more specific proposals are judged for acceptability. It is characterized by behavioural consistency and repetitiveness on the part of those who make it and those who abide by it.

This definition refers to decisions made over time. Similarly, policy has been conceived as a web of decisions (Easton 1953) and a process of decisions (Widavsky 1979). We might also conceive of different competing and interacting policies or systems of policy making. Analysis of content seeks to describe and explain the genesis and development of particular policies. Much of the UK academic study of social policy has been conducted in this way. The process of identification of social problems which social policies address is an identifiable area of study in itself (Manning 1985). Changes in policy over time can be plotted in a number of areas.

The nature of the 'social liquor' problem, for example, has changed significantly over time (Makela and Viikari 1977). Late nineteenth and early twentieth-century concerns – motivated *inter alia* by attempts to instil bourgeois self-discipline in the newly industrialized working class (Harrison 1971; Gusfield 1963; Blocker 1976) – culminated in early twentieth-century temperance movements which aimed to restrict and control alcohol as a product. Following the political failure of prohibition, the emphasis shifted to the individual aspects of the problems associated with addiction. A concern for 'alcoholism' characterized policy from the 1930s to the mid-twentieth century. By the late twentieth century, a 'post addiction' approach had emerged, drawing upon behaviourally and environmentally conceived problems and fitting within a public health perspective on alcohol problems (Room 1981; Berridge 1989). Policy on illicit drugs has gone through a similar transformation (Stimson 1987), though shifting significantly in the 1980s and 1990s in response to policy on HIV/AIDS (Berridge 1990). Further policy changes occurred in response to changing consumption patterns in the 1990s and the reputed 'pick-and-mix' style of illicit drug use. The emergence of new drugs such as ecstasy associated with dance cultures has brought new, arguably more liberal policy responses in the UK (South 1999; Shiner and Newburn 1997; Parker *et al.* 1995). Concern has focused on the relatively wide-scale recreational use of illicit drugs as well as problematic use. The nature of the 'social problem' of drug misuse changes over time. Such change can be found in many areas of healthy public policy.

Policy analysis also focuses on the stages through which policy action passes, attempting to account for the influences on these processes which may be societal, governmental, organizational, or even individual. Any analysis of the policy process can be broken down into component parts. A sevenfold typology is preferred by several authors (Hogwood and Gunn 1981; Gordon *et al.* 1977; Ham and Hill 1984), referring to policy content, policy process, policy outputs, evaluation studies, information for policy making, process of advocacy, and policy advocacy.

- *Policy content* seeks to describe and explain the genesis and development of particular policies. Much of UK social policy has been conducted in this way.
- *Policy process* focuses on the stages through which policy action passes and attempts to assess influences upon this process. Such analysis may be directed at organizational, governmental, or societal processes.
- *Policy outputs* seek to explain the variety of levels of expenditure or service provision. Policies may be examined as dependent variables influenced by social, economic, technological, and other variables (Dye 1976).
- *Evaluation or impact studies* are concerned with the impact policies have on a population.
- *Information for policy making* is the method of amassing information to assist policy makers in reaching decisions. This may be carried out by government departments, academics, or other organizations.
- *Process of advocacy* refers to attempts to improve the nature of the policy-making system, particularly the machinery of government through the development of planning systems and new approaches to co-ordination which involve the analyst in pressing for specific options and ideas in the policy process, either on their own behalf or via a pressure group.

Within this sevenfold typology, a distinction can be made between policy analysis, which provides a more academic or objective understanding of policy (the first three), and one that provides more committed analysis for policy development (the latter three). On the whole the literature on healthy public policy falls into the category of committed policy analysis.

Understanding the implementation process is central to understanding any policy development. The adoption of particular policies by different groups and subcultures will depend on how such policies are conceived, how they are introduced, the group's commitment to them, the local resources available to assist their introduction, and a range of other socio-economic factors. Policies and strategies can be modified and altered, often substantially, during development. The presence of powerful interests can have an obstructive or 'watering down' effect in such cases (Hawks 1990). It has become apparent that policy introduction conceived of only as a 'top-down' process is very limited in health promotion (Donati 1988). Policy development can also be generated from the 'bottom-up' and success might depend upon a combination of top-down and bottom-up approaches (Sabatier 1986). Context will affect all implementation, and an understanding of macro and local power structures within the socio-political environment is central to success (Barrett and Hill 1984; Milio 1987).

Central to the implementation of healthy public policy is the development of co-ordinating mechanisms to facilitate multi-sectoral involvement and community participation. Co-ordination might be achieved by the establishment of a central body or organization or, alternatively, by enabling local bodies working on single issues. In any co-ordination there will be key decision-makers and resource allocators to be identified and key 'stakeholders' who will influence the course of policy co-ordination. Analysis of the policy process must take account of these factors in building a picture of the policy context.

A large number of factors come to bear on the policy process. Analysis of these policy contexts will be central to assessing the feasibility of developing healthy public policy. Such an analysis can clarify the limitations and constraints placed on any policy development. Social policy would appear to have much to offer health promotion here. However, as a discipline or field of study, social policy is not a single entity but contains competing perspectives which any introduction must consider. Interpretation of macro and micro social, political, and economic structural process is complex and within social science there are a variety of approaches or perspectives.

Perspectives

Whilst differences in perspective have always been apparent in social policy, these seem to have been accentuated in the latter twentieth and earlier twenty-first centuries, which have been characterized by much theoretical ferment. This change, in part, is in response to a rapidly changing social environment.

Debates about the appropriateness of state interventions date back to 1960s social policy. Some favoured 'universal' provision of social welfare as a basic right of citizenship (Townsend 1968; Titmuss 1968; Redding 1970), whilst others argued for more limited 'selective' interventions for the needy only (Friedman 1962; Gray and Sheldon 1969). A basic consensus on the central role of the state intervention had, by the early 1970s, begun to break down. Questions were raised about the very principles of social care mechanism, including: How far had social welfare policies succeeded? Who benefited most from them? Whose interests they had serviced? What had influenced their operation? This discussion coincided with broader socio-political change and what has been referred to as a 'crisis' in welfare. Economic changes and problems of the mid-1970s – inflation, recession, and low growth – had affected many Western societies and forced a rethink of welfare provision and in some cases an attack on the welfare state. There had been a tacit retreat from a commitment to welfare in Britain as early as the 1960s. Labour Party policy had withdrawn from Keynesian approaches to economic regulation as the USA, Canada, and much of Europe was also to do in the face of a world economic recession (Loney *et al.* 1988). Public spending received substantial cuts.

Neo-conservative policies dominated the political agenda in Britain and the USA, providing ideological support for removing state spending and introducing measures to reduce what was seen as unnecessary state encroachment into the market and the lives of individuals. Income taxation was reduced, markets de-regularized, and state monopolies removed. A period of 'neo-liberal' government had begun which saw a changed role for the state, characterized by a rolling back of the state and a promotion of entrepreneurship and the market. There was a renewed belief in the market as a rational organizing principle which could successfully produce services sensitive to the needs of the consumer and successfully generate employment. Emphasis was placed upon self-reliance and initiative and avoidance of what was seen as the 'dangers' of dependency upon state provision. Neo-liberal concerns have been reflected in more recent social policy. The transformation in the social and economic underpinnings of welfare posed new problems and unearthed new study areas for the discipline. New sources of theory were drawn upon from sociology and political science in particular, which led to greater differences in perspective.

George and Wilding (1976) were amongst the first UK social policy analysts to describe different ideologies of welfare in social policy. Prior to this, differing 'value positions' had been recognized, yet these positions had not been patterned nor had their relevance been brought to the forefront of study. Analysis of ideology introduced the idea that social policies were the outcome of conflict and interests, and authors such as George and Wilding were critical of previous, often unacknowledged, consensus models of society where it was often assumed that policy developed rationally towards largely agreed upon objectives. This approach to public policy may be described as a 'rational deductive' and/or an 'incrementalist' approach (Ziglio 1987). By contrast, Marxist political, economic, conflict, and pluralistic approaches were being put forward to provide understanding of the policy process.

There are a number of ways of representing the different ideological groupings of social policy analysts. George and Wilding's book is a good source of these, though there are others (Lee and Raban 1983; Williams 1989; O'Brien and Penna 1998). Understanding of these is an essential component to understanding social policy. One of the most common themes in such descriptions is pro- and anti-state position. Analysts can be placed along a continuum according to these positions. George (1981) has identified a number of analysts constructing such types.

A variety of positions are portrayed, ranging from out-and-out free market individualists at one extreme to out-and-out collectivists in favour of the command economy at the other. More or less liberal and socialist collectivists in favour of the welfare state are arranged in the middle of the continuum. Each ideological grouping spells out a different set of expectations of and obligations upon both states and citizens in the working of welfare provision and policy. Each set of prescriptions can be found in various forms in contemporary policy discussions. All approaches to policy, however, will adopt a particular theoretical perspective (or set of perspectives) either explicitly or implicitly. A lack of awareness of the diversity in perspective may itself be a barrier to policy planning and implementation (Pederson *et al.* 1988). Different groups may promote different policies at different times and for different reasons. Understanding this diversity is part of understanding the policy environment.

PRO-STATE

ANTI-STATE

Anti-Collectivism	Reluctant Collectivism	Fabian Socialism	Marxism[1]
Market Liberals	Political Liberals	Social Democrats	neo-Marxists[2]
Classical Economic Theory	neo-Mercantilism	Marxisms[3] 'its socialist derivatives'	
Residual	Institutional	'Normative' or 'Socialist'[4]	
Conservatism	Positive State	Social Security State	Social Welfare State — Radicalism[5]

Figure 6.1 Typologies of welfare ideologies

Notes:
1 George and Wilding (1976).
2 Room (1979).
3 Pinker (1979).
4 Mishra (1977: 35–6) and George and Manning (1980), after Titmuss (1974: Ch. 2).
5 Furniss and Tilson (1977).

Source: Lee and Raban (1983)

Though useful as an outline, we must be aware that more subtle differences exist even within the various positions on this continuum. A useful distinction has been made between types of state intervention, between the state as a financer of welfare provision, a deliverer of welfare, and a regulator of welfare (Le Grand 1982). These analytic distinctions make ideological categorization a potentially complex exercise. Moreover, ideological sketches such as these tend to reproduce a basic opposition between those who support state intervention and those who favour market solutions and freedom of choice in services, a feature of 1990s social care provision.

The opposition of market and state-sponsored solutions to health and welfare may be seen as rather simplistic, however. Both means of service delivery have come under critical scrutiny and currently most political parties would appear to accept a more modest role for the state in the regulation of national economies and welfare. Indeed, during the 1980s and 1990s some of the fundamental 'collectivist' or 'modern' ideas of welfare were fundamentally challenged. The basic values of 'altruism' that were held to underlie social insurance and collective responsibility for others identified by founders of the discipline, such as Titmuss (1970) were being challenged by those of self-interest and the market logic. It has been suggested that social relationships underlying social welfare have undergone such significant transformation in recent decades that a qualitatively different era of social policy is characteristic of 'post-' or 'late-modern' principles (Carter 1998).

Several social theorists have suggested that the turn of the twenty-first century can be characterized by a newer, more 'reflexive modernity' in which many traditional and familiar aspects of our lives are open to change, negotiation, and choice. As the pace of social and technological change has increased, individuals are presented with less certainty in most areas of their lives. Traditional identities, based on production relationships, for example, are less binding, as employment patterns are less predictable and stable. Individuals' increasingly experience life as characterized by risk and uncertainty. Analysts such as Ulrich Beck (1992) and Anthony Giddens (1991) have argued that we now live in a 'risk society' in which we must increasingly reflect upon, choose, and construct our life-styles and our identities. An element of risk society is its 'individualizing tendency'. In the past, certain social problems were experienced as collective problems requiring collective solutions – such as unemployment or poor wages, for example, which the Labour movement fought to combat. More recently, the risks of life, whether they be unemployment or problems of housing, are experienced as subjective and the result of inadequate personal risk-management. Ideologies of self-reliance and self-management that accompanied neo-liberal social policies have, it is argued, constructed new 'enterprising' citizens, who attempt to guarantee their own security rather than rely upon that previously provided by the state. Private pensions, insurance against the risks of life are increasingly individual rather than collective contracts. Health professionals in the employment of the state, similarly, increasingly focus less on the delivery of services to individual clients as to the management of populations at risk (Castel 1991). Risk appears to turn what was previously a collective 'social' matter into a 'private' concern.

The self-empowered citizen depicted in much of behavioural health promotion programmes would appear to fit this description of individualized risk manager (Culpitt 1999). Under conditions of reflexive modernization, individuals are expected to be less reliant upon the support of the state to combat the uncertainties of life and must make arrangements with other private or community organizations to reduce risk. The development of an increasingly 'risk-oriented', individualized society has profound social, political, and economic ramifications, and the expectations of 'social' policy are changing. The emergence of newer forms of social policy may be associated with such reflexivity.

Since the early 1980s there has been increasing interest in how public–private partnerships and related forms of governance contribute to policy processes. Alternatives to marketized solutions to welfare, on the one hand, and state provision, on the other, have turned increasingly to governance (Amin and Hausner 1997). The concept of governance has addressed various problems related to the perceived failures of both governments and markets. There have been calls for more flexible responses to contemporary problems and the alignment of the agendas of the apparently competitive sectors (private and government) by negotiated, long-term consensual projects which co-ordinate the combined activities of multiple, interdependent actors (Kooiman 1993). There is a shift towards commitment to dialogue and exchange, aligning partners into a range of interdependent decisions – a process that is: dialogic rather than monologic, pluralistic rather than monolithic, heterarchic rather than either hierarchic or anarchic. (Jessop, B. (1997) 'Capitalism and its Future: Remarks on Regulation, Government and Governance' *Review of International Political Economy*, 4(3), 435–455). This complex, reflexive process involves interpersonal networking, inter-organizational negotiation, and intersystemic steering. These are different modes of co-ordination than those found in traditional 'modern' approaches to governance associated with, for example, traditional, top-down, single sector professional public health practice. Healthy public policy may be seen as a species of such policy approaches. In many ways, such approaches attempt to step outside the assumption in much traditional social policy of a fundamental opposition between the needs of capital and of health and welfare. Different perspectives would suggest different approaches to policy development and this diversity is identifiable in many healthy public policy initiatives.

We will now examine such differences with reference to substance misuse policy. Some approaches to policy on substance misuse are characterized by assumptions of conflicting interests and dispute, whilst others would seem to adopt a more consensual view of policy planning and implementation.

Varieties of healthy public policy

Conflict

Most contemporary perspectives on drug misuse are associated with the 'new public health' and place emphasis on primary care, prevention, and health promotion as well as crime prevention and social care. Problems are usually the outcome of various mixes of host, agent, and environment or, alternatively expressed, people, products, and settings (Robinson 1989). A problematic interrelation of these three elements results in drinking and driving, for example. Solutions to problems take place on a broad front and calls are made for an increasingly ambitious range of interventions (Chapman-Walsh 1990), some methods having a more proven track record than others (Grant 1989). Most of the current efforts have been geared to reducing consumption by depressing demand, though efforts have also been directed at supply (WHO 1988a). Though there are many potential ways for health promotion related to drug misuse, those working within the field tend to prefer and emphasize one approach and in doing so reveal particular theoretical orientations and assumptions about the way they see the world.

A conflict or political economy approach to policy is more likely to favour state interventionist solutions to the problems relating to substance misuse. Conflict models assume fundamental oppositions of interests as a necessary part of the social order. Conflict theory has flourished in sociology (referred to in Thorogood's chapter) and has contributed much to the analysis of social policy. It has contributed greatly to the sociology of health and illness (Navarro 1976, 1982, 1986; Waitzkin 1983; Gerhardt 1989) and highlights oppositions of interests between producers and suppliers on the one hand and consumers on the other. This obvious division of interest is most starkly highlighted in relation to policy development on illegal drugs. Most societies have formulated policy on substance use that rests on assumptions of a fundamental opposition of interest between producers and consumers. Typically, this involves identifying some psychoactive substances that may legitimately be used and others that may not, without being subjected to sanction or punishment. There is great variety in the drugs brought under policy regulation in this way, even within Western societies. There are levels of agreement internationally however, witnessed by international efforts to suppress the use of heroin since the turn of the twentieth century (Hartnoll 1989). Subsequent efforts have been made to introduce control mechanisms. Efforts are made nationally and internationally to prevent production and distribution (or 'trafficking'). Steps have been taken to seize financial assets of producers and distributors (or 'dealers'). A number of international bodies involved in the control of certain types of drugs have emerged, including the Commission on Narcotic Drugs (CND), the Division of Narcotic Drugs (DND), The International Narcotics Board (INCB), the United National Fund for Drug Abuse Control (UNFDAC), and Departments of the World Health

Organization. Interpol and other international law enforcement mechanisms have also appeared.

Individual countries have developed policies, research studies, and enforcement mechanisms based upon a need to protect consumers or potential consumers from the dangers of exposure to specific sets of substances. Australia and the United Kingdom have both developed comprehensive drug strategies which have exhibited this exclusionary or restrictive policy. Opiates have been singled out for such restriction from most countries, though other substances, such as cannabis, have more frequently received a more lenient or liberal form of regulation (MacGregor 1989). There is some indication that efforts to reduce HIV/AIDS infection have had a liberalizing effect on policy towards injectable drugs in the UK (Berridge 1990; MacGregor 1989).

Public health policies on substance misuse have generally incorporated control and exclusion statements. The statement endorsed by the Adelaide Conference on healthy public policy is one such example (WHO 1988a). Whilst calling for measures to reduce demand, such as restriction of advertising and price increases, it also recommends regulating or eliminating the production of psychoactive substances and restricting availability of alcohol, tobacco, and other drugs through methods such as liquor licensing, street-level law enforcement, and rational prescribing practices.

Tobacco production is another area in which opposing interests and conflict in the policy process have been identified, representing a mismatch of interest between consumer and producer. World manufacture of tobacco products is controlled by a handful of multinational companies – the transnational tobacco conglomerates (TCCs) such as British American Tobacco and Imperial Tobacco. These few companies effectively control most aspects of the business process – from leaf production to marketing and distribution of the final products (Booth *et al.* 1990). TTCs have interests in paper mills, shipping, oil companies, retail networks, and are able to use all of these networks to ward off competition, to enter and develop new markets, and to influence price and quality. With such large corporate interests at stake, the potential for creating health-promoting environments may seem highly problematic. The power of tobacco producers and their ability to thwart efforts of advocates of public health policy have been well documented (Taylor, D., 1984). Such analysis has often called for state intervention to curtail the play of market forces (whether these are seen as 'free enterprise' or monopolistic). The need to counterbalance the powers of the producer in the name of public health has also been well documented in relation to alcohol misuse.

Whilst many contemporary analysts of public policy on alcohol have tried to distance themselves from the highly centralized control of the temperance period, concern for aspects of production and distribution of alcohol has remained important to public health advocates (WHO 1988a). Debate about the role of the state in the regulation of production has pointed to fundamental conflicts of interest (Koskikalio 1979; Makela and Viikari 1977; Parker 1977). States must balance economic interests on the one hand against public health concerns on the other. This is not simply the opposition between commercial and public interest; the state itself is often a beneficiary of tax revenue from sales on alcohol. There may be internal conflict between different government departments. Despite state intervention, measures have been recommended on a wide number of fronts, including: increasing relative price; restricting distribution to certain times, places, or social groups (e.g. age limits); increasing probability of detection and punishments for alcohol-related crime infringements (e.g. drinking and driving or public drunkenness); and numerous other policy measures (Grant 1989; Royal College of Physicians 1987; Home Office 1987a). Some countries have attempted to solve such conflicts by placing production and distribution of alcohol in the hands of the state monopolies, notably Sweden and Norway (Davies and Walsh 1983).

Substance misuse, then, would seem to highlight one area of healthy public policy where intransigent interests are a major obstacle to policy development. Consumer movements and co-operatives with aims closer to those of public health advocates frequently encounter the full force of such interests (Senoda 1990). Other areas of conflict of interests have been identified, however. Fundamental inequalities in resources and power in society will continue to undermine attempts to work to agreed healthy public policy targets. Rhetoric on healthy public policy may have underestimated underlying conflict in this respect (Pederson *et al.* 1988) and could be accused of the idealism found in other Health For All statements (Strong 1986). Whilst such statements offer a positive starting point to policy development, there is a danger of glossing over differences in perspective that will imply differences in policy content, process, evaluation, and advocacy.

Some areas of healthy public policy may be appropriately placed within a combative or 'war oriented' model of policy making (Van der Kamp 1990). Many recent conflicts in interest have arisen in relation to the environment. The decision in 2001 by the USA not to honour the Kyoto Agreement on the restriction of 'greenhouse gases' illustrates conflicts within the states, who may be torn between the interests of consumers world-wide and local industrial interests. Structural conflicts may be so fundamental to a social system that capital will almost always confront state and/or public interests. Inequalities in resources between state, capital, and civil society (including consumers and producers) may be such that policy options for health are severely limited. The social policy environment may be such that resource allocation prevents groups becoming involved in the policy-making process.

Recent UK trends towards greater differences between the rich and the poor is likely to exclude many people and groups from participation, or at least bias any input to the policy process (Farrent and Taft 1990). In other words, structural inequalities may shape and influence the policy process. In such circumstances, healthy public policy development may be less about challenging such inequalities than about developing better coping strategies and mechanisms, such as stronger community lobbies (Legg and Sylvan 1990). Analysis of these structures will largely determine the nature of one's perspective. As well as being caused by structural inequality and imbalances of power, conflict can be generated by oppositions between forces of change and resistance to social innovation. Much health promotion effort is geared towards developing techniques to enhance 'persuasive strategies' and to involve potential co-operators in policy change. In all the above senses, conflict may prove to be an important part of health promotion.

Consensus

The combative approach to healthy public policy is certainly not universal. For theoretical and empirical reasons, a number of analysts have emphasized the role of co-operation and collaboration. Much of the work on healthy public policy has demonstrated the potential for the pooling of efforts. It has been argued that a different style and culture of public policy are emerging in health and social care which are pluralistic in approach and involve a greater number of actors than previously. 'Public' increasingly means more than state, and administrative planning is increasingly emerging from outside professional, government, or commercial quarters. Such thinking is implied in approaches to governance that are broader than the state, discussed above. They have been apparent in the UK policy perspective described as a 'Third Way' politics.

'Third Way' politics attempts to build new relationships between the individual, the community, and the state involving partnerships and co-operation. Such thinking seeks to revive civic culture and looks for synergy between public and private sectors to provide health and welfare solutions, using market dynamics for the public interest (Giddens 2000). Such approaches suggest that a policy strategy is possible which does not oppose the interests of capital and social justice, and that the traditional political oppositions between left and right are less relevant. 'Third Way' politics seek a framework for policy-making that takes account of recent changes in social relationships and attempts to transcend both an old-style, social democratic 'welfarism' on the one hand and the 'hands off' approach to welfare that has been sought by neo-liberalism. It assumes that social and economic policy are intrinsically connected and that it is possible to respond positively to the rapid changes occurring locally and globally within a 'mixed economy of welfare'. Third Way strategies are one attempt to deal with issues of pluralism and diversity and newer patterns of inequality that 'modern welfare' had difficulties accommodating. In doing so, it redefines the rights and obligations of citizens, states, communities, private corporations, and other agencies.

In many ways the ethos of the sentiments of the Ottawa Charter (WHO 1986b) would appear to fit within 'Third Way' policy thinking. The Charter calls for involvement and partnerships in promoting health and suggests ways of marrying private and public sector efforts for health gain. There has been considerable work in this area in previous years. More recent statements on health promotion policy such as the Jakarta Declaration (WHO 1997) continue to stress the broader social and policy determinants of health and the need to 'invest' in health and solutions that favour complex, multi-sectoral strategies of governance. Many health promotion initiatives may be seen as prototypes for such policy development. Policy on substance misuse provides useful examples here, often stressing the potential for efforts at the margins of economic and political institutions. Research in the field of alcohol policy, and UK policy on alcohol misuse in particular, can illustrate such an approach.

UK policy on substance misuse in the 1980s and 1990s specified a multi-sectoral, locally co-ordinated approach. In 1987, for example, an inter-departmental Ministerial Committee on Alcohol Misuse was established to co-ordinate government strategy (Home Office 1987b). There followed a government circular calling for locally co-ordinated, multi-sectoral action to assess the extent of alcohol misuse and design methods of combating it, drawing upon local resources (DHSS 1989). The circular matches healthy public policy's exhortations to multi-sectoral, multi-actor efforts. A feature of the government response has been the encouragement of involvement by the drinks trade to take steps to combat alcohol misuse, attempting to step up voluntary agreements on regulation and to introduce innovative schemes. This policy position reinforced earlier statements that talked of alcohol misuse being 'everybody's business' (DHSS 1981: 40). The principles of these locally governed partnerships are enshrined in more recent drug misuse policy in the UK, such as *Tackling Drugs Together* (HMSO 1995) and the more recent (Cmmd 1998) *10 Year Strategy for Tackling Drugs*. Calls for the establishment of local drug prevention teams have attempted to recruit the efforts of communities and encourage them to resist and deal with the use of illegal drugs in a variety of ways. The progression of this type of drug policy might be seen as moving away from the highly centralized and 'socialized' solutions and towards local governance.

Such approaches assume certain levels of consensus can be achieved by drawing together different organizations and agencies with different interests and agendas through a process of 'partisan mutual adjustment' (Lindblorn 1965; Harrison and Tether 1990). Agreements may be reached through negotiation, bargaining, and manipulation. Diverse inter-organizational interests can be picked and matched to approximate something like overall policy.

The task of social policy in such research work is to explore areas of potential 'mutual adjustment' in order to maximize prevention potential in the cause of healthy public policy. This may well mean an extensive exploration of the complexity of the complete policy networks – from exploration of government departments and sub-departments and their responsibilities and decision-making powers (Harrison and Tether 1990) to the structure of the brewing trade (Booth *et al.* 1990; Grant 1989). The relative effectiveness of different regulatory mechanisms would need to be assessed within the policy complex, such as the consequences of: restrictions of advertising;

fiscal controls; the differences between voluntary agreements and statutory mechanisms to regulate production, promotion and distribution; different types of crime prevention measures. A picture can be constructed of the gains and the losses – health, financial, and organizational – of each policy option for each participant in the policy process and the likely political will to change. Use of Policy analysis can be used to manipulate the consensual policy-making process. Organization networks may be manipulated by a number of persuasion techniques: information dissemination, incentives, and sanctions (Sharpe 1978). Such an approach need not opt simply for consensual, non-governmental, local policy preferences; instead it might draw up a menu of policy options to be considered against overall objectives, whilst building up a knowledge of the network of organizations, alliances, and decisions that make up the complex policy environment. Only by thoroughly exploring the webs of decision making, and the potential gains and losses to different parties, can the potential for mutual adjustment be discovered.

In the study of healthy public policy on substance misuse, then, there exist differences in perspective; and the adoption of a particular approach has implications for the study and the development of policy. Adopting an out-and-out conflict perspective might run the risk of over-pessimism and a failure to make use of existing policy resources. On the other hand, the naïve assumption of consensus could seriously underestimate the structural impediments to successful policy development. Each approach will favour a particular range of policy options. Conflict approaches are likely to favour state intervention to address issues of structural inequality. Consensual approaches are likely to stress more local, non-state interventionist methods (though this is by no means universal). Clearly, no approach to policy development is without limitation and unintended consequence. Study of social policy and healthy public policy involves developing a reflexive aware-ness of the range of policy perspectives, within academic study and within the everyday policy environment.

Conclusion

Social policy has been, and is likely to remain, central to health promotion. Healthy public policy developed as a fundamental element of health promo-tion and drew upon social policy conceptually and empirically. Social policy provides knowledge of how to 'do' healthy public policy: how to develop policies for health gain. The field of social policy can provide vital reflective knowledge on the origin of health promotion itself and its emergence as a newer type of health policy. The rhetoric of healthy public policy implied new ways of thinking about health and government policy and anticipated a new policy environment with new mechanisms for policy development. Such approaches might be seen to be commensurate with 'neo-liberal' government policy and/or to more recent 'Third Way' thinking. Understanding the policy environment is central to both. Social policy as a field of study has undergone considerable change and development over recent decades, reflecting broader social change.

Social policy comprises diverse perspectives which reflect different assumptions about the nature of the social world. Healthy public policy can be seen to fall into similarly diverse perspectives. Substance misuse policy provides examples of such diversity – even though most will be working within a public health perspective. Conflict and consensus perspectives can be identified within this literature. Analysis of these perspectives provides an understanding of the complexity of the study of, as well as the actual, social policy environment. Diversity in perspective is a feature of social policy and healthy public policy.

The study of social policy will contribute greatly to health promotion. It will continue to provide an understanding of: how healthy public policy features in today's policy environment; the role of the state, the citizen, and the community in policy development; the process and possibility of developing visions of healthy public policy; the scope for inter-sectoral co-operation; the scope for co-ordination of healthy public policy; and how the 'public good' might be reconciled with individual and other interests in fostering healthy public policy (Pederson *et al.* 1988). Such programmes of study are as pertinent to the development to social policy as they are to healthy public policy, allowing us to consider health promotion as social policy.

References and bibliography

Amin, A. and Hausner, J. (eds) (1997) *Beyond Market and Hierarchy: Interactive Governance and Social Complexity*, Cheltenham: Edward Elgar.

Ashton, J. and Seymour, H. (1988) *The New Public Health*, Milton Keynes: Open University Press.

Barnes, C. (1996) 'Institutional discrimination against disabled people and the campaign for anti-discrimination legislation,' in I. Taylor (ed.) *Critical Social Policy: a Reader*, London: Sage.

Barrett, S. and Hill, M. J. (1984) 'Policy bargaining and structure in implementation of theory: towards an integrated perspective', *Policy and Politics* 12 (3): 219–40.

Baum, F. (1993) 'Healthy cities and change: social movement or bureaucratic tool?', *Health Promotion International* 8 (1): 31–40.

Beattie, A. (1991) 'Knowledge and control in health promotion: a test case for social policy and social theory', in J. Gabe, M. Calnan, and M. Bury (eds) *The Sociology of the Health Service*, London: Routledge.

Beck, U. (1992) *Risk Society. Towards a New Modernity*, London: Sage.

Bell, D. (1960) *The End of Ideology*, New York: The Free Press.

Berridge, V. (1989) 'History and addiction control: the case of alcohol', in D. Robinson, A. Maynard, and R. Chester (eds) *Controlling Legal Addictions*, Basingstoke: Macmillan.

—— (ed.) (1990) *Drug Research and Policy in Britain*, Aldershot: Avebury.

Beveridge, W. (1942) *Social Insurance and Allied Services*, London: HMSO.

Blocker, J. S. (1976) *Retreat from Reform: The Prohibition Movement in the United States 1890–1913*, Westport, MA: Greenwood Press.

Blum, H. L. (1981) *Planning for Health: Genetics for the Eighties*, New York: Human Sciences Press.

Bocock, R., Clarke, J., Cochrane, A., Graham, P., and Wilson, M. (1987) *The State or the Market? Politics and Welfare in Contemporary Britain*, London: Sage in association with Open University Press.

Booth, M., Harticy, K., and Powell, M. (1990) 'Industry structure, performance and policy', in A. Maynard and P. Tether (eds) *Preventing Alcohol and Tobacco Problems*, vol. 1, Aldershot: Avebury.

Booth, T. (1981a) 'Collaboration between the health and social services: Part I, a case study in joint care planning?', *Policy and Politics* 9 (1): 23–49.

—— (1981b) 'Collaboration between the health and social services: Part II case study in joint finance', *Policy and Politics* 9 (2): 205–26.

Boulding, K. (1967) 'The boundaries of social policy', *Social Work* 12 (1).

Brown, M. (1983) 'The development of social administration', in M. Loney, D. Boswell, and J. Clerke (eds) *Social Policy and Social Welfare*, Milton Keynes: Open University Press.

Bruce, M. (1961) *The Coming of the Welfare State*, London: Batsford.

Brundtland Report, The (1987) *Our Common Future*, Oxford: Oxford University Press/World Commission on Environment and Development.

Bruun, K. E. (1985) 'Formulating comprehensive national alcohol policies', in M. Grant (ed.) *Alcohol Policies*, European Series No. 18, Copenhagen: WHO Regional Publications.

Bruun, K., Edwards, G., Lumio, M., Makela, K., Pan, L., Popham, R., Room, R., Schmidt, W., Skog, O., Sulkunen, P., and Osterberg, E. (1975) *Alcohol Control Policies in Public Health Perspective*, Finland: The Finnish Foundation for Alcohol Studies.

Bunton, R. (1990) 'Regulating our favourite drug', in P. Abbott and G. Payne (eds) *New Directions in the Sociology of Health*, Basingstoke: Falmer.

—— (1992) 'More than a woolly jumper: health promotion as social regulation', *Critical Public Health*, (Summer) 2: 4–11.

Bunton, R., Nettleton, S., and Burrows, R. (1995) *The Sociology of Health Promotion and the New Public Health*, London: Routledge.

Cahill, M. (1994) *The New Social Policy*, Oxford: Blackwell.

Carter, J. (ed.) (1998) *Post-modernity and the Fragmentation of Welfare*, London: Routledge.

Castel, R. (1991) 'From dangerousness to risk', in G. Burchell, C. Gordon, and P. Miller (eds) *The Foucault Effect: Studies in Governmentality*, London: Harvester Wheatsheaf.

Chapman-Walsh, D. (1990) 'The shifting boundaries of alcohol policy', *Health Affairs*, summer.

Chu, C. (1994) 'Integrating health and environment: the key to an ecological public health', in C. Chu and R. Simpson (eds) *Ecological Public Health: from Vision to Practice*, Toronto: Canada and Aus. Inst. of Applied Environ. Research Griffith University and Centre for Health Promotion.

Coburn, D. (2000) 'Income inequality, social cohesion and the health status of populations: the role of neo-liberalism', *Social Science & Medicine* 51: 135–46.

Crossland, C. A. R. (1956) *The Future of Socialism*, London: Cape.

Culpitt, I. (1999) *Social Policy and Risk*, London: Sage.

Davies, P. and Walsh, D. (1983) *Alcohol Problems and Alcohol Control in Europe*, London: Croom Helm.

DHSS (1981) *Drinking Sensibly*, London: HMSO.

—— (1989) *Interdepartmental Circular on Alcohol Misuse*, HN (89) 4 LAC (89) 6. WOC 8/89 WHC 89 (14).

Donati, P. (1988) 'The need for new social policy perspectives in health behaviour research', in R. Anderson, J. Davies, I. Kickbusch, D. McQueen, and D. Turner (eds) *Health Behaviour Research and Health Promotion*, Oxford: Oxford University Press.

Donnison, D. (1979) 'Social policy since Titmuss', *Journal of Social Policy* 8 (2): 178–87.

Dorn, N. (1987) 'Drink and political economy', in C. Heller *et al.* (eds) *Drug Use and Misuse: A Reader*, Chichester: Wiley in association with Open University.

Doyal, L. (1981) *The Political Economy of Health*, London: Pluto.

Draper, P. (ed.) (1991) *Health through Public Policy: the Greening of Public Health*, London: Green Print.

Duhl, L. J. (1986) *Health Planning and Social Change*, New York: Human Sciences Press.

Dye, R. R. (1976) *Policy Analysis*, Alabama: Alabama University Press.

Easton, D. (1953) *The Political System*, New York: Knopf.

Elston, M. A. (1991) 'The politics of professional power: medicine in a changing health service', in J. Gabe *et al.* (eds) *The Sociology of the Health Service*, London: Routledge.

Evans, R. and Stoddart, G. (1990) 'Producing health, consuming health care', *Social Science & Medicine* 31(12): 1347–63.

Evers, A., Farrent, W., and Trojan, A. (eds) (1990) *Healthy Public Policy at the Local Level*, Colorado: Westview Press.

Farrent, W. and Taft, A. (1990) 'Building healthy public policy in an unhealthy climate: a case study from Paddington and North Kensington', in A. Evers, W. Farrent, and A. Trojan (eds) *Healthy Public Policy at the Local Level*, Colorado: Westview Press.

Fitzgerald, T. (1983) 'The new Right and the family', in M. Loney, D. Boswell, and J. Clark (eds) (1988) *Social Policy and Social Welfare*, Milton Keynes: Open University Press.

Freidson, E. (1970) *Profession of Medicine*, New York: Dodd, Mead.

Friedman, M. (1962) *Capitalism and Freedom*, Chicago, IL: University of Chicago Press.

Furniss, N. and Tilton, T. (1977) *The Case for the Welfare State*, Bloomington, IN: Indiana University Press.

George, P. (1981) 'Ideology and the Welfare State'. Unpublished paper delivered to the Annual Conference of the Social Administration Association, Leeds University, July.

George, P. and Manning, N. (1980) *Socialism, Social Welfare and the Soviet Union*, London: Routledge & Kegan Paul.

George, P. and Wilding, R (1976) *Ideology and Social Welfare*, London: Routledge & Kegan Paul.

—— (1985a) *Ideology and Social Welfare*, 2nd edn, London: Routledge & Kegan Paul.

—— (1985b) *The Impact of Social Policy*, London: Routledge & Kegan Paul.

Gerhardt, V. (1989) *Ideas about Illness: An Intellectual and Political History of Medical Sociology*, London: Macmillan.

Godfrey, C. and Robinson, D. (eds) (1990) *Preventing Alcohol and Tobacco Problems*, vol. 2, Aldershot: Avebury.

Giddens, A. (1991) *Modernity and Self-Identity: Self and Society in the Late Modern Age*, Cambridge: Polity.

Giddens, A. (2000) *The Runaway World Debate: Third Way Politics* www.lse.ac. uk\text\RWDThirdWayDef[1](1).htm

Ginsburg, N. (1998) 'postmodernity and social Europe', in J. Carter (ed.) *Postmodernity and the Fragmentation of Welfare*, London: Routledge.

Gordon, I., Lewis, J., and Young, K. (1977) 'Perspectives on policy analysis', *Public Administration Bulletin* 25.

Grant, M. (ed.) (1985) *Alcohol Policies*, European Series No. 18, Geneva: WHO Regional Publications.

—— (1989) 'Controlling alcohol abuse', in D. Robinson, A. Maynard, and R. Chester (eds) *Controlling Legal Addictions*, Basingstoke: Macmillan.

Gray, H. and Sheldon, A. (1969) *Universal and Selective Social Benefits*, London: Institute of Economic Affairs.

Gusfield, J. R. (1963) *Symbolic Crusade*, Urbana, IL: University of Illinois Press.

Ham, C. and Hill, C. (1984) *The Policy Process in the Modern Capitalist State*, Brighton: Wheatsheaf Books.

Hancock, T. (1982) 'Beyond health care', *The Futurist*, August 4: 13.

Harrison, B. (1971) *Drink and the Victorians: The Temperance Question in England, 1815–1872*, London: Faber.

Harrison, L. and Tether, P. (1990) 'Tax policy: structure and process', in A. Maynard and D. Tether (eds) *Preventing Alcohol and Tobacco Problems*, vol. 1, Aldershot: Avebury.

Hartnoll, R. (1989) 'The international context', in S. MacGregor (ed.) *Drugs and British Society: Responses to a Social Problem in the 1980s*, London: Routledge.

Hawks, D. V. (1990) 'The watering down of Australia's health policy on alcohol', *Drug and Alcohol Review* 9 (1): 91–5.

Heller, T., Gott, M., and Jeffery, C. (eds) (1987) *Drug Use and Misuse: A Reader*, Chichester: Wiley in association with the Open University.

Hogwood, B. W. and Gunn, L. A. (1981) *The Policy Orientation*, Strathclyde: Centre for the Study of Public Policy, University of Strathclyde.

Home Office (1987a) *Young People and Alcohol: Report of the Working Group of the Standing Conference on Crime Prevention*, London: Home Office.

—— (1987b) *The Licensing Act 1964. Government Proposals for Reforms*, London: Home Office.

Jacobson, B. (1981) *The Lady Killers*, London: Pluto.

Jones, K. (1954) *Lunacy, Law and Conscience*, London: Routledge & Kegan Paul.

Kooiman, J. (ed.) (1993) *Modern Governance. New Government–Society Interactions*, London: Sage.

Koskikailio, I. (1979) 'Socio-economic functions of Finnish restaurants', *British Journal of Addiction* 74: 67–78.

Lavis, J. and Sullivan, T. (1999) 'Governing health', in D. Drache and T. Sullivan (eds) *Health Reform: Public Success, Private Failure*. London: Routledge.

Lee, P. and Raban, C. (1983) 'Welfare and ideology', in M. Loney, D. Boswell, and J. Clerke (eds) (1988) *Social Policy and Social Welfare*, Milton Keynes: Open University Press.

Legg, D. and Sylvan, L. (1990) 'Community participation in health: the Consumers' Health Forum and the Victoria District Health Council Programme', in A. G. Evers, W. Farrent, and A. Trojan (eds) *Healthy Public Policy at the Local Level*, Colorado: Westview Press.

Le Grand, J. (1982) *The Strategy of Equality*, London: Allen & Unwin.

Levine, H. G. (1978) 'The discovery of addiction: changing conceptions of habitual drunkenness in America', *Journal of Studies on Alcohol* 39: 143–74.

Lindblorn, C. (1965) *The Intelligence of Democracy*, New York: The Free Press.

Loney, M. (ed.) (1987) *The State or the Market?*, London: Sage.

Loney, M., Boswell, D., and Clerke, J. (eds) (1988) *Social Policy and Social Welfare*, Milton Keynes: Open University Press.

MacGregor, S. (eds) (1989) *Drugs and British Society: Responses to a Social Problem in the 1980s*, London: Routledge.

Makela, K. and Viikari, M. (1977) 'Notes on alcohol and the state', *Acta Sociologica* 20: 155–79.

Makela, K., Room, R., Single, E., Sulkunen, R., and Walsh, B. (1981) *Alcohol, Society and the State*, Vol. 1, Toronto: Addiction Research Foundation.

Manning, N. (1985) 'Constructing social problems', in N. Manning (ed.) *Social Problems and Welfare Ideology*, Aldershot: Gower.

Marshall, T. H. (1975) *Social Policy*, 4th edition, London: Hutchinson.

Marshall, T. H. and Rees, A. M. (1985) *T. H. Marshall's Social Policy*, London: Hutchinson.

Maynard, A. and Robinson, D. (1990) 'Preventing alcohol and tobacco problems', in C. Godfrey and D. Robinson (eds) *Preventing Alcohol and Tobacco Problems*, Vol. 2; Aldershot: Avebury.

Maynard, A. and Tether, P. (eds) (1990) *Preventing Alcohol and Tobacco Problems*, Vol. 1, Aldershot: Avebury.

Milio, N. (1986) *Promoting Health through Public Policy*, Ottawa: Canadian Public Health Association.

—— (1987) 'Healthy public policy: Issues and scenarios'. Unpublished paper prepared for a Symposium on Healthy Public Policy, Yale University, 5 October.

Mishra, R. (1977) *Society and Social Policy*, London: Macmillan.

—— (1984) *The Welfare State in Crisis*, London: Wheatsheaf.

Navarro, V. (1976) *Medicine under Capitalism*, London: Croom Helm.

—— (1982) 'The crisis of the international capitalist order and its implications for the welfare state', *International Journal of Health Services* 12 (2): 169–90.

—— (1986) *Crisis, Health and Medicine: A Social Critique*, London: Tavistock.

O'Brien, M. and Penna, S. (1998) *Theorising Welfare, Enlightenment and Modern Society*, London: Sage.

Parker, D. (1977) 'Alcohol control policy and the fiscal crisis of the state', *Drinking and Drug Practices Survey* 13 (December): 3–6.

Parker, H., Measham, F., and Aldridge, J. (1995) *Drugs Futures: Changing Patterns for Drug Use amongst English Youth*, London: Institute for the Study of Drug Dependence.

Pascall, G. (1986) *Social Policy: A Feminist Analysis*, London: Tavistock.

Pederson, A. P., Edwards, R. K., Kelner, M., Marshall, V. W., and Albson, K. R. (1988) 'Coordinating healthy public policy: an analytic literature review and Bibliography', Health Services and Promotion Branch Working Paper HSPB 88–1, Toronto: Health and Welfare Canada.

Pinker, R. (1979) *The Idea of Welfare*, London: Heinemann.

Redding, M. (1970) 'Universality and selectivity', in W. Robson and B. Crick (eds) *The Future of Social Services*, Harmondsworth: Penguin.

Rein, M. (1970) *Social Policy: Issues of Choice and Change*, London: Random House.

Rex, J. (1978) 'British sociology's war of religion', *New Society*, 11 May.

Rhodes, T. and Hartnoll, R. (eds) (1996) *AIDS, Drugs and Prevention: Perspectives on Individual and Community Action*, London: Routledge.

Robinson, D. (1989) 'Controlling legal addictions: "taking advantage of what's there"', in D. Robinson, A. Maynard, and R. Chester (eds) *Controlling Legal Addictions*, Basingstoke: Macmillan.

Robinson, D. and Maynard, A. (1990) 'Preventing alcohol and tobacco problems', in C. Godfrey and C. Robinson (eds) *Preventing Alcohol and Tobacco Problems*, Vol. 2, Aldershot: Avebury.

Robinson, D., Maynard, A., and Chester, R. (1989a) *Controlling Legal Addictions*, Basingstoke: Macmillan.

Robinson, D., Tether, R, and Teller, J. (1989b) *Preventing Alcohol Problems: A Guide for Local Action*, London: Tavistock.

Rodgers, B. N. *et al.* (1968) *Comparative Social Administration*, London: Allen & Unwin.

Room, G. (1979) *The Sociology of Welfare*, London: Blackwell.

Room, R. (1981) 'The case for a problem prevention approach to alcohol, drug and mental problems', *Public Health Reports* 96: 26–33.

Royal College of Physicians (1987) *A Great and Growing Evil*, London: Tavistock.

Sabatier, P. A. (1986) 'Top-down and bottom-up approaches to implementation research: a critical analysis and suggested synthesis', *Journal of Public Policy* 6 (l): 21–48.

Senoda, K. (1990) 'Health promotion and consumers' cooperative movements in Japan', in A. Evers, W. Farrent, and A. Trojan (eds) *Healthy Public Policy at the Local Level*, Colorado: Westview Press.

Sharpe, L. J. (1978) 'The social scientist and policy making in Britain and America: a comparison', in M. Bulmer (ed.) *Social Policy Research*, London: Macmillan.

Shiner, M. and Newburn, T. (1997) 'Definitely, maybe not? The normalisation of recreational drug use amongst young people', *Sociology*, 31 (3): 511–29.

Small, N. (1988) 'AIDS and social policy', *Critical Social Policy* 21 (Spring): 9–29.

South, N. (ed.) (1999) *Drugs: Cultures, Controls and Everyday Life*, London: Sage.

Stacey, M. (1988) 'Strengthening communities', International Conference on Health Promotion, Ottawa, Canada: Selected Conference Proceedings, Ottawa: WHO, Health and Welfare Canada, and Canadian Public Health Association.

Stimson, G. (1987) 'British drug policies in the 1980s: a preliminary analysis and suggestions for research', *British Journal of Addiction* 82: 477.

Stokols, D. (2000) 'The social ecological paradigm of wellness promotion', in M. Schneider Jamner and D. Stokols (eds) *Promoting Human Wellness*, Berkeley, CA: University of California Press.

Strong, P. M. (1986) 'A new modelling of medicine? Comments on the WHO's regional strategy for Europe', *Social Science and Medicine* 22 (2): 193–9.

Sulkunen, R. (1985) 'International aspects of the prevention of alcohol problems: research experiences and perspectives', in M. Grant (ed.) *Alcohol Policies*, Copenhagen: WHO.

Taylor, D. (1996) (ed.) *Critical Social Policy: a Reader*, London: Sage.

Taylor, R. (1984) *Smoking Ring*, London: Bodley Head.

Tether, R. and Robinson, D. (1986) *Preventing Alcohol Problems: A Guide for Local Action*, London: Tavistock.

Titmuss, R. M. (1968) 'Address to the Social Administration Association', quoted in M. Brown (1983).

—— (1968) *Commitment to Welfare*, London: Allen & Unwin.

—— (1970) *The Gift Relationship*, London: Allen & Unwin.

—— (1974) *Social Policy*, London: Allen & Unwin.

Townsend, R. (ed.) (1968) *Social Services for All?*, London: Fabian Society.

—— (ed.) (1975) *Sociology and Social Policy*, London: Allen & Unwin.

Van der Kamp, J. (1990) 'Managing health promotion as an open process: holistic and ecological tools for managing and marketing of innovations', in A. Evers, W. Farrent, and A. Trojan (eds) *Healthy Public Policy at a Local Level*, Colorado: Westview.

Van Lennep, E. (1980) 'From the welfare state to the welfare society', *OECD Observer* 107: 19–20.

Waitzkin, H. (1983) *The Second Sickness: Contradictions of Capitalist Health Care*, New York: Free Press.

Waitzkin, H. and Waterman, B. (1974) *The Exploitation of Illness in Capitalist Society*, New York. Bobbs-Merrill.

Walker, A. (1983) 'Social policy, social administration and the social construction of welfare' in M. Loney, D. Boswell, and J. Clerke (eds) *Social Policy and Social Welfare*, Milton Keynes: Open University Press.

Walsh, B. and Grant, M. (1985) *Public Health Implications of Alcohol Production and Trade*, Geneva: WHO.

WHO (1985) *Targets for Health For All*, Copenhagen: WHO Regional Office for Europe.

—— (1986a) *Intersectoral Action for Health; the Role of Intersectoral Cooperation in National Strategies for Health For All*, Geneva: WHO.

WHO (1986b) *The Ottawa Charter for Health Promotion*, WHO: Health and Welfare Canada and Canadian Public Health Association.

—— (1988a) *Health Policies to Combat Drug and Alcohol Problems*, A Satellite Conference to the Healthy Public Policy Conference, Sydney and Canberra, Australia, 24–31 March 1988. Consensus Statement prepared by WHO Expert Working Group, Geneva: WHO.

—— (1988b) 'The Adelaide Recommendations', *Healthy Public Policy*, Copenhagen: WHO/EURO.

—— (1992) *Action for Public Health Conference on Supportive Environments for Health*. 3rd International Conference on Health Promotion held in Sundsvall, Sweden in 1991. Geneva: WHO.

—— (1997) *The Jakarta Declaration on Leading Health Promotion into the Twenty-first Century*. Adopted at the Fourth Conference on Health Promotion, July 21–5 1997. Geneva: WHO.

Widavsky, A. (1979) *Speaking Truth To Power: The Art and Craft of Policy Analysis*, Boston: Little Brown.

Wilding, P. (1982) *Professional Power and Social Welfare*, London: Routledge & Kegan Paul.

—— (ed.) (1986) *In Defence of the Welfare State*, Manchester: Manchester University Press.

Williams, F. (1989) *Social Policy: a Critical Introduction*, Cambridge: Polity Press.

—— (1994) 'Social relations, welfare and the post-Fordist debate', in R. Burrows and B. Loader (eds) *Towards a Post-Fordist Welfare State*, London: Routledge.

Wilson, E. (1983) 'Feminism and social policy', in M. Loney, D. Boswell, and J. Clerke (eds) *Social Policy and Social Welfare*, Milton Keynes: Open University Press.

Wittrock, R. and De Leon, P. (1986) 'Policy as a moving target: a call for conceptual realism', *Policy Studies Review* 6 (1): 44–60.

Ziglio, E. (1987) 'Policy making and planning in conditions of uncertainty: theoretical considerations for health promotion policy', Draft Working Paper No. 7, Edinburgh: Research Unit in Health and Behavioural Change.

7 Health promotion and politics

Dominic Harrison

Introduction

Access to the material conditions necessary for health is a human right, and while health, at least at a population level, has long been understood to be secured through social organization – it is itself determined by the political process (Evans *et al.* 1994; Levin and Ziglio 1996; Harrison and Ziglio 1998). Despite this widespread understanding, the view that population health promotion might require intervention in the domain of social organization still tends to be presented as innovatory, radical, contested, or litigious. Within both public policy making and the training of professionals employed to work in the field of public health, 'political skills' are rarely mentioned by name, while public health action that requires political intervention mostly remains part of the 'hidden history' of public health success. A significant effect is that people die from the consequences of actions not taken and much progress in public health practice is delayed. Understanding the causes and consequences of the delay requires an exploration of politics – both as a discipline and as an embodied reality both within social organization and the management and conception of public health itself.

This chapter explores some broad illustrative domains of contemporary political concern as applied to health promotion and public health. Focusing on what is often referred to as the 'New World Order', the central thesis is that the political process and the nature of social organization have been transformed by globalization and that this in turn must drive changes within the nature of public health practice as a form of progressive social change. The chapter argues that it may no longer be tenable to hold health promotion and public health as distinct territories of separate professional expertise. The political project for what might be called 'the health development disciplines' is to locate emergent and more complex notions of progress in population health within the wider, unified, but networked discipline of 'sustainable human development'. An underpinning theme throughout the chapter is the 'politics of integration' – an approach that this chapter will adopt in its own exposition.

The politics of definition

Even to attempt a description of politics is itself a political act, as the definition, nature, and scope of politics are what Gallie (1955–6) has described as 'essentially contested concepts' – the descriptive parameters requiring conceptual differentiation amenable only to choice of a political nature. Following Heywood (2000), this chapter proposes a fourfold classification of what politics is concerned with:

1   Politics is primarily associated with the art of government and the activities of the state.
2   Politics is primarily concerned with the conduct and management of a community's affairs in pursuit of the notion of the (Aristotelian) 'good life'.
3   Politics is concerned with the generation and resolution of conflict through compromise, conciliation, negotiation, and other strategies.
4   Politics is about the production, distribution, and use of resources in the course of social existence, the nature of which is exercised through power relations.

The significance of accepting the last definition is that there is generally a politics of everything. As the feminist author Kate Millett observed in 1970, 'politics is about power-structured relationships, arrangements whereby one group of persons is controlled by another'.

In 1920 Winslow famously defined public health (at least for his own century) as:

> The science and art of preventing disease and prolonging life, and promoting physical and mental health and efficiency, through organized community efforts. . . . And the development of the social machinery which will ensure to every individual in the community a standard of living adequate for the maintenance of health.

Any purposeful activity to create health – especially that which engages 'the social machinery' – may well require political acts under all four domains of definition. This was something that did not trouble the post-war consensus that defined Article 25 of the Universal Declaration of Human Rights enacted on 10 December 1948 by the General Assembly of the United Nations, which states that:

> Everyone has the right to a standard of living adequate for the health and well-being of himself and of his family, including food, clothing, housing and medical care and necessary social services, and the right to security in the event of unemployment, sickness, disability, widowhood, old age or other lack of livelihood in circumstances beyond his control.

The politics of parties

Ideology is generally used in its neutral sense to refer to a distinctive set of ideas of any group or class (as discussed in Chapter 6). At first glance it would appear easy to place the ideology of health promotion and public health practice within traditional 'left-wing' party political values. Seminal publications such as the WHO Ottawa Charter (1986) are explicit as to their underpinning values and strategies which involve: equity, inter-sectoral collaboration, peace, building a stable eco-system, social justice, building healthy public policy, creating supportive environments for health, strengthening community action, and developing personal skills. Left-wing governments have traditionally been distinguished by (often imperfectly defined) ideological or value differences relating to freedom, equality, fraternity, rights, progress, reform, and internationalism. Right-wing governments in turn are traditionally attached to ideas such as authority, hierarchy, order, duty, tradition, reaction, and nationalism (Heywood 2000).

However, differentiation across such 'left and right' politics is probably already redundant. Most world democracies of the Northern and Western political communities have become a largely indistinguishable version of social democracy, following 'contingent' or pragmatic agendas characterized by a 'we do what works' approach. Despite their claims, these are not un-ideological in nature, as they almost universally operate within a neo-liberal economic paradigm (i.e. one tending to promote market individualism and government authoritarianism). Fukuyama (1992) suggests this 'post-Cold War' trend signifies 'the end of all viable alternatives to market capitalism, as the basis of economic organization, and liberal democracy as the basis of political organization'. The late 1990s did see a 'third way' – post or 'renewal' social democratic tradition, as espoused by Clinton in the US and Blair in the UK. Its provenance is not entirely clear, but as Giddens (1999) maintains, the concept probably relates to a general acceptance of market and globalized capitalism, qualified by a communitarian emphasis upon social duty and the reciprocal nature of rights and responsibilities. Since, or perhaps because of, 'post social-democratic third-way politics', participation in party politics is declining fast. Yet participation in a wide variety of new social movements is increasing. Typically, as Frankel (1987) comments, peace activists, gays, feminists, animal rights activists, anti-consumerists, etc. 'do not have a unified identity as a social movement'. However, as Dobson (2001) points out, this is hardly the point: 'The crucial project would not be to manufacture an identity between hetero-geneous groups, but to identify that group (or groups) whose project most profoundly questions the presuppositions on which present social practices depend.' One such illuminative example of the collaborative yet diverse coalition developing an articulate pre-election intervention was evidenced in the UK in 1996, when 'The Real World Coalition' clearly captured the political mood at the end of nearly two decades of conservative government. This was an alliance of over 40 national and international civic bodies, charities, non-governmental organizations and agencies, covering issues such as poverty, community, economics, environment, pollution and development. In a book called *The Politics of the Real World* (Jacobs 1996), they expressed the dissatisfaction with the formal party political system and expressed concerns that now stand as a powerful precursor to the growing world 'anti-capitalist or anti-globalization' movement of the new century. They said

> Many people today feel that something has gone wrong . . . the quality of life seems to be declining, crime soars, traffic and pollution spiral, mass unemployment is undiminished, many people experience stress and insecurity at work, poverty is growing and inequalities have left many people excluded from mainstream society . . . everywhere a sense of community is breaking down. There is global environmental degradation and the future of the planet is uncertain. Yet the political system seems barely to register what is happening.

This movement is a broad church – its demonstrations are against the global democratic deficit, the World Trade Organization, the global financial and cultural hegemony of 'Corporate America', and a host of other related dissatisfactions. It has set an international and local political agenda outside traditional political parties and single nation states. The unifying idea that political systems seem unresponsive and that they fail to address related, integrated, and global problems is central to the 'new politics'. This politics is concerned with all four of the political domains identified above and is primarily concerned with issues of authority, law, power, governance, and participation within the globalized world. The response of civil society – a term most commonly used to refer to a realm of autonomous and self-regulating groups, pressure groups, and associations operating separately from the authority of the state – is starting to grow dramatically. It is a major ally to those concerned with improving the health of populations.

The politics of authority and law

The authority of government – often seen as a form of legitimate power – is enshrined in its capacity to make law, defined as a set of public and enforceable rules that apply to any political community. If politics is, 'in its broadest sense, the activity through which people make, preserve and amend the general rules under which they live' (Heywood 2000), then the social goal of enshrining in law the promotion of the public's health must be a fundamental task. This idea is not new. A stone inscription still above the door of the public health department in London's Southwark, quotes Cicero saying: 'The health of the people is the highest law'. This is symbolically placed high above the eye-line of the building's users, and it omits to mention how the highest law might be enforced or who is to be the enforcer. More contemporary lawmakers do not have this problem. Into the inspirational interstices, global corporations, themselves barely 200 years old, have now erected 'free trade' as the *de facto* highest law of the people. This 'highest law', practically, symbolically, and legally is enforced by the World Trade Organization (WTO), with the sometimes reluctant support of the governments of elected democracies throughout the industrialized world. The WTO is the best funded, best enforced and largest, supra-national global agency of transworld governance in history. The promotion of public health is definitely not on its agenda. As it is not an elected body, neither individuals nor the institutions of civic society can easily change it, but without change it will remain the most significant global generator of 'risk conditions' and structurally generated health inequality for populations across the world.

The politics of governance

This democratic deficit of the WTO reflects shifts in the balance of power brought about by processes of globalization. Power itself is defined by Boulding (1989) as 'the ability to influence the behaviour of others in a manner not of their choosing' but it is not a 'zero sum'. Both politicians and professions, with wider interests and constituencies than the WTO, who see economic growth as a means to an end and not an end in itself, have a very important contribution to make – especially perhaps those concerned to improve the health of the public.

If all governments, at least those in the industrialised north and west of the globe, are operating on neo-liberal economic paradigms, then perhaps participation in party politics and the process of government becomes a secondary activity for levering political change – especially for health. The locus of political action necessarily transfers to the operational domain. This is concerned with how change in the management and organization of the institutions of daily life might be effected. The collective cultural response to this agenda has been the development of 'governance systems' – a growing industry of pandemic proportions. Both public and private organizations have been developing new systems of public participation, consumer responsiveness, or citizen involvement to cope with the twin phenomena of public disaffection with party politics and the demand for a greater say in effecting change. Osborne and Gaebler (1991) suggest that governance may be defined as

> the process by which we collectively solve our problems and meet society's needs. As such, it is different from government, which is the instrument we use. They suggest the instrument is outdated and the process of re-invention has begun.

This descriptive challenge moves away from more determinist notions that social structures alone determine individual and community 'life chances'. The 'agent' *can* change the structures through which they experience life and may be more or less facilitated to do so by empowering and transparent social systems. The promotion of good governance, one that allows 'the exercise of political, economic and administrative authority to manage a society's affairs' has emerged as a key approach by the United Nations Development Program and is framed as the central locus for fostering the overarching goal of 'Sustainable Human Development' (UNDP 1997).

It is probably within this framework that future leverage and advocacy on the wider determinants of population health might best be pursued at local, regional, national, and global levels. To be effective, this must take account of globalization and canalize the trends that may support progressive social change for health.

The politics of globalization

According to Scholte (2000), the causal dynamics of globalization are multi-layered. At its root is an increasingly rational, secular, and anthropocentric view of the world concerned to address a global public through technological innovation involving increased air transport, electronic communication, and dismembered but connected communities of interest. Driven primarily by the interests of global capital, the world's industrial communities have had to secure international frameworks of law for property rights, cross-border movements of money, investments, trade, and procedural standardization. The core thesis is that globalization is a transformation of social, and perhaps psychological geography, marked by the growth of supra-territorial spaces and the simultaneous actions of increased fragmentation and connectivity within persons, systems, structures, organizations, and relationships. But these affects are both contested and differentiated. Those that are identified are spread unevenly across the north and south of the globe as well as between the professional / unskilled and between the young /older members of communities. Whilst globalization has not entirely changed the underlying social dynamics of government, the state and communities, it has produced important changes. Scholte and others such as O'Meara *et al.* (2000) argue that there are winners and losers. Positively, globalization has encouraged additional loci of governance besides the state, the spread of additional forms of community, and the development of diverse types of knowledge besides the rational. It has supported cultural regeneration, decentralization of power, and has increased economic efficiency – at least for some. Negatively, it has through its implicit adoption of neo-liberal economic policy rapidly increased ecological degradation and poverty. It has worsened working conditions and supported cultural hegemony and colonialization. It has widened various inequalities and deepened democratic deficits. Scholte (2000) argues it is 'neither good nor bad – its outcomes depend on human decisions which can be debated and changed'. This provides a clear challenge to public health, which must engage with this wider social and cultural transformation. If it is to be concerned with the promotion of public health and reduction of health inequalities within a globalized world, it must be a key political player in developing 'health competent' instruments of social governance across all sectors and levels.

The politics of health promotion and public health

Rather uncomfortably, towards the end of the last century, it was realized that neither the health services nor indeed the provision of health promotion services make much difference to the health of populations. There is simply no relationship at a population level between national spending on health services and the health of populations (World Bank 1993). The rather more complex reality is that adequate population approaches to the prevention of multi-factorial disease and the promotion of the public's health simply cannot be easily purchased as an 'additive commodity' – to be bought from *health-directed* expenditure (i.e. health care system expenditure) (see Buse and Walt 2000; Levin and Ziglio 1996; Evans and Stoddart 1990).

Like human development, population health is really an outcome of 'emergent capacity' arising from the integrated effects of *health-related* social, economic, and cultural activity and investment. Nominated health promotion budgets in the UK amounted to only 1 per cent of the 7 per cent of GDP for the National Health Service in 1997. This could never make any serious impact on health at a whole population level – the services provided and resources invested are at best symbolic. A wider and more consistent approach, congruent with the evidence as to where health is created, is to acknowledge that every decision and investment, in every sector, may either improve the health of populations or damage it. What is needed is an overarching policy, planning and investment, approach that integrates health development into all social, economic, cultural, health, and other planning. The World Health Organization's Investment for Health programme has been exploring these concepts since 1997 and considerable progress has been made at the conceptual level.

One unpredicted effect of both these new understandings and the globalization process has been to dissemble and deconstruct the known territories of professional expertise of those groups professionally involved in public health. There is a micro-politics of health promotion that is largely concerned with its own history as a discipline, its status and its relationships to the more powerful tribes of paid medical professionals. But the new century has widened the professional stakeholders in social progress. The profession of health promotion may now, for instance, be expanded to include all those people employed in area-based regeneration and development programmes, almost all of which may have population health improvement as an implicit and predicated outcome. The implications of such an integrated perspective on health, regeneration and development may well go beyond issues of professional delimitation. In a seminal publication, Tengs *et al.* (1995) – a multi-disciplinary group of North American academics writing for the journal *Risk Analysis* – sought to develop a common methodology to compare 'five hundred life-saving interventions and their cost-effectiveness'. Table 7.1 below compares the cost per life year saved of a range of common clinical, preventive, engineering, and social interventions.

The inconsistency of social investments in health protection, disease prevention, and disease treatment across all sectors makes a strong case for just the kind of integrationist approaches advocated in this chapter. The implementation of such an approach would require a commitment to health investment equality amongst risk-exposed populations, an open, integrated, rational and democratically governed decision-making process, the pooling of cross-sectoral budgets and disinvestments in high-technology medical intervention – as well as a range of other equally difficult 'political deliverables'. It is significant that although the benefits are wider, the currency of benefit is rooted in the domain of health (as longevity). This perhaps demonstrates that the health of the public is rapidly becoming both a strategic instrument and a cultural metaphor for social justice, environmental quality, and 'good governance'.

The promotion of health is indeed the business of everyone and whilst it may now be said that 'health promotion is an activity not a profession', it is also true that 'public health is a social objective and not just a branch of medicine.'

Both professions may ultimately need to consider themselves contributory sub-disciplines to the wider social movement or collective profession of sustainable human development. The political levers for this wider focus on the determinants of health are outside of health care and are systemic in nature. They require concerted, sophisticated, and integrated political action

Table 7.1 Cost per life year saved of a range of common clinical, preventive, engineering, and social interventions

Intervention	Cost per life year saved US$
Screening blood donors for HIV	14,000
Neonatal intensive care for low birthweight infants	270,000
Influenza vaccine for high-risk people	570
2 vessel coronary artery bypass graft surgery	75,000
Mammography every three years for women aged 50–65	2,700
Fire detectors in homes	50
Random motor vehicle safety inspections	1,500
Coal-fired power plant emission control	50
Ban Amitraz pesticide on apples	50
Terminate sale of all three-wheeled all-terrain vehicles	50
Seat belts for all passengers in school buses	2,800,000
Flammability standard for children's sleepwear, ages 0–6	50

Source: Tengs *et al.* (1995) 'Five hundred life-saving interventions and their cost effectiveness', *Risk Analysis* 15 (3).

to bring about change and they require professionals concerned with public health to engage with the politics of systems and organization through processes other than the management of departments and dedicated public health budgets.

The politics of systems and organization

The process of global disaggregation and fragmentation has to some extent facilitated the growth of new systems and professional relationships. There are many definitions of systems but in general terms

> a system is anything that takes its integrity and form from the ongoing interaction of its parts . . . Systems are defined by the fact that their elements have a common purpose and behave in common ways, precisely because they are interrelated towards that purpose.
>
> (Roberts and Kleiner 1999)

Organizations, political communities, sectors, and professions at each of the levels of social governance – global, global regions, national, regional, sub-regional, local, neighbourhood/community – are rapidly restructuring and establishing new competencies to act, but they are finding it difficult to keep up. The collective ability to create systems of appropriate governance and the institutional capacity to meet the challenge to connect people, stakeholders, policies, and purpose, may well be the central determinant of future social and organizational effectiveness. It will also be a significant determinant of capacity to intervene to promote health. These changes have brought with them a need to ask questions *collaboratively* about the structure, 'fitness for purpose', subsidiarity, resourcing, and governance of health within all social systems.

It is salutary to reflect that in 1866 Florence Nightingale was asked to open the Manchester Children's Hospital and, in a strongly worded – even political letter – she refused, saying 'building more children's hospitals is not the proper remedy for infantile mortality and sickness – the true remedy lies in improving children's homes' (Brierly 1970). Today, Manchester still has one of the poorest housing stocks in Europe, continuing to contribute to admissions to the children's hospital. Indeed, 135 years after Florence Nightingale's comments, systems of governance and institutional capacity are only just emerging that may have some prospect of addressing the challenge to improve rather than simply recover population health in that city. Such integrated systems for health development, as a social product themselves, have suffered from under-investment in research and development and are generally, intellectually 'undercapitalized'. They also suffer from poor leadership, little clear ownership, and no immediate market. Yet the generic policy issue that underpins the challenge of integrated population health development is receiving significant attention at an international level. The

Organisation for Economic Co-operation and Development OECD(B) (2000) suggests that the newly acquired need and capacity to address cross-cutting issues, of which health is only one, is a response to wider societal challenges arising from globalization:

> More than a simple transition from one more or less 'stable state' to the next, the present period seems to be one of continuing, global change, of which the most visible manifestation is the shifting and breaking down of boundaries and conceptual categories. Governments are challenged to critically examine the rigidities in their policy-making systems, and to seek ways to make them more flexible.

Characterizing the challenge as one of policy coherence, the OECD(B) (2000) however warns 'excessive efforts to enhance coherence can result in a high degree of central control, and a consequent loss of flexibility in the policy-making system'. They recommend:

> As policies become more interconnected, and as the policy context continues to change rapidly, there is a greater risk of incoherence arising among policies during their implementation phase, even among policies that seemed mutually compatible when they were first decided upon. . . . To reduce this risk, governments need to be able to adjust policies as new information is generated in the course of implementation. In order to be responsive to the context, existing mechanisms to coordinate the implementation of policies (i.e., lead ministers, inter-ministry coordination committees or secretariats) increasingly need to rely on direct feedback from actors outside of government, including the private sector, non-governmental organizations, the media, and special interest groups.

These reflections are particularly cogent for a knowledge-based activity such as health development. Both knowledge production and knowledge management are at the core of any integrated mission to develop population health and reduce inequalities. What may generate the real inequality between the economies of the North and South in the future is not knowledge itself, but the capacity to generate new knowledge. This capacity is embedded in relationships and networks both inter-sectoral and trans-hierarchical. These capacities need to be strengthened by new forms of organizational and social governance.

Similarly, it has become increasingly recognized that long-term economic growth is dependent on investment in knowledge production and diffusion. Barro (1991), OECD(A) (2000a), and Florida (1995) have emphasized the significance not just of individual learning but of the learning that takes place within and between organizations. However, knowledge *in itself* does not contribute to economic growth or health development. Crucially, it has to be incorporated into the production of goods and services, decisions, and resource allocation in all sectors. Hence, educated and skilled individuals not only have to be produced (via the education and training system) but also their knowledge and skills have to be used – their work needs to be organized in ways that ensure the real utilization of their competencies. Such understandings have significant implications for the systems and professions involved in the promotion of the public's health. Networked organization is a prerequisite for effective knowledge production and the management of cross-cutting policy and strategy for health. Ferlie and Pettigrew (1996) argue that hierarchies, markets, and networks are the three archetypal modes of organization, each requiring different forms of organizational structure and management style – (management style in networked organizations is characterized as 'diplomatic' rather than 'military' or 'entrepreneurial').

They argue that

> the network perspective redirects our attention away from formal structure and policy to the importance of patterns of social relationships within organisations, including (perhaps especially) informal ties. It conceptualises market processes in highly relational and socially embedded terms. ... Within the public sector, questions of inter-agency co-operation and networks are also assuming greater importance as it has become clear that the implementation of many policies requires agencies and tiers of government to co-operate.
>
> (Ferlie and Pettigrew 1996)

They argue that network forms of organization are functional for types of workflow characterized by the following:

- an increased requirement for flexibility and learning
- dynamic, unstable, uncertain, working environments
- requirements to co-produce products, services or knowledge
- knowledge-based, innovative, high-tech, de-layered, team-based work
- work requiring the management of intra-organizational and cultural diversity.

Ferlie and Pettigrew also draw attention to some of the advantages and challenges of networking, recognizing that in resolving some difficulties, network organizations can generate others. Challenges include the fact that network organization is long-term, emergent, and developmental task. Network organization can find itself in difficulty in wider organizational contexts where the dominant management and cultural paradigms are limited to short-term goals (or political cycles!). Network organizations are highly dependent on inter-personal relationships and so can be vulnerable to staff movements and difficulties in relationships.

However, on the positive side, network organizations have a greater capacity to bring in new stakeholders and players, which is particularly important to equity and knowledge based production. Based on mutual orientation and reciprocity, network organizations may fit better with demands emerging from rapid and paradoxical influences of globalization. The public health community must embrace the challenge to regroup and respond to this emergent context using the many organizational, technical, and analytical skills it has acquired during the past 150 years of its own professional development. There may also be costs, political risks and losses – both professional and emotional – to be faced if it is to be done well.

The politics of distance

Involvement with the 'social machinery', 'new social movements', and new organizational forms carries a further significant political risk that must be managed by the public health community and it is one held in common with the international development community. Chambers (1997) defines this as the risk of 'embedded error'. For Chambers, embedded errors in international development reflect 'widely held views that are generalised in professional practice, particularly because they fit what powerful people want to believe . . . and are sustained'. These arise also because most of the powerful in professions, those who have risen to the top in careers, those writing books, teaching, accrediting practitioners, or commissioning research are old men – long since out of touch with any reality 'on the ground'. Stark and ageist as this statement might seem, the veracity of the analysis might not be too difficult to establish also within the world of public health. Citing disastrous case studies of the failures of international development projects since the 1950s, he lays at least some of the blame at the door of professional structures, distance, and power:

> Professionalism is concerned with our knowledge, and how we learn, analyse and prescribe. In all these examples the erroneous beliefs were embedded in the concepts, values, methods and behaviour normally dominant in disciplines and professions. Those who were wrong had had a long education and training whether as macro-economists, engineers, agrionomists, foresters, administrators or social scientists. Most were highly numerate. Most were specialists. All were linked with other professional colleagues around the world. Through letters, the telephone, workshops, conferences, professional journals and papers, they were in touch with their professional peers and with current dominant values and beliefs. Their learning was then more likely to come laterally or from above than from below, and to follow current ideologies and fashions.

Of distance, he wrote:

Distance blocks, blurs and distorts vision and distance is institutionalised. Most of those who were wrong were physically, organisationally, socially and cognitively distant from the people and conditions they were analysing, planning and prescribing for and making predictions about. Physically, they were centrally based in headquarters, in offices, in laboratories and on research stations far from local complex, diverse, dynamic and unpredictable rural realities. Organisationally they were trapped by norms of behaviour, by routines and by resources (or their lack) which kept them in central places and rewarded them for working there. Socially they were different and apart from rural people. Their contact if any was confined to short special occasions as development tourists. Cognitively they were distant, having different categories, criteria, values and life experiences. Being distant they relied on secondary data. They calculated with the figures that were to hand and treated the numbers as reality.

Of power:

Power hinders learning. Those who were wrong were powerful. They were senior, almost all men, mostly white and influential, whether through age, professional authority, control of funds or position, or hierarchy. Their power conditioned their perceptions and prevented them from learning. The realities of life and conditions are elusive: they are local complex, diverse, dynamic and unpredictable. Central professionals are pervasively ignorant, out-of-touch, and out of date about such realities.

Such insights resonate strongly with many of the known political causes of public health failure such as New Variant CJD/BSE (Mad Cow Disease) – particularly within the UK.

The politics of risk

The management of risk consequences through mediation and social reconciliation is a key new role for health promotion and public health professionals (as discussed in Chapters 5 and 6 in this volume). From pre-history, risks have been managed by prayer, sacrifices, or other rituals. Scientific method, especially when aligned to vested interests, manages little better. Government discourse on risk is generally inadequate at exposing framing assumptions, or revealing who carries the burden of the risk consequences that might be experienced throughout communities.

With 'risk analysis technology', governments and industry have – assisted by the positivist risk management industry – sought to assess, quantify, manage, and communicate risks on the public's behalf. Assumptions underpinning such activities are that:

- There are rational means through which quantitative methods can be developed to make decisions about risk – including and especially 'health and environmental risks'.
- All risks are discoverable and measurable.
- All risks can be controlled with the requisite skill and expertise.

Such beliefs are inherent in both the pure engineering view and what is known as the 'psychometric' tradition. From this perspective there *are* real risks which may or may not be understood by the public according to a range of discoverable psycho-social factors that can be mapped (and presumably manipulated) to 're-align' public risk perception to an appropriate understanding of 'real risk'. From such assumptions certain research questions become prescient. Bennett and Calman (1999: 6), for instance, review the literature on 'fright factors', asking 'why do some risks trigger so much more alarm, anxiety or outrage than others, seemingly regardless of scientific estimates of their seriousness?' They contend that the top five 'fright factors' that tend to make risks more worrying, (and less acceptable) if perceived, include:

1 That the risk is involuntary (e.g. exposure to pollution) rather than voluntary (such as smoking).
2 That the risk is inequitably distributed (some benefit whilst others suffer the consequences).
3 That the risk is inescapable by taking precautions.
4 The risk arises from a novel or unfamiliar source.
5 That the risk results from man-made rather than natural sources.

They also point out in this review that the public may have difficulty understanding concepts of probability and thus will overestimate the 'true risks' of some events. They argue that trust is a key feature and that the media, principal amongst others, serve to exaggerate health risks through a process described as the 'social amplification of risk'.

However, this attribution of cause and proposed solutions to risk management is diametrically opposed to the analysis of Ulrich Beck, a German sociologist who developed the concept of a 'risk society' (1992). Central to his thesis was that modern society not only produces products, goods and wealth but also risks (bads). Traditional 'welfare societies' redistribute wealth, whereas modern risk societies redistribute risks. Beck argues that there is now a world of hazard and risk that is more complex and insidious than can be described by traditional understandings of risk, which attributes simple numbers or percentages to the likelihood of a future risk event. Beck (1992: 28) argues that our risk society is not an option that can be chosen or rejected in the process of political debate. Instead it is a basic structural condition of advanced industrialization where potential hazards undermine and /or cancel the established safety systems of the provident state's existing risk calculation. Beck argues environmental and health risks now created cannot be limited to time and space and are irreversible systematically produced hazards, which are balanced beyond the insurance limit.

Thus, as Douglas (1986) comments:

> Risks are subject to interpretation and risks are first and foremost risks if we cannot accept them. Thus social legitimation and acceptance of risk have become decisive for understanding the significance of risks for the social order. This in turn leads to conflicts about risks emerging as conflicts about knowledge or 'knowledge and definition struggles'.

The definition of what may or may not be a risk is thus left to the process of what Beck calls 'sub-politics'. Risks and their acceptable limits are 'defined by technocrats and politicians at international conferences, government and industry funded researchers who, from such closed debates eventually reveal risks, options for action or standards of acceptability' (Beck 1992). However, as Adam and Van Loon (2000) argue, most progress might be made by going beyond realist–absolutist versus constructionist–relativist positions. We may need to overlook the diversion of exact calculation (of 'real' risk) and to focus on uncovering 'that which is hidden' in the public communication of risks and work on the development of 'technologies of mediation'. In focusing on widening the collective responsibility and governance for risk, the mediation of all described risk, and the exposition of the uncovered and unequal risk consequences of decisions, we might promote greater individual and global health equity.

The events of September 11, 2001, focused the world's attention on the fault lines of structural inequality, poverty, and injustice and have raised the profile of risk management through a largely public health discourse. Following the collapse of the twin towers of the World Trade Center in New York, the subsequent threats and counter-threats to individual, community, regional, national, and global health are emergent and explicit. These risks are expressed through social, economic, and cultural pathways and challenge the public's health profoundly.

However, as Table 7.2 below demonstrates, the global burden of terror on September 11 was by no means confined to America. Terrors of different and equally devastating consequence affected other men, women, and children across the world on that day.

One of the consequences of September 11 may be that the social, political, and professional management of risk consequences will become a key public health function. In delivering this, mediation and social reconciliation processes, as yet unsystematized and unmanaged, may become primary roots to secondary prevention of harm arising from community-wide risk events. Primary prevention must be the promotion of equity on a global scale. Equity, a central public health value, requires that action be taken on those differences or inequalities that are systematic, unfair, unjust, and avoidable. The war against terrorism announced by President Bush and endorsed by America's

Table 7.2 On September 11, 2001

	Number
People (mainly Americans) who died in the terrorist attacks	3,000
People who died of hunger on September 11, 2001	24,000
Children killed by diarrhoea on September 11, 2001	6,020
Children killed by measles on September 11, 2001	2,700
(*Assuming annual deaths are evenly distributed*)	
Also on September 11:	
Malnourished children in developing countries	149 million
People without access to safe drinking water	1,100 million
People without access to adequate sanitation	2,400 million
People living on less than $1 per day	1,200 million
African children under 15 living with HIV	1.1 million
Children without access to basic education	100 million
Illiterate adults	875 million
Women who die each year in pregnancy and childbirth	515,000
Annual average number of people killed by drought and famine 1972–96	73,606
Annual average number of children killed in conflict 1990–2000	200,000
Annual average number of children made homeless by conflict 1990–2000	1.2 million

Source: New Internationalist

allies, has opted for military and diplomatic strategies for the containment of the risk consequences of terrorism, but as yet, it shows little sign of addressing the causes. Quoting 'state failure, and lack of development', *The Lancet*'s (2001) October editorial suggested a more sustainable response would be 'that foreign policy goals should incorporate health, development and human rights as key strategic objectives . . . attacking hunger, disease, poverty and social exclusion . . . Public health is an undervalued measure of our future global security.'

Conclusion: the politics of integration

For the last 30 years or so, health promotion and public health professionals have differentiated their skills, capacities, and professional objectives from the wider project of sustainable human development and social regeneration. But there is now a growing understanding that the integrated outcome of the population's 'well-being' is a shared social objective. It could be argued that the profession of public health evolved its practice on a 'deficit model' of analysis and intervention. It began as a response to problems and it has generally focused its gaze on health needs, with the inevitable outcome that remedial or ameliorative action – often in the form of health services – has been proscribed as the solution. Those involved with the promotion of the public's health have been encouraged to focus on the consequences of problems – usually problems arising from underdevelopment. They have been trained to conceptualize 'that which things are done about' as diseases, vulnerable population groups, risk behaviours, and the management of public health programmes (often of little sustainable effect). The claim that even most of these were preventive does not overcome the criticism.

The alternative and emergent approach is to examine 'capacities or assets' of individuals and communities and to plan supportive, integrated, and sustainable development / social regeneration as the future pathway to population health improvement. This approach brings new actors and agencies to the forefront of public health practice. There are many entry points to this approach and many professional and lay capacities to be liberated in its delivery. It is also open and creative – such an approach could focus, for instance, on spatial or cultural development pathways to health improvement such as 'rivers' or 'friendship'! It would be just as easy to construct quite different programmes of health improvement and regeneration around these foci, whose outcomes may be more effective in the improvement of population health, the regeneration of communities, and the mobilization of public participation. Health development, health improvement, health promotion, disease prevention, health protection, and communicable disease control may still, on occasion, require programmes to address specific issues. But the need for such action is largely determined by the causal nature of any given population's risk exposure – which itself is determined by the state of human development within any particular community. Thus there is a need collectively to create an integrated model of sustainable human development, which includes social regeneration and public health improvement – both as key constituents and as strategic instruments – for the delivery of the population's well-being.

Regeneration and development professionals already associate their work with wider societal goals. Public health (the profession) is just re-learning to do that and is sharpening up the conceptual development of integrated public health practice. Professionals employed to improve the population's health are increasing their understanding of the complexity of their role and realizing that to improve health in an environment transformed by globalization is to act against 'a syndrome or a complex' and not a single bacteria, disease, or problem. To pursue the medical metaphor, public health (the social objective) addresses different but connected symptoms and usually requires multiple social medications. Most of those that are effective and sustainable are to do with regeneration and development.

As Demos (1997) has identified, the new politics is:

- *holistic* – integrated across all sectors;
- *preventive* – moving away from curing to preventing problems;
- *outcome-orientated* – focused on outcomes not measures of activity; and
- *culture changing* – concentrated around persuasion and information rather than coercion and command.

Cross-functional outcome measures that determine the quality of life where people live and work require integrated and networked inputs. If the health of the public is to be the highest law, then public health must engage with the political processes implicit in globalization and realize it is not itself outside of the reality it may wish to change. Fragmentation, de-construction and de-centralization of power may be features of its own political and professional future. In addition, globalization may be delivering new and unexpected challenges. The social management of equity and risk consequences are under-conceptualized social processes whose cultural expression is most often focused on population health outcomes.

The health development professions must ally themselves with civic society in the development of systems of health governance at each level of social and economic administration. They must network their knowledge and skills across all levels, systems, sectors, and professions. They must politically intervene within the 'social machinery' of the state and within all forms of social organization and systems where decisions are made and resources allocated. They must join in the wider social project of sustainable human development at every level, from local to global. Finally, they must be careful to avoid 'embedded error' in the development of their practice, to learn from other domains, and not to become too attached to the contemporary practice of 'policy-based evidence-making' for public health.

References

Adam, B. and Van Loon, J. (2000) 'Introduction: repositioning risk; the challenge for social theory', in B. Adam, U. Beck, and J. Van Loon (2000) *The Risk Society and Beyond Critical Issues for Social Theory*, London: Sage, p. 2

Barro, R. J. (1991) 'Economic growth in a cross section of countries', *Quarterly Journal of Economics* 106: 407–43.

Beck, U. (1992) *Risk Society. Towards a New Modernity*, London: Sage.

Bennett, P. and Calman, K. (1999) *Risk Communication and Public Health*. Oxford: OUP.

Boulding, K. (1989) *Three Faces of Power*, Newbury Park, CA: Sage.

Brierly, J. K. (1970) *A Natural History of Man*, London: Heinemann.

Bureau for Development Policy (1997) *Strengthening Capacity for People-Centred Development. Decentralised Governance Programme*. Bureau for Development Policy, UNDP. http://magnet.undp.org/docs/dec/decen923/decenpro.htm – 5 September 2000

Buse, K. and Walt, G. (2000) 'The United Nations and Global Public–Private Health Partnerships: in Search of "Good" Global Health Governance'. Workshop on Public–Private Partnerships in Public Health, Endicott House, Dedham, Mass. April 7–8.

Cabinet Office (2000) *Wiring It Up: Whitehall's Management of Cross-Cutting Policies and Services*. A Performance and Innovation Unit Report. London: HMSO.

Chambers, R. (1997) *Whose Reality Counts? Putting the First Last*, London: Intermediate Technology.

Demos (1997) *Holistic Government*, London: Demos.

Dobson, A. (2001) *Green Political Thought*, London: Routledge.

Douglas, M. (1986) *Risk Acceptability according to the Social Sciences*. London: Routledge, Kegan & Paul.

Evans, R. G. and Stoddart, G. L. (1990) 'Producing health, consuming health care', *Social Science and Medicine* 31(12): 1347–63.

Evans, R., Morris L. *et al.* (1994) 'Why are some people healthy and others not?', *The Determinants of Health of Populations*, New York: de Gruyter.

Ferlie, E. and Pettigrew, A. (1996) 'Managing through networks: Some issues and implications for the NHS', *British Journal of Management* 7 (special issue): 581–99 (March).

Florida, R. (1995) 'Toward the learning region', *Futures* 27 (5): 527–36.

Frankel, B. (1987) *The Post Industrial Utopians*, Oxford: Polity Press.

Fukuyama, F. (1992) *The End of History and the Last Man*. London: Hamilton.

Gallie, W. B. (1955–6) 'Essentially contested concepts', *Proceedings of the Aristotelian Society*, 56: pp. 157–97.

Giddens, A. (1999) *The Third Way: The Renewal of Social Democracy*, Cambridge: Polity.

Harrison, D. and Ziglio, E. (eds) (1998) 'Social determinants of health: implications for the health professions'. *Forum: Trends in Experimental & Clinical Medicine*, Suppl. No. 4. Italian National Academy of Medicine. Available on *http://www. accmed.net/hpi*.

HDA (2001) *http://www.hda-online.org.uk/downloads/pdfs/Short_Report.pdf*

Heywood, A. (2000) *Key Concepts in Politics*, London: Macmillan.

Jacobs, M. (1996) *Politics of the Real World: Meeting the New Century*. Written and edited for the Real World Coalition, London: Earthscan Publications.

Lancet (2001) Editorial: 'Public Health: a neglected counter terrorism measure', *Lancet* 358, (6 October): 1112–13.

Levin, L. S. and Ziglio, E. (1996) 'Health promotion as an investment strategy: considerations on theory and practice', *Health Promotion International* 11(1): 33–40.

Millet, K. (1970) *Sexual Politics*, London: Virago.

OECD (2000a) *Cities and Regions in the New Learning Economy*. OECD *www.oecd.org* – June 2000.

OECD (2000b) *Strategic Governance and Policy Making Section of the OECD/ PUMA* web-site updated: 21–07–00 *www.oecd.org*

O'Meara, P., Mehlinger, H. D. and Krain, M. (2000) *Globalisation and the Challenges of a New Century: A Reader*, Bloomington, IN: Indiana University Press.

Osborne, D. and Gaebler, T. (1992) *Reinventing Government*, London: Plume.

Roberts, C. and Kleiner, A. (1999) 'Five kinds of systems thinking', in P. Senge *et al. The Dance of Change: The Challenges of Sustaining Momentum in Learning Organizations*, London: Nicholas Brierly Publishing.

Scholte, J. A. (2000) *Globalisation: A Critical Introduction*, New York: Palgrave, p. 106.

Tengs, T. *et al.* (1995) 'Five hundred life-saving interventions and their cost effectiveness', *Risk Analysis* 15 (3): 369–90.

The Real World Coalition (1996) *The Politics of the Real World*, London: Earthscan.

Winslow C-E.A (1920) 'The untilled fields of Public Health', *Science* N.S. 51 (1306): 923–33.

World Bank (1993) *World Development Report: Investing in Health*. World Development Indicators. New York: Oxford University Press.

8 Using economics in health promotion

David Cohen and Janine Hale

Introduction

A belief that health promotion will reduce health care costs has led many to see health promotion as a way of saving money, and economics as the discipline to highlight where these savings can be made. This shows a lack of understanding both of the objectives of health promotion and of the role that economics can play in the pursuit of those objectives. While it is possible that money may be saved through health promotion, this is not normally its primary objective. Indeed, if saving money were the sole objective, then any health gains which could be achieved only at positive cost would not be pursued. Since virtually all programmes of treatment and cure achieve health gains at some positive cost, such a restriction on health promotion would clearly be illogical.

Economics provides the framework for considering how efficiently health promotion achieves its objectives and how health promotion resources can be used most cost-effectively. Economics also provides an analysis of health-promoting behaviour and of the incentives that exist to prevent ill health or to engage in activities that damage health. Such appraisal and analysis can produce essential information for devising, planning, implementing, and evaluating health promotion programmes. To appreciate how economics can play these roles, this chapter begins by explaining basic economic principles, highlighting the fact that economics is first and foremost a way of thinking. This is followed by a discussion of how economics offers an alternative analysis of health-affecting behaviour and the implications this can have for health promotion policy. The set of techniques that have been developed from the economic way of thinking are then described, followed by an illustration which shows the way that economic appraisal can help with decision making in health promotion.

Economics as a way of thinking

Economics is the study of how society chooses to use its scarce resources to produce various outputs (goods and services). It is also about who benefits from those outputs. In economics, the term 'resources' refers to those things that contribute to production, such as land, labour, and equipment. Money only contributes to production if used to rent land, hire labour, buy equipment, and so on. In other words, money gives a command over resources, but is not itself a resource.

Within the formal health care sector, the production of 'better health' requires the input of various health service resources such as doctors, nurses, drugs, dressings, and operating theatres. In the case of much prevention, better health can also be viewed as something produced by individuals combining their own time with various other inputs. The starting point of economics is that resources are scarce relative to the demands made on them. On a national level, it is not possible to double the output of all goods and services because of an insufficiency of available resources. Scarcity means that large increases in any one type of output may be achieved only by shifting resources away from the production of other outputs, thus sacrificing what would otherwise have been produced. In economic thinking, the cost of any production is perceived in terms of these sacrifices, i.e. what has been forgone by not using the resources in another way. This is called 'opportunity cost' and is a different concept from money cost.

Opportunity cost is also a relevant concept when viewing the individual as a producer of his or her own health improvements. The time available to put into health production is finite, and the money available to command the other needed resources is also limited. A programme of exercise may not involve any monetary expenditure, but since the time spent exercising means forgoing benefits from work or leisure time, there is an opportunity cost. Scarcity means that choices must be made about how to allocate resources between competing alternatives. While there can be no single basis on which all choices should be made, it is at least possible to identify a number of criteria for choice. The criterion most used in economics is 'efficiency', which is about attempting to maximize the benefits from available resources. According to this criterion, it is unwise to devote resources to A if more benefit could be obtained by using the resources in B. Similarly, if C and D produce the same level of benefit, but C does so using fewer resources, then C is the more efficient. One activity can never be said to be more efficient than another purely on the basis of being more beneficial or purely on the basis of being less costly. The efficiency decision must involve both. Of course, maximizing benefits from available resources is not the only noble social objective. Inefficient policies can legitimately be pursued if other criteria, such as equity or political expedience, can justify them. Comparing programmes in terms of their efficiency, however, forces explicit identification and consideration of these other criteria if less efficient programmes are to be defended.

Economics and health-affecting behaviour

As other chapters in this book demonstrate, theories have developed within various disciplines to explain health-affecting behaviour. Though economics is not conventionally thought of as a behavioural science, it contains a well-developed set of theories on what influences consumers' demand for various goods and services. If health-affecting behaviour is regarded as the demand for health-affecting goods and services, then economic theories of demand can provide an alternative explanation for such behaviour. Unfortunately, preventive goods (including preventive health care) and hazardous goods have attributes which complicate matters when they are analysed in terms of conventional demand theory.

In economic theory, goods and services are demanded for the 'utility' (satisfaction) which they provide. Most health care services, however, do not directly yield positive utility. Health care can be unpleasant (can yield negative utility) and, unless we all have Munchausen syndrome, there must be some other explanation why people demand these services. Economists have postulated that the demand for health care is a 'derived demand'. People do not demand a health care service for its own sake. Rather, the demand for health care is derived from people's demand for health.

Clearly, the commodity 'health' is not something that only health care professionals can produce. In the preventive sense, individuals can produce health by combining their own time with various other resource inputs such as vitamin tablets, jogging shoes, or high-fibre cereals. (Note that in this context these goods are considered to be resources because they are contributing to production of something else.)

Based on the seminal work of Michael Grossman (1972), economists have developed models that view individuals as *producers* of health (for example, Cropper 1977; Ippolito 1981; Muurinen 1982). These are based on what is called the 'human capital' approach, in that individuals are seen as making new investments in their own health. These models have helped to increase our understanding of human behaviour regarding the demand for various preventive and hazardous goods. For example, while conventional demand theory explains and predicts how demand for a hazardous good such as cigarettes (or any other good) depends on its price, Ippolito's model shows how this demand is also dependent on whether the hazard is constant (i.e. has a fixed probability of death per unit consumed) or cumulative, as in the case of cigarettes. Cohen (1984) has developed a model of preventive behaviour which differs from those above in its recognition that many preventive goods (and all hazardous goods) are not demanded for preventive reasons at all. According to this model, preventive or hazardous goods provide two types of utility – that derived directly from the use value of the good (e.g. the good taste of wholemeal bread or the pleasure of smoking), and that derived from the knowledge that consuming the good alters the risk of future illness or injury. This model provides messages for policy concerning the most effective way of manipulating the demand for preventive or hazardous goods. For example, the model suggests that advertising messages which address the use value of goods may be more effective than health education, which focuses on risk attributes if the former are shown to dominate the decision to consume. In the case of smoking, this may mean making smokers feel guilty about the annoyance they cause to non-smokers, rather than making them worry about their own future health.

In recent years, the technique of conjoint analysis, initially developed in market research, has been used by health economists to assess the relative importance of different characteristics in the way goods or services are provided. An estimate of the total utility an individual gains from a good or service with particular characteristics can also be calculated, which could be used to forecast the likely uptake if a new health promotion programme were introduced. This technique has been used to a limited extent in health promotion (van der Pol and Ryan 1996; Spoth 1989, 1991, 1992; Spoth and Redmond 1993) and there is scope for further work in this area.

As a means of explaining health-affecting behaviour, economics has not had a particularly great impact on the development of health promotion. This may in part be due to the presence of well-developed theories from other disciplines in this area. However, economics is having a major influence on health promotion in terms of evaluation.

Economic appraisal

The cost-benefit approach, which is the foundation of economic appraisal, is outlined in Figure 8.1. The diagram shows that all policies/programmes/activities involve the use of resources. Whether these are resources diverted from other uses or made available for a specific use is irrelevant, since either the resources could have been used in another way or the money used to pay for them could have been used to control other resources. The benefits of these other potential uses will be forgone if the programme in question is pursued. This sacrifice of benefits is the cost. At the same time something good must be expected to result. This is the benefit.

The cost-benefit approach is about weighing gains against sacrifices. Something passes the cost-benefit test if the value of the gains exceeds the value of the sacrifices. If it fails the test, the implication is that the required resources could produce greater benefit if used in another way. The trade-off is between benefits gained and benefits forgone, not between benefits gained and cash. Only in an ideal world of infinite resources could everything that produces benefit be pursued. Costs can be defined as all resources which have alternative uses – hence involve an opportunity cost. Benefits can be defined as all things of value which emerge. Non-resource costs such as anxiety or pain can be treated as negative benefits. Resource savings can be treated as negative costs. Not all exponents of the cost-benefit approach classify costs and benefits in quite this way (see, for example, Drummond 1980; Mooney *et al.* 1986). Nevertheless, there is no dispute about what factors need to be taken into account in an economic appraisal. How one separates costs and benefits does not matter to the end result of the appraisal, so long as nothing of importance is omitted and the correct sign (+ or –) is applied.

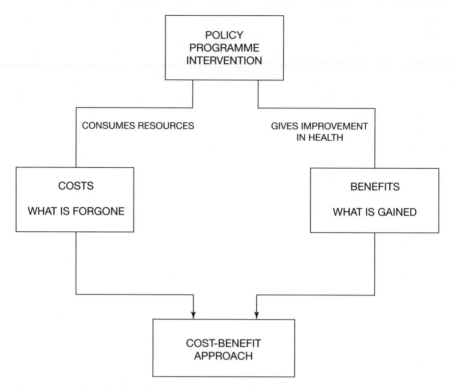

Figure 8.1 The cost-benefit approach
Source: Adapted from Drummond (1980)

The major problem of putting this theoretical framework into practice is of course that costs and benefits are not normally measured in common units. A list of costs and benefits will include such things as hours of doctor time, number of doses of a drug, and number of life-years gained. As each of these is measured in different units, summing costs and benefits and then weighing one sum against the other is not possible unless a common unit can be found in which all can be described. Since, by definition, all costs and benefits have the common feature of being of value, and since the £ symbol represents relative value, it is possible (in theory at least) to express each in terms of its value and sum them accordingly.

Valuation is relatively straightforward when market prices are attached. If an ounce of gold sells for ten times more than an ounce of silver, it is normally accepted that gold is valued ten times more highly than silver. But how can a year of life be added to this comparison of values? To many, the idea of even trying to put money symbols against benefits such as lives saved or pain relieved is at best distasteful. However, the view of those who argue that pain relief or human life is beyond considerations of cost (i.e. of infinite value) cannot be reconciled with observed reality. If human life were of infinite value then society would be unwilling to trade anything off in exchange for it, i.e. society would be willing to pay an infinite amount to save it. Given the multiplicity of human wants, this cannot be. It is known, for example, that the number of expected traffic fatalities could be reduced if crash barriers were built between the carriageways of every motorway, a flyover built at every dangerous intersection, and if all sharp bends in roads were straightened. The fact that not all motorways have crash barriers and that dangerous bends and intersections still exist is proof that society, or its representatives who make such decisions, does not put an infinite value on human life. The opportunity cost of doing all the above is judged to be too high.

Even at an individual level, observed behaviour shows that human life is not of infinite value. People do make trade-offs. Smokers who are aware of the health hazard of smoking trade off the risk of future illness or death against their present satisfaction and pleasure. The same is true of people who willingly accept the risk of injury or death by crossing the road at a busy intersection rather that take the extra minute to walk to the pedestrian underpass down the road. As Cullis and West (1979) point out,

> Few people, if any, seek to maximise their health and life expectance per se. To do so involves sacrificing opportunities to eat, drink, play games, drive, etc. that at the margin may be a greater source of utility than an additional (expected) minute or hour of life.

Inevitably, choosing a value to put on something like human life will be controversial, but such valuations cannot be avoided. Economists point out that they are made implicitly every time a decision either to do or not to do something is made. For example, if a motorway crash barrier programme is rejected on grounds of cost (say £X), and it is estimated that if it were constructed Y lives could be saved, then it is implied that the value of a life is less than £X/Y since this is what it would have cost on average to save each life.

Table 8.1 lists various implied values of life in different situations. In no case was this value made explicit at the time the decision was taken, yet the decisions implied values none the less. Since the people who may die in another Ronan Point disaster are unknown, i.e. they are statistical lives, and since the same is true for the babies not yet conceived whose lives could be saved by screening of pregnant women, it must be asked why society is willing to spend £20 million to save a life in one area but unwilling to spend £50 to save a life in another. If the objective is to save the greatest number of lives (strictly it should be life-years) from the resources dedicated to life saving, then society's pursuit of this efficiency objective will be aided by this sort of information being available.

Table 8.1 Some implied values of life

Source	Implied value of life £
Screening of pregnant women to prevent stillbirth	50
Government decision not to introduce childproof containers for drugs	1,000
Motorway driving behaviour	94,000
Legislation on tractor cabs	100,000
Proposals for improved safety on trawlers	1 million
Change in building regulations following collapse of Ronan Point high-rise flats	20 million

Source: Adapted from Mooney (1977)

Cost-benefit analysis

Cost-benefit analysis (CBA) begins by identifying and measuring in physical or other units all of the resources used or saved by the programme and all the positive or negative valued outcomes which result. It adopts what is called a 'social welfare' approach in which all costs and benefits are considered, irrespective of who bears the costs or who receives the benefits. It then attempts to place money values on each. This allows CBA to answer the question of whether and to what extent any programme or policy should be pursued.

When market prices are available, they are normally used to value costs and benefits. When market prices do not exist, money values can still be applied by any of a variety of methods. The way in which money values can be placed on human life illustrates this. The earliest method of valuing human life equated the value of a life with the productive potential of the individual. Narrow interpretation of this approach means that a value of zero must be placed on the lives of the elderly, the mentally handicapped, housewives, and others. The fact that health services (which have opportunity costs) are not withheld from these groups demonstrates that society clearly places a positive value on their lives. Use of earning potential can, however, be defended by noting that one of the objectives of health care is to increase people's productivity. Valuations based on earning potential can then be viewed as minima. If someone who is kept alive and healthy will contribute £X to the economy, then society ought to be willing to pay at least £X to keep him or her alive to do it. This should not be interpreted as meaning that society should not be willing to spend £X + 1.

A second method of assigning money values to human life is based on people's willingness to pay for small reductions in risk. While conceptually pleasing because it attempts to tease out the values of those actually at risk, the approach can be criticized on several grounds. For one thing, the valuations that emerge are normally much higher than those estimated by other means (Jones-Lee 1976). For another, it is questionable whether individuals can attach any real meaning to a risk reduction from say 1 in 100,000 to 1 in 110,000 (Cohen 1981). Additionally, it is not clear whether consumer-based values are appropriate in health care valuation (Mooney 1986). A third method is to use implied values, as discussed above, or to use the amounts that courts have awarded in compensation for accidental death. This method has merit in that it is based on existing decision-making procedures and value structures. The problem, as seen above, is that the range of values can be enormous.

Differential timing of costs and benefits

Shifting resources from one area to another, in particular from treatment to health promotion, can involve major changes in the timing of costs and benefits. Any shift from treatment to health promotion will involve forgoing current benefits for benefits that will arise in the future.

In financial appraisal, explicit recognition is given to the idea that society appears not to be indifferent to the timing of costs and benefits, preferring to delay costs as long as possible and receive benefits as soon as possible. This is expressed in the form of positive interest rates in financial markets. Discount rates (the inverse of interest rates) are applied to all future costs and benefits to express them in terms of their 'present values'. The Treasury sets an official discount rate for all formal cost-benefit appraisals in the public sector. The rate is currently 6 per cent per annum in real (after adjusting for inflation) terms.

In theory, the same adjustment process is required for health costs and benefits. There is no dispute among economists on the validity of the discounting process, although there is considerable disagreement between economists as to what the most appropriate discount rate for health benefits ought to be. In the United States the 'Panel on Cost Effectiveness in Health and Medicine' recently recommended that a 3 per cent discount be used (Gold *et al.* 1996).

In the case of health promotion, the implications of applying the 6 per cent Treasury rate need to be carefully considered. Applying this rate has the effect of reducing the present value of benefits which arise more than 50 years in the future to virtually zero. If the medical model is applied, and the benefits of health promotion are seen as reductions in future morbidity and mortality, such a severe adjustment can be argued to be inappropriate. If, however, the short-term benefits of health promotion which feature more prominently in other models are considered, then the effect of discounting can be far less pronounced. Non-economists may take a stronger line, arguing that the whole process of discounting is unjustified (West 1985). Failure to discount, however, implies a 0 per cent discount rate which must be defended. This would require arguing that society is indifferent to when benefits are received, willingly sacrificing ten lives today in exchange for the saving of ten lives in the distant future. This is inconsistent both with logic and with observed behaviour.

Dealing with uncertainty

Estimation of the benefits of health promotion programmes requires the use of assumptions – sometimes fairly heroic assumptions. Since the only thing certain about the future is that it is uncertain, this is inevitable. But what if these assumptions prove to be wrong? Clearly, it is not possible for any technique to remove the problem of uncertainty. No technique can make the unknowable known, but, if it can indicate the extent to which getting each variable right matters, then much of value is gleaned.

Sensitivity analysis is a technique used within the cost-benefit framework to test how sensitive conclusions are to any changes in assumptions. It is applied by identifying those variables around which most uncertainty exists and altering their values. Essentially this means redoing the analysis using these altered figures. In many cases, such changes make little difference to the overall result. In other cases, changes can radically alter the original conclusion. For example, by using a range of discount rates (including zero) in sensitivity analysis, the impact that discounting has on the results can be assessed (Tolley 1993). Sensitivity analysis gives an indication of the degree of confidence one can have in the conclusions. Additionally, it identifies which estimates and assumptions may require further investigation before a decision is taken.

Alternatives to cost-benefit analysis within the framework

Given the difficulties of assigning money values to intangibles, it is not surprising that full cost-benefit appraisals are rare. There are, however, a number of other techniques under the cost-benefit umbrella which are simpler to apply in practice. Inevitably, these are more restrictive in terms of how their conclusions can guide policy.

Cost-effectiveness analysis

By weighing gains against sacrifices, CBA directly addresses the question of whether or to what extent any programme should be pursued. It questions the worth of the objective. Often, however, the question of whether to undertake or expand a programme is not at issue. A decision may already have been taken. The issue is no longer 'should we?', but '*how* should we?' In such cases a simpler technique under the cost-benefit approach is available.

Cost-effectiveness analysis (CEA) accepts that there are normally alternative ways of pursuing any objective and seeks the alternative that either produces most benefit for a given cost or that achieves a given benefit at least cost. This is known as '*technical efficiency*'. Again a 'social welfare' view can be adopted and the same definitions of costs and benefits applied. However, since an assessment of whether benefits *exceed* costs is not required, there is no need to place money values on benefits. Thus if a breast cancer screening programme is to be undertaken, CEA can indicate whether mammography using mobile units is more *cost-effective* than at fixed sites. CEA cannot say whether society's scarce resources should be allocated to breast cancer screening.

While addressing a much narrower question, a major advantage of CEA is that benefits need only be expressed in 'units of effectiveness'. This means, however, that CEA can only compare alternatives that produce that specific unit of effectiveness. Specifying the unit of effectiveness is often not a problem since many programmes have very precise and clearly defined objectives. A breast cancer screening programme, for example, which has a specific objective to detect pre-symptomatic cancers, will measure effectiveness in terms of 'true positive cases of pre-symptomatic cancers detected'. A CEA will identify the method with the lowest cost per true positive case of pre-symptomatic cancer detected. It would *not* seek the lowest cost per woman screened, since 'women screened' would only be the appropriate unit of effectiveness if the sole objective of the programme were to screen women with no concern regarding whether or not any cases were detected.

In the case of much health promotion, however, there can be more than one objective, with changes in different outcomes being achieved with different time scales. Nutbeam (1998) has identified three levels of outcome – health promotion outcomes such as increased health literacy; intermediate health outcomes such as the adoption of healthier lifestyles; and health and social outcomes such as improvements in quality of life or reductions in mortality. Thus, for example, an anti-smoking health promotion campaign may have the objectives of (i) increasing knowledge and awareness (health literacy) to allow consumers to make more informed choices, (ii) reducing smoking prevalence (healthy lifestyles) in addition to (iii) future (discounted) reductions in smoking-related morbidity and mortality. A policy to increase tobacco duty may have the sole objective of reducing smoking prevalence (ignoring any incentives the government may have to raise more revenue). Comparing the two solely in terms of cost per quitter (objective ii) is arguably inappropriate as it ignores the additional value of knowledge-based informed choice from the health promotion route. CEA cannot handle multiple objectives.

This limitation should not imply that CEA has no place in the appraisal of health promotion. There are instances within health promotion where single objectives exist, and CEA can be very informative in these instances. Also, if it is accepted that the *principal* objective of health promotion is to achieve a healthier population, health promotion can be compared with alternative means of achieving health gains. Any additional benefits which health promotion may confer can be dealt with in two ways. If a health promotion programme is shown to be a more cost-effective way of achieving a health gain, then any additional benefits need not be considered since their inclusion would only reinforce the conclusion already reached. If health promotion is shown to be less cost-effective at achieving a health gain, then the implied value principle can now be employed. Anyone who still argues in favour of the health promotion programme must now explicitly value the additional benefits from the health promotion route at more than the difference in cost between the two programmes.

For example, if increasing taxes has a cost per quitter of £100 and the health promotion programme has a cost per quitter of £120, then anyone arguing in favour of health promotion must be placing a value of at least £20 on the benefit of increased knowledge. What the 'correct' value for increased knowledge ought to be is not easily answered, but the appraisal has at least forced explicit consideration of this issue. If the tax route is chosen, it will be implied that increased knowledge is worth less than £20. If the health promotion route is chosen, it will be implied that it is worth at least £20. Note that this question of 'worth' is a cost-benefit not a cost-effectiveness issue. Further, economic appraisal does not answer the question. It merely provides the information to others who will make the decision.

Cost-utility analysis

The problem with cost-effectiveness analysis is that it can only compare programmes that produce the same units of effectiveness. It is thus arguably of value only within narrowly defined areas of activity. However, the broader the chosen unit of effectiveness, the wider the applicability of the results. For example, both breast cancer screening and anti-smoking campaigns have an ultimate objective of saving lives (or more precisely years of life saved). Use of life-years gained as the unit of effectiveness allows the cost per life-year in the two programmes to be compared. Moreover, the results can further be used in comparison with the cost per life saved of any other life-saving programme.

While this broadening of cost-effectiveness analysis is useful, there remain two weaknesses. First, comparison is still limited to programmes whose benefits come in the form of life saving. Second, and perhaps more important, comparison by cost per life-year gained assumes that a year of life bedridden and in pain is equivalent to a year of life in perfect health. This problem could be overcome by using a 'global' measure which can describe the benefit from any health intervention. However, because the thing being measured (health gain) is multidimensional and value laden, it will never be possible to derive a perfect global measure. It must be remembered, though, that the trade-off between health gains in one activity and health gains in another is unavoidable. If addressing the nature of these gains and losses by means of imperfect measures results in better decisions being taken, then the measures are of value. What is being sought is improvement not perfection.

In theory any effective intervention produces health along one of two basic dimensions. It either makes people live longer or it improves the quality of their life, or some combination of the two. Thus in theory all interventions produce Quality Adjusted Life Years (QALY) (Rosser and Kind 1978). If the output of all programmes were measured in QALY terms, then comparison of cost/QALY would allow a complete generalization of cost-effectiveness analysis. This type of CEA using QALYs (or related output measures) is called cost-utility analysis (CUA).

Whilst CUA provides a useful way of comparing all programmes, its application to health promotion is not at all straightforward and, arguably, the QALY measures that have been developed to date are not sensitive enough to pick up changes arising due to a health promotion programme (Cribb and Haycox 1989).

A practical example of economic appraisal: general practitioner advice to quit smoking

Cigarette smoking is a major cause of preventable morbidity and mortality. It has been associated with an increase in deaths from various cancers (mouth, oesophagus, pharynx, larynx, lung, pancreas, bladder), from chronic obstructive pulmonary disease and other respiratory diseases, from vascular diseases and from peptic ulcers (Doll *et al.* 1994). Smoking during pregnancy is associated with low birth-weight babies and a range of other complications including sudden infant death syndrome (Di Franza and Lew 1995). Second-hand or passive smoking has been shown to increase risk of lung cancer and ischaemic heart disease in non-smokers (Hackshaw *et al.* 1997) and of respiratory illness in children (Margolis *et al.* 1997; Stoddart and Miller 1995). Smoking is estimated to cost the NHS between £1.4 billion and £1.7 billion per year and costs British industry about 50 million lost working days, valued at some £1,710 million (Health Education Authority 1997). The potential benefits from reduced cigarette smoking appear to be very large indeed.

The fact that potential benefits are large, however, is not sufficient reason to increase effort in this area. Evidence on a programme's ability to produce these benefits is required, as is information on the cost of producing them. Some preventable outcomes may not be major in terms of potential benefits, but if the benefits can be achieved at very small cost, then programmes in this area may be more efficient than programmes directed at the larger morbidity and mortality areas.

The issue of reducing smoking prevalence can be addressed from either a cost-benefit or a cost-effectiveness approach. The former examines the extent to which anti-smoking measures are an efficient use of scarce resources: i.e. should more resources be directed to anti-smoking programmes? The second takes it as given that anti-smoking is a worthwhile pursuit and seeks to identify the most cost-effective way of reducing smoking prevalence.

By the mid-1980s evidence was emerging to show that advice to smokers by their general practitioners on why and how they should quit could be an effective way of reducing smoking prevalence (Russell *et al.* 1979; Woods *et al.* 1980; Stewart and Rosser 1982; Wilson *et al.* 1982; Jamrozik *et al.* 1984; Richmond *et al.* 1986). The available evidence suggests that brief advice to smokers by their general practitioners on why and how they should quit could be an effective intervention (Buck 1997). Such advice, however, is not costless as it requires scarce general practitioner time, particularly if a repeat visit is part of the advice regime.

Approach 1: cost-benefit analysis

A cost-benefit analysis of GP advice to stop smoking would identify all the resource costs of the programme. Based on current knowledge of the relationship between smoking and smoking-related diseases, an estimate would be made of the expected reductions in these diseases. The benefits (and negative costs) of such reductions would be calculated under three broad headings:

1   *resource savings* from having to treat less smoking-related disease, and possibly from having to fight fewer fires – and the resulting losses of property and life;
2   *productivity gains* because the people not acquiring smoking-related diseases will not lose work and leisure time; and
3   *the intangible benefits* of living a longer life and not suffering the pain and misery of illness.

Expressing all costs and all benefits in money terms allows the cost-benefit test to be applied.

Smoking is a complex issue, however, and there are numerous problems in applying cost-benefit analysis in practice. Aside from the difficulty of assigning money values to the items under 3 above, a number of other questions arise. Should the 'utility loss' (the forgone pleasure) of ex-smokers be included? Should the annoyance caused to non-smokers by cigarette smoke be taken into account and what value should be placed on it? Does smoking increase cleaning costs? If reduced smoking causes jobs to be lost in the tobacco industry, do they have to be included as well?

Because of these and other complicating factors no one has yet produced a comprehensive cost-benefit study of anti-smoking programmes. It is not surprising, therefore, that GP advice in particular has not been put to the cost-benefit test.

Approach 2: cost-effectiveness analysis

General practitioner advice to stop smoking has the same objective as all other anti-smoking measures – to achieve a reduction in smoking prevalence which will bring about a reduction in smoking-related morbidity and mortality. There are many other means of pursuing this same objective, including:

• increased taxation
• stronger health warnings on cigarette packets
• restrictions on who can purchase cigarettes

- mass media anti-smoking campaigns
- direct measures such as quit smoking classes, contests, etc.

There are arguments for and against each of these. Increased taxation is known to be effective. Grossman and Chaloupka (1997) estimated that a 10 per cent increase in the price of cigarettes through taxation would lead to a 7 per cent reduction in the number of teenage smokers and a 6 per cent reduction in the amount consumed. Whilst it is recognized that adult smokers do not react to price changes to the same extent as teenagers, a reduction in the number of adult smokers would also be expected alongside a reduction in their daily consumption levels (ibid.). On the other hand, an argument against increased taxation is that tobacco duty is a 'regressive tax' which hurts the poor far more than the rich.

Mass media health information campaigns have the advantage of reaching a large number of people at relatively low cost. The evidence on the effectiveness of such campaigns suggests that the resulting change in behaviour from a pure information campaign is not that great (Buck 1997). There is evidence, however, to suggest that when combined with a social support component, they can be a cost-effective method of promoting smoking cessation (Ratcliffe *et al.* 1997).

Arguments for and against each of the above methods can be made from many perspectives, including the sociological, psychological, ethical, and political. The economic perspective is not advocated as a superior way of thinking. It is only an alternative, but one which together with other perspectives can make a major contribution to health promotion. Under the cost-effectiveness perspective the cost of each of the measures is estimated, followed by estimates of the effectiveness of each in reducing smoking prevalence. A comparison is then made in terms of cost per quitter. The method with the lowest cost per quitter is the most cost-effective.

In the United States, Altman *et al.* (1987) compared the cost-effectiveness of three smoking cessation programmes aimed at smokers who had expressed a desire to quit: a self-help quit smoking kit; a smoking cessation contest with prizes; and a smoking cessation class. The quit rates achieved were 21 per cent for the kit, 22 per cent for the contest, and 35 per cent for the class. The marginal costs per quitter were $45, $61, and $266 respectively. Sensitivity analyses indicated that even if the effectiveness of the kit were to drop to a 6 per cent quit rate, it would still be the most cost-effective option. The clear implication was that, given a limited budget, a sufficient number of interested smokers, and an objective of maximizing the number of quitters, then spending the budget on the self-help kit would achieve the maximum smoking cessation.

Broadening the objective

While such analyses can be of much assistance in choosing between anti-smoking programmes (and in the above case only between anti-smoking programmes aimed at smokers who have expressed a desire to quit), cost-effectiveness analysis is no more than a ranking of alternative ways of achieving a given objective; in this case getting smokers to quit. In any ranking one alternative must come out on top. The ranking tells us nothing about how efficient anti-smoking is *vis-à-vis* programmes that produce other types of benefits.

As explained above, however, broadening the objective – say to life-years gained – is one way of overcoming this weakness. If the alternative anti-smoking measures are compared in terms of cost per life-year gained, then the cost-effectiveness of each can be compared with the cost-effectiveness of any other programmes that produce benefits in the form of life-years gained.

A study by Cummings *et al.* (1989) measured the effectiveness of GP advice to stop smoking in terms of life-years gained. The cost per life-year from an original brief advice session ranged from $705–988 for men, and from $1,204–2,058 for women, depending on the assumptions used. The authors were able to compare this with the cost-effectiveness of other preventive measures which had been appraised in cost per life-year terms, including treating moderate hypertension ($11,300), treating mild hypertension ($24,408), and treating hypercholesterolemia ($65,000–108,000). Thus, a cost-effectiveness study using this broader unit of effectiveness allows comparisons beyond the specific area of non-smoking.

Further broadening the objective

While this broadening of cost-effectiveness analysis is useful, there remain the two weaknesses described earlier, viz. comparison is still limited to programmes whose benefits are in the form of life saving and there is an implied assumption that life-years of different quality are valued equally.

To overcome this, a cost-utility analysis of GP advice to stop smoking was undertaken by Williams (1990), which estimated the marginal cost per QALY (from reduced coronary heart disease alone) to be £167. One objective of this study was to exemplify the QALY approach, and despite his acknowledged need to make some fairly heroic assumptions, Williams was able to compare this figure with other programmes which have been appraised in terms of cost per QALY, such as pacemaker replacement for heart block (£700), kidney transplantation (cadaver) (£3,000), heart transplantation (£5,000), and hospital haemodialysis (£14,000).

It is important to stress that cost/QALY information is intended to assist, not replace decision making. It advises that resources shifted *on the margin* from high to low cost/QALY programmes will allow an overall increase in benefit at no additional resource cost, i.e. there will be an efficiency gain. Cost/QALY figures will vary as programmes are expanded or contracted and a high figure must not be interpreted as calling for an end to that pro-gramme. Williams' results imply that additional resources would be far more efficiently used to increase GP advice to smokers than to expand the hospital haemodialysis programme.

Broadening the objective beyond the individual

Economics has traditionally adopted an individualistic framework – regarding social welfare simply as the sum of the welfare of the individuals within society. Health promotion, however, has increasingly been focusing attention on the issue of community development, which suggests that the traditional economics view may not be the most appropriate way for economists to participate in this area (Shiell and Hawe 1996).

In recent years, however, economists have been developing the related concept of 'social capital' which measures aspects of 'society' as feelings of belonging and trust. The general economics literature is investigating how an increase in social capital can lead to improved economic performance (e.g. Knack and Keefer 1997) while the health economics literature has been extending this to explore the relationships between social capital and health (e.g. Lomas 1998). There is at present a paucity of evidence about the cost-effectiveness of community health promotion programmes involving multiple strategies (Dunt *et al.* 1995; Buck *et al.* 1996). Further work in this area may bring the disciplines of health promotion and health economics closer together.

Conclusion

The main message from economics is that health promotion may well be a good thing but it should not be blindly pursued. The expected benefits of health promotion may be attractive, but no benefits are achieved without sacrifices. As this book shows, health promotion comes in many forms and guises. As a discipline, economics contributes to health promotion by identifying which forms of health promotion are worthwhile and which are not. It provides a framework which enables identification of where the benefits of health promotion justify the cost and to what extent. Economics is about informed choice not evangelism.

This is an important aspect of health promotion because properly conducted economic appraisals present reasoned and justifiable arguments as to why more resources should be directed towards health promotion generally. In terms of dealing with competing health promotion programmes, economics can show how resources can be most cost-effectively allocated to ensure the maximum health gains from whatever level of resources is secured for these activities. As a behavioural science, economics can also make an important contribution to health promotion by increasing our understanding of what affects health-promoting behaviour. There is much scope for increasing this contribution of economics in future.

References

Altman, D. G., Flora, J. A., Fortmann, S. P., and Farquhar, J. W. (1987) 'The cost-effectiveness of three smoking cessation programs', *American Journal of Public Health* 77: 162–5.

Atkinson, A. B. and Skegg, J. L. (1973) 'Anti-smoking publicity and the demand for tobacco in the UK', *Manchester School of Economics and Social Studies* 41: 265–82.

Buck, D. (1997) 'The cost effectiveness of smoking cessation interventions: What do we know?', *International Journal of Health Education* 35: 44–52.

Buck, D., Godfrey, C., Killoran, A., and Tolley, K. 'Reducing the burden of coronary heart disease: health promotion, its effectiveness and cost', *Health Education Research*. 11: 487–99.

Chen, Y., Li, W., and Yu, S. (1986) 'Influence of passive smoking on admissions for respiratory illness in early childhoods', *British Medical Journal* 293: 303–6.

Cohen, D. R. (1981) *Prevention as an Economic Good*, Health Economics Research Unit, Discussion Paper No. 02/81, University of Aberdeen.

—— (1984) 'The utility model of preventive behaviour', *International Journal of Social Economics* 10: 52–62.

Cohen, D. R. and Henderson, J. (1988) *Health, Prevention and Economics*, Oxford: Oxford Medical Publications.

Cribb, A. and Haycox, A. (1989) 'Economic analysis in the evaluation of health promotion', *Community Medicine* 11: 299–305.

Cropper, M. L. (1977) 'Health, investment in health, and occupational choice', *Journal of Political Economy* 86: 1273–94.

Cullis, J. G. and West, P. A. (1979) *The Economics of Health: An Introduction*, Oxford: Martin Robertson.

Cummings, S. R., Rubin, S. M., and Oster, G., (1989) 'The cost-effectiveness of counseling smokers to quit', *Journal of the American Medical Association* 261 (1): 75–9.

Di Franza, J. R. and Lew, R. A. (1995) 'Effect of maternal cigarette smoking on pregnancy complications and sudden infant death syndrome', *Journal of Family Practice* 40: 385–94.

Doll, R. (1983) 'Prospects for prevention', *British Medical Journal* 280: 445–53.

Doll, R., Peto, R., Wheatley, K., Gray, R., and Sutherland, I. (1994) 'Mortality in relation to smoking: 40 years observations on male British doctors', *British Medical Journal* 309: 901–11.

Drummond, M. F. (1980) *Principles of Economic Appraisal in Health Care*, Oxford: Oxford Medical Publication.

Dunt, D. R., Crowley, S. and Day, N. A. (1995) 'Is prevention really better than cure? Parameters of the debate and implications for programme design', *Health Promotion International* 10: 325–34.

Engleman, S. R. and Forbes, J. (1986) 'Economic aspects of health education', *Social Science and Medicine* 22: 443–58.

Fujii, E. T. (1980) 'The demand for cigarettes: further empirical evidence and its implications for public policy', *Applied Economics* 12: 479–89.

Gold, M. R., Siegel, J. E., Russell, L. B., Weinstein, M. C. (1996) *Cost Effectiveness in Health and Medicine*, New York: Oxford University Press.

Grossman, M. (1972) 'On the concept of health capital and the demand for health', *Journal of Political Economy* 80: 223–55.

Grossman, M. and Chaloupka, F. J. (1997) *Cigarette Taxes – the Straw to Break the Camel's Back*. Public Health Reports 112: 290–7.

Hackshaw, A. K., Law, M. R., and Wald, N. J. (1997) 'The accumulated evidence on lung cancer and environmental tobacco smoke', *British Medical Journal* 315: 980–8.

Health Education Authority (1997) *Cost-Effectiveness of Smoking Interventions*, London: HMSO.

Ippolito, P. M. (1981) 'Information and the life cycle consumption of hazardous goods', *Economic Inquiry* 19: 529–58.

Jamrozik, K., Vessey, M., Fowler, G., Wald, N., Parker, G., and Van Vanakis, H. (1984) 'Controlled trial of three different antismoking interventions in general practice', *British Medical Journal* 288: 1499–503.

Johnson, J. (1980) 'Advertising and the aggregate demand for cigarettes: a comment', *European Economic Review* 14: 117–25.

Jones-Lee, M. W. (1976) *The Value of Life: An Economic Analysis*, London: Martin Robertson.

Knack, S. and Keefer, P. (1997) 'Does social capital have an economic payoff? A cross-country investigation', *Quarterly Journal of Economics* 112 (4): 1251–88.

Lomas, J. (1998) 'Social capital and health: Implications for public health and epidemiology', *Social Science and Medicine* 47 (9): 1181–88.

Margolis, P. A., Keyes, L. L., Greenberg R. A. *et al.* (1997) 'Urinary cotinine and parent history as indicators of passive smoking and predictors of lower respiratory illness in infants', *Paediatr. Pulmon.* 23: 417–23.

Metra Consulting Group Ltd (1979) *The Relationship between Total Cigarette Advertising and Total Cigarette Consumption in the U.K.*, London: Metra Consulting Group.

Mooney, G. H. (1977) *The Valuation of Human Life*, London: Macmillan.

—— (1986) *Economics, Medicine and Health Care*, Brighton: Wheatsheaf.

Mooney, G. H., Russell, E. M., and Weir, R. D. (1986) *Choices for Health Care*, 2nd edition, Basingstoke: Macmillan.

Muurinen, J. M. (1982) 'Demand for health: a generalised Grossman model', *Journal of Health Economics* 1: 5–28.

Nutbeam, D. (1998) 'Evaluation health promotion: progress, problems and solutions', *Health Promotion International* 13: 27–44.

Peto, J. (1974) 'Price and consumption of cigarettes: a case for intervention?', *British Journal of Preventive and Social Medicine* 28: 241–5.

Ratcliffe, J., Cairns, J., and Platt, S. (1997) 'Cost-effectiveness of a mass media led anti-smoking campaign in Scotland'. *Tobacco Control* 6: 104–10.

Richmond, R. L., Austin, A., and Webster, I. W. (1986) 'Three year evaluation of a programme by general practitioners to help patients to stop smoking', *British Medical Journal* 292: 803–6.

Rosser, R. and Kind, P. (1978) 'A scale of valuations of states of illness: is there a social consensus?', *International Journal of Epidemiology* 7(4): 347–58.

Russell, M. A. H. (1973) 'Changes in cigarette price and consumption in men in Britain, 1946–71: a preliminary analysis', *British Journal of Preventive and Social Medicine* 27: 1–7.

Russell, M. A. H., Wilson, C., Taylor, C., and Baker, C. D. (1979) 'Effects of general practitioner advice against smoking', *British Medical Journal* 2: 234–5.

Sheill, A. and Hawe, P. (1966) 'Health promotion community development and the tyranny of individualism', *Health Economics* 5: 241–7.

Spoth, R. (1989) 'Applying conjoint analysis of consumer preferences to the development of utility responsive health promotion programs', *Health Education Research* 4: 439–49.

Spoth, R. (1991) 'Smoking cessation program preferences associated with stage of quitting', *Addictive Behaviours* 16: 427–80.

Spoth, R. and Redmond, C. (1993) 'Identifying program preferences through conjoint analysis: illustrative results from a parent sample', *American Journal of Health Promotion* 8: 124–33.

Stewart, P. J. and Rosser, W. W. (1982) 'The impact of routine advice on smoking cessation from family physicians', *Canadian Medical Association Journal* 126: 1051–4.

Stoddart, J. J. and Miller, T. (1995) 'Impact of parental smoking on the prevalence of wheezing respiratory illness in children', *American Journal of Epidemiology* 141: 96–102.

Stjernfeldt, M., Berglund, K., Lindsten, J., and Ludvigsson, J. (1986) 'Maternal smoking during pregnancy and risk of childhood cancer', *Lancet* i: 1350–2.

Sumner, M. T. (1971) 'The demand for tobacco in the U.K'., *The Manchester School* 39: 23–36.

Tobacco Advisory Council (1981) *Advertising Controls and Their Effects on Total Cigarette Consumption*, London: TAC.

Tobin, M. V. *et al.* (1987) 'Cigarette smoking and inflammatory bowel disease', *Gastroenterology* 93: 316–21.

Tolley, K. (1993) *Health Promotion: How to Measure Cost-Effectiveness*, London: HEA.

van der Pol, M. and Ryan, M. (1966) 'Using conjoint analysis to establish consumer preferences for fruit and vegetables', *British Food Journal* 98: 5–12.

Wald, N. J., Nanchahal, K., Thompson, S. G., and Cuckle, H. S. (1986) 'Does breathing other people's tobacco smoke cause lung cancer?', *British Medical Journal* 293: 1217–22.

West, R. R. (1985) 'Valuation of life in long run health care programmes', *British Medical Journal* 291: 1139–41.

Williams, A. (1990) 'Screening for risk of CHD: is it a wise use of resources?', in M. Oliver, M. Ashley-Miller, and D. Wood (eds) *Strategy for Screening for Risk of Coronary Heart Disease*, London: Wiley.

Wilson, D., Wood, G., Johnston, N., and Sicurella, J. (1982) 'Randomized clinical trial of supportive follow-up for cigarette smokers in a family practice', *Canadian Medical Association Journal* 126: 127–9.

Woods, O. J., Cullen, M. J., and Dorrnan, R. H. (1980) 'The prevention of coronary heart disease in general practice', *Journal of the Royal College of General Practitioners* 30: 52–7.

9 Communication theory and health promotion

Gordon Macdonald

Communication is an essential building block for health promotion; without actual communication little could be done to improve population health whether one adopts a lifestyle or structuralist approach to public health improvement. Communication also forms the bedrock of innovation-diffusion theory, which in turn is one of the most tested and applied theories in health promotion practice. This chapter discusses communication ideas before describing and critiquing innovation-diffusion theory. It provides some applied examples of how the theory has helped health promotion practice.

Communication at its very simplest involves a communicator or communication event, a message, and a recipient. This communication act is the basic building block for all social relationships. It is the means by which all information and knowledge are transmitted. The communicator uses a series of signs or symbols which he or she encodes in a message. The recipient, once his or her attention is aroused, decodes the message and, if motivated, acts on the information received. In essence the communication event is to do with the conveyance of meaning. The effectiveness of any given message influences the degree to which it is decoded and acted upon. Communication used in this sense is as much to do with persuasion as it is to do with informing: it is not therefore to be confused with communication in an educational sense (see Chapter 5). It is more akin to training (as in education and training) since it attempts to develop certain attitudes and forms of behaviour. A great deal of research has gone into the development of persuasive communication and a useful bibliography lists over 25,000 studies (Lipstein and McGuire 1978).

The simplistic model of communication noted above is developed into something much more substantial by McGuire (1978). In his persuasion/communication matrix he cites five communication or input variables (see Figure 9.1) which further develop the three outlined above. Each of these five input variables – source, message, channel, receiver, and destination – can be subdivided again into four, five, or even six further dependent variables. The variables contributing to source, for example, could be credibility, likeability, power, quantity, and demography; or to message they could be appeal, style, organization, and quantity; to channel they would be mass media, directness (essentially one-to-one), and human sensory modes; to receiver they would

Input: Communication variables	Source					Message				Channel	Receiver	Destination
Output: Steps in being persuaded	Credibility	Likability	Power	Quantity	Demographics	Appeal	Style	Organization	Quantity	Mass media Directness Human sensory modes	Demographic characteristics Personality traits Receiver attitudes/belief characteristics	Cognitive/behavioural traits Product- or practice-based impact
Exposure Simple exposure Attention to communication												
Emotional Response Aroused Affect					(See text for details of columns and rows subdivisions)							
Encoding Attention to content Perception Learning Remembering												
Acceptance												
Overt Behaviour												
Consolidation												

Figure 9.1 The communication/persuasion matrix, indicating the divisions on the output (persuasion) side
Source: Lipstein and McGuire (1978)

be demographic characteristics, personality traits, and receiver attitude/belief characteristics; and finally to destination (in the sense of the ultimate goal of the communication) they would be cognitive/behavioural targets and whether the final impact was product or practice based.

On the vertical axis of the matrix, six output variables are listed which are a great deal less controllable than the input variables. These independent variables include exposure to the message (if the communication is to have any persuasive impact at all); second, information perception; third, the essentials of the communication must be encoded (comprehended and stored); fourth, the message must be acceptable; fifth, overt behaviour in line with the communicator's intent must follow; and finally there should be some form of post-behavioural consolidation. The matrix may be viewed in terms of the vertical axis representing the persuasion output and the horizontal axis representing the communication input. In very general terms and accepting a non-linear progression, the further down and to the right the communication goes, the more successful it becomes. In other words, when the communication has reached the consolidation/destination intersection then it has reached the intended extent of the message originator.

McGuire's persuasion/communication matrix represents a scheme for understanding the psychological, physical, and spatial considerations associated with communication even though it may be criticized for breaking up what is a continuous and on-going process into fragmented boxed sections. This process is of crucial importance if the communication is concerned with a new idea, practice, or product since it is the intention of the communicator to promote adoption of the innovation. Effective communication and the diffusion and adoption of new ideas and practices should be essential features in all health promotion programmes. Innovation-diffusion theory as a distinct branch of wider communication theories can offer a valuable contribution to the theoretical base for health education and health promotion. This chapter will describe the critical features of innovation-diffusion theory, propose some criticism of it, and yet show, with the aid of one or two examples, how it can be of use in the broader development of health promotion as a discipline.

Lipstein and McGuire were concerned with establishing a framework for communication for public health lifestyle changes, and this has been built upon by other theorists and academics in more recent times. Public health communication is not only concerned with lifestyle changes *per se*, but with how individuals receive and perceive public health messages in relation to risk. The debate between the so-called social dimension or 'amplification' of risk and the more cognitive/psychological lifestyle perception of risk communications is illustrated by Pidgeon *et al.* (1999). They argue for the case that puts communication about risk within a social context that allows for what went before (the risk communication) but also pays attention to the content of the risk communication and its possible cognitive interpretation.

Others (for example, Guttman 2000) have been more concerned with the moral and ethical dilemmas facing public health authorities when formulating and disseminating public health measures. Guttman argues that public health messages are not value free and in many instances 'persuade' individuals and communities to question or alter their own values. Little of these issues relating to risk communication and ethical dilemmas facing public health communicators are evident in most research reporting on innovation-diffusion programmes. More of this later; first we need to describe the theory.

Innovation-diffusion theory

The origins of innovation-diffusion research and discipline development can be traced back to the nineteenth century when British and German social anthropologists developed forms of diffusion theory in attempting to explain why a particular society adopts new practices and ideas. These theories were picked up by the French sociologist Tarde (1903) who pioneered the 'S'-shaped diffusion curve and the idea of the pivotal role of opinion leaders. However, it was not until the middle of the twentieth century that a truly new paradigm emerged with the publication of a study on the diffusion of a new hybrid corn in Iowa by Ryan and Gross (1943). This study is referred to again later in this chapter, but it is worth noting at this stage that, although diffusion research is a particular type or branch of communication research, it mostly developed in academic departments, such as psychology, anthropology, and sociology. Until the 1960s there were few, if any, departments specializing in communication studies anywhere in the world. The classical 'model' developed for the communication of innovations identifies four key elements, namely an innovation (1) which is communicated through certain channels (2) over a period of time (3) to members of a social system (4) (Schramm and Lerner 1978).

An innovation has been defined (Rogers 1995) as an idea or practice or object perceived as new by an individual. It is the perceived newness of the idea that largely determines the individual's reaction to it. It matters little to the individual just how objectively new an idea or practice is. Robertson (1971) however attempted to define degrees of newness or innovation. A continuous innovation causes the least disruption of the conventional consumption patterns of a community or individual. Examples of a continuous innovation, in the context of health promotion, are adding fluoride to toothpaste or reducing sugar content in jam. A dynamically continuous innovation involves more disruption than a continuous innovation; it need not involve new consumption patterns but it often involves a new product that alters behaviour in some way, for example an electric toothbrush. Finally, a discontinuous innovation is one that involves a new product or practice and involves new consumption patterns and forms of behaviour. Examples here might be exercise bicycles, television, or aerobics.

This categorization of Robertson's is more applicable to commercial products rather than to innovation in terms of behaviour related to health.

Even the distinction by Brown (1981) between a consumer innovation like a television set and a technological innovation like robotic production lines does little to clarify the situation. In relation to this chapter, the author is far more interested in an innovation that concerns new forms of behaviour and practices, particularly in how they apply to health, as opposed to product innovation, although the latter may well accompany new forms of lifestyle. Innovation-diffusion theory and practice can then be related back to basic communication theory.

Innovation requires communication. In the basic model of source – message – recipient, outlined at the beginning of the chapter, the message element as well as the recipient becomes of paramount importance. With an innovation there is introduced a degree of uncertainty since to the individual recipient, the message is the innovation and therefore subjectively new. This is the unique and peculiar nature of the diffusion of innovations.

Diffusion, on the other hand, is the process by which an innovation is communicated. The diffusion is communicated by a variety of channels over a period of time within a social system or community. It is a process of convergence rather than divergence; that is, it is concerned with a two-way flow of communication between the source of the innovation and the recipient of it. Diffusion is, as a result, concerned with social change, since when new ideas are forthcoming and disseminated they are either adopted or rejected, both of which lead to certain consequences, and social change is likely to occur.

The classical model of diffusion (briefly referred to above) identified four main elements or constituents of diffusion. These four elements are common to all diffusion research. They are (i) the innovation, (ii) the communication channels, (iii) the time lapse, and (iv) the social system or community (Figure 9.2).

Similarly, any communication of innovations is subject to generalization relating to the nature of the communication and the speed with which it is adopted, evaluated, and accepted. Rogers and Shoemaker (1971) have derived a set of 103 generalizations from major research projects on adoption-diffusion and produced an adoption model based on four functional stages. These stages, summarized below, relate to traditional approaches or models in diffusion studies.

Rogers and Shoemaker	*Traditional*
1 Knowledge	1 Awareness
	2 Information
2 Persuasion	3 Evaluation
3 Decision	4 Trial adoption
4 Adoption (or rejection)	5 Adoption

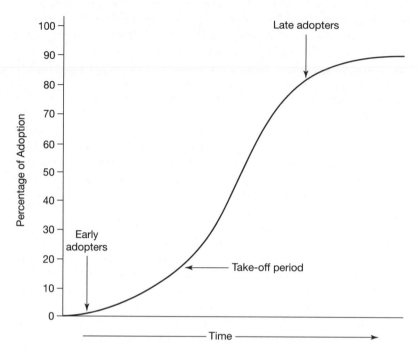

Figure 9.2 The S-shaped diffusion curve

The traditional model first conceptualized by rural sociologists at Iowa State University (Ryan and Gross 1943) consists of five stages. The awareness stage for the individual is characterized by the fact that s/he first learns of the innovation, but has no detailed knowledge. At the second stage the person seeks further information about the innovation and possibly considers usage. The evaluation stage could mean the mental adoption by the individual. This would involve weighing up the pros and contra-indications for adoption. The next stage includes the trial of the innovation (in some small way) to determine its value. At the final adoption stage the individual would decide whether to use the innovation on a large scale or not.

Rogers and Shoemaker's model makes one or two modifications. First, their knowledge stage is essentially a combination of the awareness and information process from the traditional model. Second, the persuasion stage is characterized by the individual attempting to form favourable or unfavourable attitudes towards the innovation. The recipient then engages in activities designed to test the acceptability of the idea (decision stage) and this loosely relates to the trial adoption stage, but it is at the fourth stage that Rogers and Shoemaker's model deviates the most radically from the traditional approaches in that they build into it the distinct possibility of rejection or discontinuity and this is a useful contribution.

Both models rely heavily on the rational conceptualization of decision making (knowledge leads to attitude shift which leads to changed practice or adoption) and not necessarily on human motivation or behaviour in the real world. The stages are not necessarily sequential, in that the individual may evaluate without first seeking knowledge or may trial adopt before going through the persuasion/evaluation stage. Similarly, an individual may lose interest and reject the innovation at any stage rather that wait until the final stage as indicated in both models. Perhaps a more realistic model is illustrated in Figure 9.3. Whilst it represents a sequential course for the individual during the diffusion, there is more flexibility in it and it does allow movement between any of the stages or indeed stage omissions.

Whichever model is adopted and whichever sequence is followed by the individual, the whole adoption process is something of a mental exercise for anyone exposed to an innovation; that is, the individual passes through a

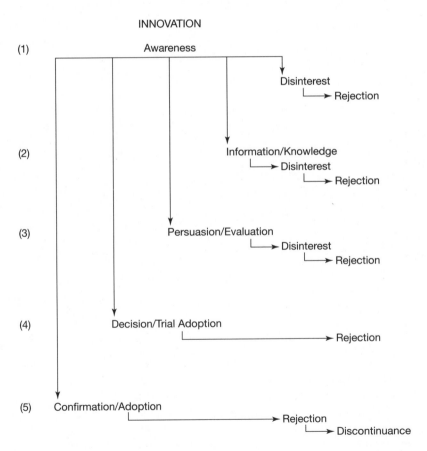

Figure 9.3 Innovation-diffusion stages

series of stages relating to adoption-diffusion from when first learning of the
new idea to its final adoption.

There are, however, three other important mitigating factors associated
with adoption-diffusion: time, information source, and acceptance variables.

For many innovations an S-shaped curve has characterized full diffusion.
Ryan and Gross demonstrated in their study of the adoption of hybrid seed
corn within a farming community that it took 14 years for the product to be
fully accepted and adopted and that the cumulative adoption percentage
followed the S-shape with a 5-year lag period between awareness and
adoption (Figure 9.4).

The information source is a second contributory factor in determining not
only the rate of adoption but also the speed of communication and credibility
attached to the innovation. Specific information sources relate more closely
to particular stages of adoption. Mass media, crucially television, play an

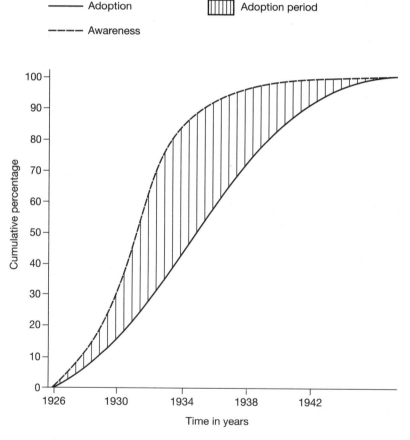

Figure 9.4 Adoption of hybrid seed corn in two Iowa farm communities
Source: Ryan and Gross (1943)

important role in the early stages concerned with information and awareness but are less significant in the later stages. Here interpersonal sources such as friends and known experts become far more important and are considered critical during the evaluation and the (trial) adoption stages. This construct was supported by Yarbrough *et al.* (1970) when they too examined rank orders of information sources reported by farmers in the Midwest of the USA. It also lends weight to the argument that mass media serve to inform and raise awareness admirably but they have limited effect in changing opinions or behaviour.

Acceptance variables that might influence the degree or rate at which an innovation is taken up are numerous, but may be divided roughly into social structure variables and individual characteristics. Social structures or systems can play a critical role in determining the speed of diffusion. If the system norm and the hierarchical structure are such that innovation is encouraged, then acceptance rates will be higher than in a more traditional static structure. Similarly, if the directive for change is imposed from the top rather than allowing a 'free market' approach to the innovation or an approach that involves consensus and elaborate conferring, then the change will be most rapid.

Individual character variables vary the rate of acceptance principally in two ways. First, if the individual perceives the innovation as having a clearly recognizable advantage over existing practices in terms of cognition and use, then acceptance and adoption are more likely. Second, individuals accept change at varying times from awareness onset depending on a whole host of economic, political, and social reasons as well as psychological ones. Nevertheless diffusion researchers (DeFleur and Ball-Rokeach 1975; Janis *et al.* 1959; Lazarsfeld 1963) have attempted to relate the normal diffusion distribution curve divided into standard deviation units with personal and psychological characteristics of adopters and arrived at five labels. Innovators (2.5 per cent) are the first to adopt, followed by early adopters (13.5 per cent), early majority (34 per cent), late majority (34 per cent), and finally late adopters (16 per cent). This categorization of adopters (and the details various researchers have attributed to their characters and personalities) needs, however, further analysis.

A final but important acceptance variable and one that relates very much to health education/promotion diffusion is the apparent importance a change agent makes. A change agent or project/research worker employed to promote or monitor an innovation practice or programme can play, and indeed perhaps should play, a positive role in diffusion and adoption. This is more likely if the agent is client-centred rather than agency-centred; that is, they can relate to and identify with the concerns of the clients and are not perceived as somehow 'different'. This is why curriculum projects for schools have a better chance of take-up and adoption if teachers are involved with both the project writing and development and the implementation in school (Becher and Maclure 1978).

The change agent may be defined as an individual (or indeed organization) who influences the recipient's (of the innovation) decisions about that innovation, particularly in the direction deemed desirable by the change agency. In the vast majority of cases, the change agent seeks to promote the adoption of new ideas, policies, or practices. Only occasionally will the change agent attempt to slow down the diffusion process or prevent the adoption.

The change agent acts as a kind of link between the change agency which developed the innovation (or promoted its dissemination) and the recipient of the innovation, often referred to as the client or client system, since it may be an organization and not an individual. However, if there were no social or technical difference between the change agency and the client system, then there would be little need for a change agent. One of the principal tasks of the change agent is to mediate and reduce the differences that exist between the agency and the client. These differences centre around the degrees of technical expertise available within the change agency compared to that available in the client system – what Rogers (1995) has referred to as heterophily. In many cases it can cause problems for the change agent since their loyalties may be divided between the change agency and the client. Nevertheless, if the innovation is to be successfully diffused, then the change agent is a key link. The agent must however display and exhibit certain characteristics if the diffusion process is to succeed. First, the change agent should attempt to reduce the degree of heterophily between agency and client by developing homophily with the client system or individuals within that system. This may mean in practice that the agent positively seeks out those individuals who are similar in class, status, and educational attainment to themselves (Roling *et al.* 1976). Second, whilst the change agent may need to empathize with clients and the client agency, the degree of success in the diffusion process is much more likely to depend on the rate of effort the agent puts into the communication activities (Fliegel 1966). Third, change agents need to make continued contact with all types of adoption categories within the client system if the diffusion process is to be comprehensive. In an agricultural diffusion study in Brazil (Rogers *et al.* 1970), contact with potential adopters was made up as follows:

Innovators	20
Early adopters	15
Early majority	12
Late majority	5
Laggards	3

Change agent contact is an important variable in innovation-diffusion. This contact does however tend to go through seven key stages no matter what the nature of the diffusion or the type of client system. The first stage is to do with developing awareness of needs in the client; there must be a need for change. The second stage is, or can be, time-consuming in that it involves building client trust in the agent. This is an essential precursor to acceptance of an innovation. Third, the change agent should convert the expressed needs of the client into some form of diagnosis to facilitate the innovation-diffusion process. The fourth stage involves promoting the intent to change, a kind of behavioural intention in the client, with the fifth stage converting that intention into action. Having introduced the adoption, the sixth stage involves ensuring its survival within the client system and preventing discontinuance. Finally, the seventh and last stage is the ending of the working relationship between change agent and client. This is difficult but should involve allowing the client to become self-reliant and, in a sense, their own change agent.

Change agents are, then, critical components of the innovation-diffusion process. But decisions centred around whether to adopt an innovation or not are also determined by the social system or context within which the decision has to be made. Those decisions can either be individual ones or made by some form of authority on behalf of individuals or groups within the system or indeed by groups themselves in the form of a collective decision. Diffusion will probably be most rapid if the decision is authority imposed (Havelock 1974). This is because the decision to accept or reject an innovation is made by a relatively few powerful individuals in a system (organization) who have some 'right' to impose the innovation. The rate of adoption is likely to be slowest with a collective decision because of the need for consensus and close co-ordinated behaviour within the group. Individual or optional decision making concerning an innovation would come somewhere in between and would be affected by such influences as social norms, peer pressure, or communication networks.

Some innovation decision-making processes are in fact a combination of all three types outlined above. For example, the introduction of seat belts in the UK was based on optional decision making: manufacturers and individual car users could decide individually whether to adopt them or not. Legislation was then introduced making car manufacturers include seat belts in cars, although most car manufacturers had already made a collective decision to do this. Finally, in 1983, an authority-based decision was taken to make the wearing of seat belts by car drivers compulsory.

Health promotion projects and innovation-diffusion

Innovation-diffusion is, then, an integral and important component of a more general body of communication theory and can play a unique bridging role in developing the health promoter's understanding of communication theory and techniques. If we consider the introduction of new health promotion curriculum material into schools, we can see the application of diffusion theory to health promotion practice. The inventor(s) or writer(s) of the material may be considered the innovator and the material itself the innovation. The method by which this is promoted to teachers or schools would act as the communication channel; the time period might be one day, one term, or even an academic year; and the social system would be the school or perhaps a local education authority (LEA), or indeed a consortium of LEAs. Each school or LEA would go through the functional stages outlined above and decide whether to adopt or discontinue with the material (the innovation). This would largely depend on support from the opinion leaders (headteachers, advisory teachers, or health promotion co-ordinators) and from the change agents (local or national health promotion agencies or advisory teachers). Ultimately, schools will exhibit the uptake characteristics outlined by Rogers (1995) and fall into one of five categories: innovators, early adopters, early majority, late majority, and laggards.

This outline was followed with the development of many school-based health promotion curriculum projects, when health education and health promotion in schools was still in its infancy. These included the Schools Council Health Education Project materials, the Free to Choose teaching pack, and more recently the Skills for Adolescence and the Drugwise packs both produced by the Teachers' Advisory Council on Alcohol and Drug Education (TACADE). A survey indicated that where good dissemination methods had prevailed, then the likelihood of continuance with the materials was high (Parcel *et al.* 1989, 1995). In this study the researchers studied the diffusion and uptake of the Minnesota Smoking Prevention Program (MSPP) in the States and found that the innovatory programme was more likely to be adopted because it was easy to understand, it appeared superior to existing smoking prevention programmes, and it generated visible results even on a trial basis. Similar claims have been made in the UK with the Family Smoking Education project (FSE) (Newman and Nutbeam 1989; Ledwith and Peers 1988; and more recently Anderson 1999). Two studies measuring school awareness of the innovation (FSE) and factors influencing the adoption of the material (Project Smoke Free Education Group) show that the adoption rate is likely to be affected by the homophily of the change agency. That is, where the material was distributed and disseminated by a local change agent, the likelihood of adoption and maintenance was high.

More recent studies in schools have tended to support these earlier findings. Whether it relates to choices and risk of unwanted pregnancies (Basen-Engquist *et al.* 1997), violence (Orpinas *et al.* 1996), or cardiovascular health (Perry *et al.* 1997), the message appears to be that well-designed innovation-diffusion programmes for schools can work, especially if teachers are involved in the development and dissemination of the materials.

There are similar claims for studies set in the health care system. Cooke *et al.* (2000) report on a programme designed to disseminate a smoking programme to pregnant women attending ante-natal classes. They argue that where clinicians have high self-efficacy, involvement with the programme development and with the dissemination of the programme, then the programme is more likely to be successfully disseminated and sustained. This mirrors the studies relating to schools. A more detailed discussion of innovation-diffusion theory and schools is developed by Macdonald (1997).

The Working with Groups (WWG) package, though developed in the early 1980s in the UK, experienced a classical S-shaped diffusion curve during its dissemination (final report TACADE 1986). The WWG was innovatory because it provided a tangible product and skill for health education and health promotion specialists at a time when there was only a limited appreciation of the need to specialize. The innovators, the authors of the training package, ran a two-day workshop designed to familiarize the attendees with the material. At this stage the potential early adopters could show lack of interest and reject the innovation, but, after evaluation and revision, the package was enthusiastically received by the original attendees. Diffusion of the materials then commenced in earnest. Regional co-ordinators for the dissemination of the package were appointed and trained; they then became, in a sense, the change agents. They were regionally (or locally) based and so exhibited a degree of homophily with potential users of the materials.

Dissemination of the training package took place over the next two years with some startling results. All regions in the UK were exposed to the material, and by the end of 1986 over 700 people had taken part in the training workshops and gone on, in turn, to run similar dissemination courses. The WWG package was adopted on a large scale by health education and promotion specialists and became one of the most popular resource materials used by this professional group. There were a few reasons why this was achieved. First, the package was easily understood and usable; second, it could be adapted to circumstance, that is, used in its entirety, in part, or in conjunction with other material; third, the role of the regional co-ordinators was vital in the cascade approach to the innovation-diffusion through the classical train-the-trainers methodology; fourth, the participatory nature of the materials made it more comprehensible (Macdonald 1986); and, fifth, the network of regional co-ordinators allowed for the sharing of experience and expertise which provided support and development.

Innovation-diffusion theory does have, then, important implications for the dissemination of health promotion projects at local and national levels but it also provides a valuable contribution to health promotion as a discipline (Portnoy *et al.* 1989). There are, however, important caveats and it might be worth considering some of the problems associated with diffusion theory and research before concluding the chapter.

Limitations to diffusion theory

Communication of innovation theory relies heavily on research studies around product diffusion, whether applied to the commercial world or within the ambit of public health policy and health promotion. Research into the dissemination and diffusion of particular health promotion materials within a community intervention programme is fraught with methodological difficulties relating to research design, measurement, and analysis. This chapter is not concerned with the relative merits of using cross-sectional, quasi-experimental, or case study research designs, since the merits of each are dealt with extensively elsewhere (Macdonald *et al.* 1996; Nutbeam *et al.* 1990; Puska *et al.* 1985; Maccoby *et al.* 1977; and indeed to some extent in this book [see Chapter 4]) but there are cautionary tales associated with research design. Essentially, because health promotion projects and programmes are by their very nature dynamic, and because there are still large knowledge gaps in the study of diffusion within health promotion programmes, it is better to use *prospective studies*, or at least a *combination of research designs*, when developing research methodology.

In relation to *measurement*, diffusion research is criterion referenced rather than norm referenced in general. That is, when researchers measure diffusion they tend to use pre-established criteria and not comparative data between social systems. For example, a health promotion intervention that was designed to promote weight loss within a community setting is normally measured in terms of how it compares to a pre-determined standard rather than how it compares to a similar intervention in a workplace setting.

Second, in relation to *analysis*, the focus tends to be on individual outcome factors (Green and Lewis 1986) rather than on larger organizational or social issues such as network analysis. Here as much attention is paid to tracing the progress of the communication of an innovation, investigating such issues as interpretation of the innovation, distortion of the communication, etc., as there is to the eventual quantitative outcome (Hannon and Zucker 1989).

There are, however, other criticisms of innovation-diffusion theory and research, and one of the most serious is the *pro-innovation bias* of researchers (Schramm and Lerner 1978). Here there is an assumption by theorists and researchers that the innovation is a 'good' thing, and should be adopted by everyone. Research methodology has been built around the assumption that innovation is good and so in a way method has followed a non-null hypothesis. Research on innovation-diffusion is often concerned with descriptive analysis of what *is* rather than what *could be*. In other words, there has been little attempt at testing alternative practices through some kind of quasi-case control study. Pro-innovation researchers also fail to take into account issues to do with lack of awareness or ignorance of the innovation, to play down discontinuance of an innovation (see Figure 9.2), or they fail to look at anti-diffusion programmes which are designed to prevent or slow down socially unacceptable new practices (e.g. drug taking). There are two principal reasons for this. First, much diffusion research, in both the USA and the UK at least, is funded by those agencies, essentially change agencies, that have an interest in promoting innovation. Second, those innovations that are highly visible or 'successful' provide a rate of adoption that the researchers can analyse. Obviously an innovation that hasn't been adopted leaves little for researchers to investigate.

Coupled with this pro-innovation bias in diffusion studies is the issue of individual blame bias or victim blaming (similar to the approach used in many early health education programmes). So pro-innovation research bias is reinforced with victim-blaming approaches to assess the adoption of innovations because it is assumed that the innovation is 'good' and should be adopted. Those that do not adopt are labelled 'inadequate' through the use of a number of variables, such as income, educational standards, social class, cosmopolitanism, or exposure to mass media. This emphasis on the individual at the expense of the system has clouded many of the diffusion studies undertaken principally in the United States (Rogers 1995). System blame (the system is responsible to some extent for the decisions behind adoption or rejection of innovations by individuals) might allow for greater objectivity in diffusion research. Caplan and Nelson (1973) argue that diffusion researchers get confused between the cause of an event or condition, which should be subject to scientific evaluation, and the blame for an event or condition, which is subject to values and opinions. Often these values and opinions are those of the researcher or investigator. Blame is more easily attributable to an individual, and as most communication research is conducted at the individual unit level (with the possible exception of anthropological studies), it is not surprising that diffusion research adopts a victim-blaming approach in cases where innovation is rejected or ignored. The problem of victim or system blaming is related to but not central to the ethical issue running through Guttman's (2000) work on values and ethical dilemmas. He concentrates on public health communication more generally but provides useful frameworks for policy makers and practitioners to monitor and evaluate their programmes against a moral background, which is something innovation-diffusion projects rarely consider.

One of the principal problems associated with the communication of innovation is *time*. In studying a process like diffusion, time is a key ingredient but also a methodological nightmare. Diffusion of innovations takes time and as such either requires well-constructed longitudinal research which pays close attention to process elements within the diffusion or relies heavily on participant recall. Unfortunately, most diffusion studies rely on the latter method (Basch *et al.* 1986).

Essentially the respondents in diffusion research are asked to recall or remember their own history of adoption of an innovation. This method inevitably suffers from recall inaccuracies and may be largely dependent on the respondent's memory or education, or the length of time since the innovation was adopted, or indeed the salience or obviousness of the innovation. One possible solution to this recall problem is to spend more time on process research and to use multiple data-collecting points over a set time period from initial diffusion to the top of the 'S' curve. At each point in time respondents are asked whether they have adopted and what influenced that decision. A good case in point would be where an industry or employer introduces a no-smoking policy: measurements or observations should be made immediately before implementation, during implementation, and immediately after the policy went into effect. Other important steps that could be taken to reduce recall inaccuracy include choosing an innovation that is salient and has been diffused rapidly; pre-testing survey questions and training interviewers; and, finally, verifying respondents' recall by using other source data (if available), for example, medical records, newspapers, and other archival records.

Consequentialism and the problem of equity

Communication of innovation theory was created in Western industrialized societies that subscribed to the idea that technological innovation was 'good' but that it was also the cornerstone to economic and social development. The classical diffusion model, developed in the United States and Europe and based on the Ryan and Gross (1943) study, paid little, if any, attention to social structure and the consequential impact of an innovation on a community. Most studies were conducted, as I have attempted to demonstrate, through empirical data-collecting methods that assumed innovation-diffusion was good and progressive, concentrated on adopters, and analysed the means or medium of communication. When the model was adopted by developing countries in the Third World in the 1960s and 1970s, researchers began to question this dominant paradigm. These Third World scholars began to question whether the classical diffusion model contributed much to economic and/or social development. The issue, they argued (Diaz-Bordenave 1974), was one not simply of adding structural variables to diffusion analyses but examining innovation-diffusion in the context of a completely different social structure. This viewpoint, accompanied by a theoretical rethinking, led to a paradigm shift in conceptions of development. At the heart of this rethinking was whether technology was the necessary prerequisite for economic development. This paradigm shift in innovation-diffusion modelling mirrors to some extent the paradigm shift discussed in Chapter 1 in relation to health promotion theory. The shift may be illustrated below.

Clearly in this 'new' paradigm greater emphasis was placed on a paced programme of development that was socially and culturally sensitive to local economies, that considered egalitarianism as a central issue, and that held developed countries equally to blame for underdevelopment in the Third World.

It produced questions that challenged the classical assumptions associated with innovation-diffusion. These questions centred around the likely consequences of an innovation in terms of employment or unemployment, the equitable distribution of incomes, socio-economic differences, and advantages and disadvantages groups. Additionally, researchers were concerned with the movement of migrant labour from the countryside to urban centres as a result of innovations. They (Beltran 1974; Grunig 1971) began to ask whether the innovation was appropriate for the country's stage of development. Is public welfare at the heart of innovation-diffusion or is it more to do with profit motivation for wealthy industrialists? Of course these concerns were voiced largely in response to technological innovations, but the 'new' paradigm holds true when examining innovation-diffusion concerned with new public policy, schools curriculum development, or a new immunization programme. The difference is that here the innovation may be less salient to the potential adopters but may have longer-term impact. The kernel in the argument of the researchers developing the 'new' paradigm is that it is the social structure which largely determines the nature and degree of adoption of an innovation rather than the individual characteristics of the adopters. Diffusion strategies need, therefore, to be aware or take account of social structures if development is to be more equitable and the consequences of the innovation-diffusion are desirable.

Classical paradigm of development	*New paradigm of development*
1 Economic growth	1 Equality of distribution
2 Capital intensive technology	2 Improving the quality of life Emphasis on relevant technology.
3 Centralized planning of development	3 Self-reliance in development at local level
4 Mainly *internal* causes of underdevelopment	4 Internal *and* external causes of underdevelopment

Source: Adapted from Rogers (1995)

Generalizations

Rogers and Shoemaker (1971) outline 103 generalizations related to the communication of innovations based on research findings over a number of years. Some academics (Downs and Mohr 1976) have questioned the reliability of these diffusion generalizations, stating that

> perhaps the most alarming characteristic of the body of empirical study of innovation is the extreme variance among its findings, what we [Downs and Mohr] call instability . . . this occurs with relentless regularity. One should certainly expect some variation in social science research, but the record in the field of innovation is beyond interpretation. In Rogers and Shoemakers' own evaluation the reliability rates vary from as low as 15–20 per cent to as high as 75–80 per cent.

Four generalizations do score well however and it might be worthwhile examining these briefly before concluding the chapter.

1   The first generalization concerns time and the adoption period. Full diffusion of most major innovations follows the S-shaped diffusion curve

as pioneered by Ryan and Gross (1943), and as outlined in Figure 9.2. Diffusion time varies from 7 years (adoption of penicillin by physicians) to 50 years (adoption of kindergartens by education authorities in the USA (Yarbrough 1981).

2   The second generalization concerns the rate of adoption and states that the rate of acceptance of an innovation varies according to (i) the characteristics of the innovation and (ii) the attributes of the individual adoption units (adopter characteristics). Innovations are more rapidly adopted if they are salient and offer a demonstrable advantage over existing practice, if they are easy to understand and use, and if they can be used on a trial basis initially. Microwave ovens might be a useful example here. Second, the characteristics of individual adopters demand more attention from communication researchers than all other aspects of diffusion theory put together; therefore the generalization that the time of adoption by individual adoption units is related to the character-istics of the adoption unit is borne out by extensive research. Since the rate of diffusion approximates to a normal distribution curve, researchers have separated the diffusion curve into standard deviation units and then examined the characteristics of the individual adopters falling into these five deviation units. The innovators who comprise the first unit are characteristically venturesome and scientific, have a high educational standard, think abstractly, and tend to be leaders in large organizations. They, unlike the last adopter unit (laggards), are typically more technically competent and have greater wealth but they are unlikely to be opinion leaders in local communities. These are much more likely to be members of the second and third units of adoption, namely early adopters and the early majority respectively.

3   The third generalization concerns the stages adopters go through in the adoption process and it states that several functional stages are involved in the diffusion process by units of adopters. In Rogers and Shoemaker's model these included knowledge, persuasion, decision, and confirmation but could be adapted to allow for a five-stage process. In many ways this generalization is borne out by personal experiences, since with any major decision surrounding the take-up of a new idea or product, we need to be aware of the innovation, be persuaded by its efficacy/usefulness, make a decision based on this, and adopt.

4   The fourth and final generalization relates to information sources and states that the further down the diffusion curve one goes, the more the source of information will change from mass media to interpersonal. Yarbrough and Klongan (1974) found that media sources served only to draw awareness of an innovation to potential adopters and indeed were the most important source of information at the knowledge awareness stage. However, during the decision adoption stage, media sources slipped to third ranking, as interpersonal contact with peers became much more important. This generalization is perhaps the most contentious and many

researchers have questioned it (Coleman *et al.* 1966; Schramm 1977; Maccoby *et al.* 1977). Nevertheless it is important to note that information sources and their impact vary with the type of innovation and the functional stages of adoption.

Conclusion

This chapter, although ostensibly concerned with communication theory, has focused on innovation-diffusion. This is for two fundamental reasons. First, innovation-diffusion research and theory is a key, if not *the* key, to more general communication theory. It is at the heart of the basic model outlined in the first paragraph of the chapter. Without an understanding of how and why new ideas and products are communicated through a community or social system over time, the general body of communication theory would be sadly lacking. Second, work around innovation-diffusion theory allows health promotion specialists to borrow ideas and practices so that programmes, projects, ideas, and policies in health promotion can more easily and readily be diffused and adopted by practitioners. These can be on a large scale like the Stanford and North Karelia programme described in Chapter 2 in this book, or they could be on a much more local scale like the introduction of a new teaching pack in a school or the introduction of a 'trim trail' in the local community. As professional researchers often plead that good research can be achieved on a low-budget small-scale project, so innovation theory can be adapted to small, locally based programmes. The theory only provides a framework for practice, or, perhaps more importantly and in keeping with the tone of this book, the practice should inform and mould the theory. As mentioned above, innovation-diffusion theory has undergone a paradigm shift that now allows it to take cognizance of social structure. Practitioners working within that social structure have the opportunity to determine the shape and nature of that shift.

References

Anderson, K. (1999) *Young People and Alcohol, Drugs and Tobacco*, Copenhagen: WHO Regional Publications. European Series No. 66.

Basch, C. E., Eveland, J. D., and Portnoy, B. (1986) 'Diffusion systems for education and learning about health', *Family and Community Health* 9 (2): 1–26.

Basen-Engquivst, K., Parcel, G., Harrist, R., Kirby, D., Coyle, K., Banspach, S., and Rugg, D. (1997) 'The safer choices project; methodological issues in school based health promotion intervention research', *Journal of School Health* 67 (9): 365–71.

Becher, T. and Maclure, S. (1978) *The Politics of Curriculum Change*, London: Hutchinson.

Beltran, L. (1974) 'Rural development and social communication: relationships and strategies', in R. Crawford and W. Ward (eds) *Communication Strategies for Rural Development*, Proceedings of Cornell-CIAT International Symposium.

Brown, L. A. (1981) *Innovation-Diffusion – A New Perspective*, London: Methuen.

Caplan, N. and Nelson, S. (1973) 'On being useful: the nature and consequences of psychological research on social problems', *American Psychologist* 28: 199–24.

Coleman, J., Katz, E., and Menzel, H. (1966) *Medical Innovation: A Diffusion Study*, New York: Bobbs-Merrill.

Cook, M. *et al.* (2000) 'The dissemination of a smoking cessation programme; predictors of programme awareness, adoption and maintenance', *Health Promotion International* 15: 113–24.

DeFleur, M. and Ball-Rokeach, S. (1975) *Theories of Mass Communication*, New York: David McKay.

Diaz-Bordenave, J. (1974) 'Communication and adoption of agricultural innovation in Latin America', in R. Crawford and W. Ward (eds) *Communication Strategies for Rural Development*, Proceedings of Cornell-CIAT International Symposium.

Downs, G. and Mohr, L. (1976) 'Conceptual issues in the study of innovation', *Administrative Science Quarterly* 21: 700–14.

Fliegel, F. (1966) 'Attributes of innovations as factors in diffusion', *American Journal of Sociology* 72: 235–48.

Green, L. W. and Lewis, F. M. (1986) *Measurement and Evaluation in Health Education and Health Promotion*, Palo Alto, CA: Mayfield.

Grunig, J. (1971) 'Communication and the economic decision-making processes of Columbian peasants', *Economic Development and Cultural Change* 19: 580–97.

Guttman, N. (2000) *Public Health Communications: Values and Ethical Dilemmas*, Thousand Oaks, CA: Sage.

Hannon, P. J. and Zucker, D. M. (1989) 'Analysis issues in school-based health promotion studies', *Health Education Quarterly* 16 (2): 315–20.

Havelock, R. (1974) *Educational Innovation in the United States*, Vol. 1, Michigan: University of Michigan Report.

Janis, I. L. *et al.* (1959) *Personality and Persuasibility*, New Haven, CT: Yale University Press.

Lazarsfeld, P. (1963) 'Mass media and personal influence', in W. Schramm (ed.) *The Science of Communication*, New York: Basic Books.

Ledwith, F. and Peers, I. (1988) 'Development and National Dissemination of Smoking Education of Schools', University of Manchester (unpublished).

Lipstein, B. and McGuire, W. (1978) *Evaluating Advertising: A Bibliography of the Communications Process*, New York: Advertising Research Foundation.

Maccoby, N., Farquhar, J. W., Wood, P. D., and Alexander, J. K. (1977) 'Reducing the risk of cardiovascular disease effects of a community-based campaign on knowledge and behaviour', *Journal of Community Health* 3: 100–14.

Macdonald, G. (1986) 'Participation is the best form of learning', *Journal of Health at School* 2: 3.

—— (1997) 'Innovation diffusion theory and its application to health education in schools', in M. Siddel, I. Jones, J. Katz, and A. Peberdy (eds) *Debates and Dilemmas in Promoting Health*, London: Macmillan.

Macdonald, G., Veen, C., and Tones, K. (1996) 'Evidence for success in health promotion; suggestions for improvement', *Health Education Research* 11 (3): 367–76.

McGuire, W. (1978) *Evaluating Advertising: A Bibliography of the Communications Process*, New York: Advertising Research Foundation.

Newman, R. and Nutbeam, D. (1989) 'The Family Smoking Education Project: what do teachers think of it?', *Health Education Journal* 48: 9–14.

Nutbeam, D., Smith, C., and Catford, J. (1990) 'Evaluation in health education: a review of progress, possibilities and problems', *Journal of Epidemiology and Community Health* 44: 83–9.

Orpinas, P., Kelder, S., Murray, N., Fourney, A., Conroy, J., McReynolds, L., and Peters, R. (1996) 'Critical issues in implementation of a comprehensive violence prevention programme for middle schools; translating theory into practice', *Education and Urban Society* 28 (4): 456–72.

Parcel, G. *et al.* (1989) 'Translating theory into practice: intervention strategies for the diffusion of a health promotion innovation', *Family and Community Health* 12 (3): 1–13.

Parcel, G. S. *et al.* (1995) 'Diffusion of an effective tobacco prevention program. Part ii: Evaluation of the adoption phase', *Health Education Research* 10 (3): 297–307.

Perry, C., Sellers, D., Johnson, C., Pedersen, S., Bachman, K., Parcel, G., Stone, E., Leupker, R., Wu, M., Nader, P., and Cook, K. (1997) 'The child and adolescent trial for cardiovascular health' (CATCH), *Journal of School Health* 60: 406–13.

Pidgeon, N., Henwood, K., and Maguire, B. (1999) 'Public health communication and the social amplification of risks: present knowledge and future prospects', in P. Bennett and K. Calman (eds) (1999) *Risk Communication and Public Health*, Oxford: Oxford Medical Publications.

Portnoy, B., Anderson, D. M., and Eriksen, M. (1989) 'Application of diffusion theory to health promotion research', *Family and Community Health* 12 (3): 63–71.

Puska, P., Nissinen, A., Tuomilehto, J. *et al.* (1985) 'The community based strategy to prevent coronary heart disease: conclusions from ten years of the Karelia Project', *Annual Review of Public Health* 6: 147–63.

Robertson, T. S. (1971) *Innovative Behaviour and Communications*, New York: Holt, Rinehart & Winston.

Rogers, E. (1995) *Diffusion of Innovations*, New York: The Free Press.

Rogers, E. *et al.* (1970) *Diffusion of Innovations in Brazil, Nigeria and India*, Michigan: Michigan State University Research Report No. 24.

Rogers, E. M. and Shoemaker, F. F. (1971) *Communication of Innovations: A Cross-cultural Approach*, New York: The Free Press.

Roling, N. *et al.* (1976) 'The diffusion of innovations and the issue of equity in rural development', *Communication Research* 3: 155–70.

Ryan, B. and Gross, N. C. (1943) 'The diffusion of hybrid seed corn in two Iowa communities', *Rural Sociology* 8: 15–24.

Schramm, W. (1977) *Big Media, Little Media: Tools and Technology for Instruction*, London: Sage.

Schramm, W. and Lerner, D. (eds) (1978) *Communication and Change: The Last Ten Years – and the Next*, Honolulu: University Press of Hawaii.

TACADE (1986) *Monitor* 3(1).

Tarde, G. (1903) *The Laws of Imitation*, New York: Holt.

Yarbrough, P. (1981) 'Communication theory and nutrition education research', *Journal of Nutrition Education* 13 (1): 16–26.

Yarbrough, P. and Klongan, G. (1974) *Adoption and Diffusion of Innovations – Research Findings in Community Dental Health – Organizing for Action*, Sociology Report No. 113, Iowa State University.

Yarbrough, P., Klonglan, G., and Lutz, G. (1970) *System and Personal Variables as Predictors of Individual Adoption of Behavior*, Sociology Report No. 86, Iowa State University.

10 Social marketing and health promotion

Craig Lefebvre

Social marketing is an orientation to health promotion in which programmes are developed to satisfy consumers' needs, strategized to reach the audience(s) in need of the programme, and managed to meet organizational objectives (Lefebvre and Flora 1988). It is a set of principles and techniques that derive from a theoretical perspective based in marketing as it has been developed and practised in the business sector; however, social marketing practitioners borrow heavily from other disciplines (many of them reviewed in other chapters of this book) in conceptualizing approaches to changing people's attitudes and behaviours.

In one respect, social marketing has existed as long as people have sought to 'win people's hearts and minds'. Social marketing is concerned with introducing and disseminating new ideas and issues (Fine 1981) and increasing the prevalence of specific behaviours among target groups. Thus, when we examine major religious and political leaders, artists and scholars, social advocates and philosophers over the years, we are looking at people who were, at one level or another, social marketers. The extent to which these people are known to us, the impact their lives had in their own time, as well as now, and the endurance of their ideas reflect as much their success – or that of their followers – to 'market' the ideas as they do their creativity, intellect, and influence on improving people's lives. However, the term 'social marketing' was formally coined by Kotler and Zaltman (1971) to define a process in which marketing techniques and concepts are applied to social issues and causes instead of products and services.

Social marketing has evolved from business practices in which a 'product' and 'sales' orientation have been supplanted by a 'consumer' one. That is, businesses are now more likely to focus on consumers' wants and needs and trying to meet them than they are on simply producing whatever they like and then trying to convince consumers to buy it. In health promotion the parallel process has been from a more traditional 'top-down' approach in which authorities prescribe, or proscribe, health and social behaviours, and perhaps launch information campaigns to support the programmes, to 'bottom-up' efforts where the needs and wants of the people are actively solicited, attended to, and acted upon in programme planning, delivery, management, and evaluation. At its most simple, social marketing is a consumer-orientated approach that creates 'win-win' situations for all parties. Yet, as this chapter will illustrate, it is a very systematic approach to health and social issues that is limited only by the imagination of the social marketing programme.

With this overview of social marketing, it is also important to state what it is not. Social marketing is not social control; it is not focused only on changing individuals' beliefs, attitudes, and behaviours; it is not simply mass media campaigns; and it is not easy. Social marketing is a method of empowering people to be totally involved and responsible for their well-being; a problem-solving process that may suggest new and innovative ways to attack health and social problems (e.g. Manoff 1985; Novelli 1984); it is a comprehensive strategy for effecting social change on a broad scale (Lefebvre and Flora 1988); and it requires careful planning, research, and management to implement effectively.

This chapter begins with a review of the eight essential characteristics of a social marketing approach as outlined by Lefebvre and Flora (1988). This will lead to a discussion of the challenges that are posed to social marketers – especially the lack of adequate research to support social marketing's utility and effectiveness. Finally, we will conclude with a review of the field and a focus on the benefits social marketing offers health promotion endeavours.

Characteristics of social marketing

Lefebvre and Flora (1988) propose eight characteristics of social marketing programmes; they are listed in Table 10.1. These components are not necessarily displayed by every programme professing to be a social marketing one, yet the authors stress their importance in the analysis, implementation, management, and evaluation of public health programmes. The next sections describe each component in some detail.

Table 10.1 Social marketing components

Consumer orientation
Exchange theory
Audience segmentation and analysis
Formative research
Channel analysis
Marketing mix
    Message/product/service
    Price
    Place
    Promotion
    Positioning
Process tracking
Management system

Source: Lefebvre and Flora (1988)

Consumer orientation

At the heart of a marketing approach are the consumers one wishes to reach and influence. Two approaches to these consumers are possible. An agency can conceive of its target audience as essentially passive and seek to understand their wants and needs in a context of 'doing something for them'. Such an orientation will often lead to a series of messages/products/services that are designed to meet these needs, but have little direct input from consumers themselves. One weakness of this approach, as will be shown later, is that while great care is given to audience segmentation and analysis, the formative research process is forsaken. A second limitation of this approach to the consumer is most apparent when social marketing programmes are applied in a community organization context. Here we find that the crucial community organization principle of citizen participation in all aspects of programme planning, delivery, and evaluation is sacrificed as well. While many social marketing programmes have met their short-term objectives of changing people's awareness, knowledge, and behaviour, these same programmes often do not address the social and institutional contours that influence individual behaviours nor do they have the community support needed to sustain them over the longer term when external funding cycles are completed (cf. Lefebvre 1990).

The second approach to the consumer is an active one; that is, assuming that consumer input to the proposed programme is a continuing process and not one that occurs at a single point in time. The emphasis of this approach to consumers is to seek to build relationships with them over time and continually offer them opportunities to interact with programme staff. In one variant of this type of approach, lay people from the community become integral parts of the programme and assist in the actual implementation next to the professional staff (Lefebvre *et al.* 1986). Such a structure allows for dialogue between staff and community resident on a daily basis. These volunteers become the representatives of the larger set of 'consumers', and can provide the immediate feedback to staff as to how proposed programmes will be accepted by the community. They can also act as the sentinels for programmes that may not be appropriate to the community, or specific segments of it, because of social, cultural, and political norms not apparent to programme planners.

A consumer orientation does not mean that all health promotion programmes must be grassroots efforts that only build from citizens' concerns. Many health programmes are launched because of epidemiological data gathered by health authorities that identify health problems of sufficient magnitude to warrant attention. In many cases, citizens may not be aware of the scope of a health problem or health risk that has been identified. Consequently, a first priority of an information campaign is to alert the public to the problem. However, it is often the next step, engaging people into the process, that is overlooked by the planners of these programmes. Citizen participation at this stage can lay the foundation for community ownership of the effort and sculpt the next phases of the programme. It is the types of programmes that do not enlist community involvement that are decried as 'experiments in social control'. For health promotion efforts in the coming decades, it is clear that the consumer (read the 'community') must be treated as, and encouraged to be, an active partner in the process.

An orientation that favours the primacy of the consumer is intuitively and philosophically appealing to health promotion professionals; yet there are barriers to them, and their organizations, immediately and wholeheartedly embracing it. Among these barriers are (1) a failure by the organization to define its mission and objectives clearly due to a lack of inter-organizational consensus and inadequate consumer assessment; (2) not identifying key target audiences which results in a lack of focus and poorly targeted needs surveys; (3) pressures that place political/territorial/professional objectives above consumer needs; (4) organizational biases that favour expert-driven programmes; (5) the influence of intermediaries who modify the programmes' messages, products, and services before they reach the target group; and (6) the sense of urgency that often accompanies new initiatives and provides a rationalization for 'short cuts' (cf. Lefebvre and Flora 1988). It is this latter point that especially requires more attention from programme planners and policy makers. Too often it is our search for the 'quick fix' or the imposition of short timelines that leads to inadequate attention to the target group. While this is not to suggest that planning should be a protracted process, time needs to be allocated to secure proper needs assessments and community participation prior to programme implementation.

An orientation to health promotion that has the consumer public at its nexus must not only focus on consumers' wants and needs prior to programme implementation, but has to consider the satisfaction of consumers with the programme after its delivery. Satisfying consumer needs is the major objective of a marketing approach; evaluations of marketing programmes should reflect these issues as much as the 'objective' or 'hard' data of behaviour and physiological change.

Exchange theory

The operational mechanism for marketing practices of all kinds is exchange theory (Kotler 1975). Whether it be an idea, a product, or a service, the offering by one agent (i.e. an individual, group, or organization) is done within a context where the other agent has the choice to 'buy' it or not. Thus, marketing is the voluntary exchange of resources between two or more parties, and includes processes of information dissemination, public relations, lobbying, advocacy, and fund raising (Fine 1981). In social marketing, the resources we seek to exchange with our target audience are usually different from the more common form of exchanges in which money is offered for goods and services (though by no means does this exclude such transactions in a social marketing programme). Rather, social marketing is the exchange of an intangible for an intangible: accepting a new idea and discarding an old custom or adopting a new behaviour and giving up a habit. It is not easy, nor desirable, to try and give monetary value to these types of transactions. However, social marketers must recognize that different economies still come into play as a consumer weighs the costs and benefits of, for example, quitting smoking or using condoms. Consumers pay a price in terms of the time it takes to learn new information or practice new behaviours; they expend cognitive and physical effort; they risk alienating family members and friends when adopting new ideas and practices; and they may be perceived by the community-at-large as being 'different'. Public health agencies, on the other hand, often do not assess their resources appropriately to facilitate such exchanges. Whether it be their financial resources, technical expertise, their ideas, products, or services, these agencies often underestimate their value. The tendency to 'give it away' needs to be examined. The image of a consumer saying 'Why should I if they don't think it's that valuable?' has to be addressed by social marketers before the question is actually asked.

Social marketing involves consumers exchanging resources for new beliefs and behaviours. It is not a simple task to define this exchange tangibly, but it often does not need to be done. Many social marketing programmes become so focused on 'making the intangible tangible' through product and service development coupled with strong advertising campaigns that it is often overlooked that exchanges can still be effected in the cognitive domain alone. The strategy is to create an awareness among consumers that they have a problem and then offer the solution. Commercial marketers have long employed this strategy as they successfully sell everything from soap to deodorants to automobiles. The problem may relate to possible social disapproval or to lowered self-esteem. It may also appeal to more positive benefits such as greater self-confidence and success.

Social marketers sometimes offer solutions to problems that are not well defined for the average consumer. Marketers can take for granted that people are aware of the prevalence and lethality of certain health risks and pose new information and behavioural prescriptions without answering the consumer's basic question: 'What's the benefit to me?' While costs often become the marketers' prime concern in developing a programme it may be the other side of the equation – the benefits – that are of at least equal importance to the consumer. Most consumer behaviour theory suggests that it is the relative balance of costs *and* benefits that leads a consumer to accept a new idea, behaviour, product, or service. While it is important to reduce costs to the consumer to make health accessible to them, it is the perceived benefits that will determine consumer's motivation to access these resources and change. As noted earlier, it is maximizing these benefits, and communicating them clearly to consumers in ways that are meaningful to them, that distinguishes good social marketing practice. Well-crafted marketing programmes meet both consumer needs and organizational objectives (win-win).

Audience segmentation and analysis

Social marketing requires knowledge of target groups, including their sociodemographic, psychological, and behavioural characteristics (Kotler and Roberto 1989). Social marketers may aim at changing attitudes and behaviours of the public-at-large, but they approach this task by selecting and targeting subgroups of this larger population that are homogeneous with respect to one or more characteristics (e.g. lower-class minority males, middle-aged males who are contemplating becoming more physically active, the food buyer for a family). It is the process of identifying and researching these segments that is the foundation, the nucleus of programme development.

Weinstein (1987) has identified four major benefits of audience segmentation and analysis. First, by understanding the unique needs of target groups, messages, products, and services can be developed that meet the needs of those groups; this reinforces the consumer orientation and enhances the prospect of meeting organizational objectives. Segmentation also helps one determine the most cost-efficient ways to promote messages/products/ services to target groups. Segmentation can also place one's programming efforts in relation to other ideas, preferences, or behaviours already held or practised by the target group (the notion of 'positioning'). Finally, segmentation allows for a systematic approach to market coverage, rather than relying on a 'shot-gun' approach to mass marketing in which many groups, often those most in need of the message, are missed.

In developing a segmentation analysis, one must have homogeneity within each segment and heterogeneity between segments on the variable(s) of interest (Weinstein 1987; Fine 1981). Segments should also be of sufficient size to warrant the allocation of organizational resources; should be relevant and meaningful for the message, product, or service to be delivered; and should suggest different marketing mixes for each segment (Weinstein 1987; Fine 1981). However, the actual approach to segmenting a population will be based on organizational objectives, theoretical tenets, and past research and experience. There is no 'right' or 'wrong' approach to segmentation as long as formative research is undertaken to assure the match of theory and experience with present realities. Some variables along which market segmentation may be conducted are shown in Table 10.2.

Market segmentation does not need to be confined to individuals; social systems are also segmentation candidates as well. Social systems are easily divided into sector 'segments' – educational, industry, government, health, etc. These sectors can be further segmented by location (e.g. urban vs. rural health departments), membership size of composite units (e.g. larger school districts vs. smaller ones), type of business (e.g. service industries vs. manufacturing vs. agricultural), current practices (e.g. businesses with active health promotion programmes for employees), organizational factors (e.g. innovativeness, leadership style, employee participation, community involvement), characteristics associated with organizational innovativeness (e.g. centralization, complexity,

Table 10.2 Market segmentation variables

Sociodemographic variables	Behavioural	Psychological
Location (community, neighbourhood)	Use of product/service	Self-esteem
Household size	Benefits sought	Readiness for change
Age	Level of physical activity	Introspective
Sex	Use of leisure time	Sensation seeker
Race	Level of sexual activity	Hedonism
Nationality	Health professional	Achievement orientated
Religion	utilization pattern	Need for independence
Marital status		Societally conscious
Education		Belongers
Occupation		Need for approval
Income		Need for power
Social class		

formalization, interconnectedness, organizational slack, size; Rogers 1983), and many other variables. In developing broad-based health promotion programmes, attention to organizational segmentation is as necessary as population segmentation techniques in crafting comprehensive intervention strategies.

Formative research

Formative research is used here to denote research activities conducted prior to full implementation of a social marketing strategy. Indeed, formative research is best utilized when it contributes to the development of the strategy itself. These research activities include studies of audience segment needs and characteristics, market analyses to determine positioning strategies, pretesting of concepts and messages, and pilot tests of message/product/service acceptability and effectiveness. There are numerous methodologies that the social marketer can employ in designing formative studies including traditional surveys, randomized designs, panel studies, focus groups, convenience samples, 'snowball' sampling (in which early participants suggest others 'like them' for subsequent contact), piggybacking on studies being conducted by other organizations, and reviews of secondary data sources – such as research studies published in scientific and marketing journals, government and private sector reports, marketing studies sponsored by industry, and epidemiological surveys.

Kotler and Andreasen (1987) underscore the importance of engaging in more, not less, market research, and identify five 'myths' that appear to dampen enthusiasm for research activities among the not-for-profit sector. These myths are:

1   *The 'big decision' myth* in which only projects that involve large invest-
    ments of money and/or staff time are deemed suitable for research effort.
    However, the costs of conducting a research project – in terms of monetary
    investment, time needed to complete it, delays in decision making – should
    be analysed in comparison to its potential benefits – improvements in
    decision making from more information, avoiding 'square wheels', possibly
    suggesting new ideas or solutions. Not all formative research involves time-
    consuming and expensive organizational outlays. Qualitative methods
    such as focus groups and consumer panels can be quite efficient in
    providing programme managers a better sense of consumer response than
    simply going with the 'best idea'.

2   *The 'survey myopia' myth* is related to the last comment. Market research
    does not need to consist of only random surveys of target groups with
    their expenses related to design, conduct, data management, analysis,
    interpretation, and report preparation – let alone time. Limited and
    modest research objectives can be met by modest and inexpensive research
    strategies. The key is to elucidate clearly the objective of the research and
    interpret the data in the context in which it was collected.

3   *The 'big bucks' myth* also builds on the first two myths: however, research
    has lower cost alternatives. While there is certainly a sacrifice of one's
    ability to generalize from qualitative research methods, in many instances
    the marketer's objective is to 'get a feel' for the target group, not to draw
    scientifically valid conclusions for the general population.

4   *The 'sophisticated researcher' myth* obscures the notion that organizations
    do not require staff with expertise in sampling design and statistical
    analyses in order to undertake a valuable market research programme.
    What is needed are (a) clear objectives (questions), (b) a strategy that will
    elicit responses from the target group's representatives (however selected)
    in a consistent manner, (c) objective documentation of respondents'
    answers and comments (i.e. audio recordings of focus groups rather than
    a facilitator's overall conclusions; questionnaires that are administered
    and tallied consistently across respondents), (d) staff and other organiza-
    tional resource allocations to fully implement the research protocol, and
    (e) timely feedback of useful information to project managers.

5   *The 'most research is not read' myth* reflects as much a manager's lack
    of interest in, or even fear of, research results as it does the fact that
    researchers and programme managers often do not communicate well
    in identifying the decision that requires additional information and
    how the information needs to be collected and analysed in order to be
    useful to decision makers. These points reinforce the observation that
    managers who are not consumer orientated, but would rather follow
    their own preconceived ideas, will not support market research. However,
    it is also the case that unless 'implementors' and 'evaluators' are working
    together in designing research protocols, the best intentions may go for
    nought.

Even if the only market research an organization does is to challenge each staff member to talk with ten representatives from a target group every week, the ability to stay in close touch with consumers is too important simply to take for granted once the initial 'problem identification' stage of programme planning is completed. For social marketing programmes to be effective, and stay effective over the long-term, a commitment to an on-going market research programme is vital.

Channel analysis

Channel analysis is the specification and understanding of communication and distribution systems as they relate to discrete target groups. Although channel analysis could be considered part of audience analysis and formative research – especially as it relates to identifying appropriate channels through which to reach target populations – it has been separated out here both to reinforce its importance in marketing programmes and also to underscore that channels of message, product, and service distribution are critical to successful programmes.

In their analysis of what constitutes a successful public information campaign, Rice and Atkin (1989) elucidate several components directly relevant to channels:

1   It is necessary to identify and understand the media habits of the target groups.
2   Characteristics of the message source and its media help determine a campaign's effectiveness.
3   The message must reach a sufficiently large proportion of the target population in order for the campaign to be successful in meeting its objectives.
4   Messages must go through multiple channels to ensure their accessibility and appropriateness to the target group.

Lefebvre and Flora (1988) presented several more components of media that need to be considered and explored in channel analysis:

1   Their relative abilities to transmit complex messages.
2   Whether the medium is electronic or print, visual or auditory (or both), and how that will affect message design and delivery as well as audience attention, comprehension, and retention.
3   Their relative costs given their expected reach and impact.
4   Their reach, frequency of message delivery, and the continuity that can be created and controlled by the sponsoring organization.
5   The number of intermediaries that the media require – the more inter-mediaries involved, typically the less control one has over final message structure and content.

6   Each medium's potential for overuse both in terms of oversaturating a market to the extent that the target group 'turns off' the message and becomes inattentive, and the degree to which excessive demands are made on media gatekeepers which then turns them against the organization and future collaborative projects.

7   Each medium's capability to build on, or multiply, the effects achieved through another medium.

In analysing channels, one assumption that is often made by social marketing programmes is to treat channels as if communication of messages is the primary objective. Some authors assert that message design and dissemination are the major tasks of a social marketing programme (Manoff 1985). In many cases this may not be the case. While message delivery may be an important aspect of health promotion, distribution of related products and services is often what achieves the desired results, yet this aspect of channel analysis usually receives little attention. For example, in the DuaLima test market study (Doremus Porter Novelli 1986), many questions about the contraceptive marketing programme revolved around more distribution-driven concerns such as 'What type of retail outlets should be used in getting a new product into the consumer market-place?' 'What margin is required to interest the retail trade in selling the brand (of contraceptive)?' Some of these issues relate to 'Place' decisions as part of the marketing mix; yet, sufficient information needs to be gathered early on in the developmental process to permit better decision making.

The marketing mix

The marketing mix refers to what are historically the four pillars of marketing programmes – the '4 Ps': product, place, price, and promotion. The 'mix' of these four elements to meet the needs of specific market segments is the operationalization of the marketing concept. While the '4 Ps' have carried marketers far in planning and implementing effective campaigns, in today's more competitive market-place (not just for products and services, but ideas as well) one must also incorporate a fifth 'P' into the mix: position. The next sections review each element of the marketing mix.

Product

Fine (1981) provides a useful definition of 'product' as it may be expressed in social marketing programmes: 'anything having the ability to satisfy human needs or wants'. He also points out that the true test of whether this 'thing' is, or is not, a product also rests on its capacity for exchangeability; simply, are people willing to trade for it (i.e. pay a 'price')? Three types of products can thus be defined for social marketers. The first, messages, or the communication of information intended to influence the receiver's attention, knowledge, motivation, and/or behaviour (McGuire 1984), are the most common type of social marketing programme. The dissemination of 'information products' comprises the major thrust of public information, or health communication, campaigns. The creation of messages that are both scientifically sound in content and possess the creative ability to capture attention and reliably communicate the content to the desired audience are necessary features of social marketing programmes. However, it is often the tension between 'science' and 'art' (the content vs. the execution strategy) that leads to less than effective message design. Most health programmes appear to favour 'science' over 'art': what this results in are scientifically sound messages that are so dense, long-winded, presented at too high a literacy level, and in styles and layouts not conducive to attention or retention, that their impact on the target group is negligible. However, this is not meant to suggest 'glitz' over substance; rather, the dynamism should result in more creative work where art is employed to present the science. Independent of the scientific content, there are other features of message design that will affect the attention, comprehension, and retention processes of the receiver. Table 10.3 presents a list of content, design, persuasion, and memorability factors identified by Manoff (1985).

It is also important to note that message dissemination in and of itself may not be sufficient to meet consumer needs or organizational objectives. Message support through the addition of 'tangible' products and services may also be required to reinforce and amplify critical features of the message that do not lend themselves to mediated activities. For instance, support groups for persons with HIV infection or video products to use for exercising at home.

Tangible products that can be used by consumers is the second product category. These products might range from condoms in family planning projects to school curricula for AIDS education to self-help materials for smoking cessation in various formats (print, electronic, video). An even broader view of products was taken by Lefebvre and Flora (1988) who characterized any tangible representation of an agency to its markets as

Table 10.3 Factors affecting message design strategy

Content	Persuasion	Design	Memorability
The problem	Reason why	The single idea	Idea reinforcement
Target audience	Empathy	Language and	Minimizing distractions
Resistance points	Concern arousal	cultural relevance	Reprise (repetition)
Solution	Action capability	Situation and	
Required action	Believability	character	
Authoritative	Creativity	identification	
source	Benefits	Distinctive message	
		style	
		Low fatigue index	

Source: Manoff (1985: 197–203)

a product; this definition would encompass posters, brochures, and other message media from which consumers might draw certain conclusions about the organization. Such an approach to products leads an agency to adopt very specific guidelines about the development of materials, including size, colour, and location of programme logotypes; uniformity in layout; and specific language to describe the organizational mission, sponsoring agencies, and similar content features. The goal of such efforts is to establish a consistent approach to the consumer market one is targeting so that programme identity is established and reinforced on each consumer exposure to the organization. This is in contrast to a less formalized approach wherein each brochure an organization puts out has a different 'look and feel' to it, rendering it much more difficult to position the organization to its market. Success (and sometimes failure!) in these efforts is seen when quick glimpses of, or short phrases from, these materials result in correct identification by consumers of the originating agency ('It looks like something from the XYZ department!').

Products have a number of properties that should be addressed in the formative stages. Among the more important attributes of products to consider are brand name (title), features (e.g. ease of use, self-directed instruction), styling and packaging (an 'upmarket' appearance, a traditional cultural appeal), colour, and size. Other more subjective product attributes from a consumer's point of view might include: efficacy, expected benefit, safety, fit with current lifestyle, possibility of trial usage, and relative value to current product usage (or non-usage).

Many health promotion programmes feature service delivery as the cornerstone of their change efforts. In the large US community heart disease prevention studies, service delivery of one type or another was deemed essential to facilitating the individual change process. Such service delivery included screening, counselling, and referral events; adult education groups on topics of nutrition, smoking cessation, and exercise; worksite health promotion consultation and programmes; and work with food retailers to implement point-of-purchase nutrition education programmes. Clearly, many other programme components fit the service mode, including hotlines, self-help groups, consultation work, individual and family counselling, and social welfare assistance. Service delivery is often the method by which organizations structure their direct, face-to-face contacts with target markets (or clients). These interpersonal encounters are found to be the most important factor in producing changes in behaviour of the target group (Rice and Atkin 1989; Rogers 1983).

The creation of services usually arises from identified needs of specific populations and is developed from any one of a variety of philosophical and theoretical perspectives. It is not the intent here to outline the 'best' way to develop services; it is sufficient here to reiterate that such services should have a consumer-driven rationale and that formative studies document their efficacy in addressing the problem. The marketing of services, once developed and tested, does offer some unique problems to be considered.

Kotler and Bloom (1984) describe several challenges unique to service marketing. These challenges include:

- Service marketers must be as attentive to 'third parties' as they are to primary target groups. Health professionals have certain ethical and practice norms that directly impact on what they can, and cannot do, in response to 'patient demand'. Government agencies and insurance companies are other 'silent' consumers who may not be directly involved in consumer-provider exchanges, but their influence does indirectly affect such factors as the scope, content, outcome, and even availability of some services.
- Services are by their very nature less capable of being evaluated by consumers before, and many times after, being used. For example, it is difficult for clients to compare rival smoking cessation programmes and assess whether the chosen programme really did reduce the chance of developing lung cancer. Thus, client education becomes an even more important issue to address when marketing services.
- Maintaining high levels of quality control becomes a core function, especially as the number of people engaging in the delivery of the service increases. Staff training and supervision require on-going organizational commitments of time and effort. The varying backgrounds of people involved in health promotion service delivery – ranging from physicians to community nurses to dietitians to lay volunteers – makes this an area particularly vulnerable to undermining if proper acknowledgement and care is not given to quality control audits and monitoring.
- Many professionals involved in service delivery have neither the knowledge, experience, time, and/or inclination to undertake marketing activities. Hopefully, as more is learned about successful marketing practice in the service sector, and health professionals shed their reluctance to become health marketers, we will witness a changing practice pattern in which ethical and socially responsible marketing practice enhances the delivery and efficacy of health services to the public.

Price

The notion of pricing can become a source of controversy among health promotion professionals. One often encounters resistance to the idea of 'pricing' because it is equated with demanding money for products and/or services – typically from people least able to afford it. This is *not* what marketers have in mind when they discuss prices. Rather, pricing reflects the exchange theory basis of marketing presented earlier; that is, the mutual exchange of resources between two or more parties. Thus, prices represent the amount of resource expenditure necessary to receive desired goods or services. Prices people might consider in deciding whether to change a health behaviour or participate in a specific health promotion programme include:

- *Geographic distance:* How far is it to travel to a programme site? How convenient is it to sign up for a particular programme? How close is a safe exercise area?
- *Social:* What will my spouse think about my quitting smoking when he still does? How will my friends react when they find out – especially the ones that smoke?
- *Behavioural:* What am I going to do to relax if I don't smoke? What will I do when I get a craving for a cigarette?
- *Psychological:* What if I fail to quit again? Will quitting smoking be worth the agony of withdrawal?
- *Physical:* What if I start having strong withdrawal symptoms – what am I going to do? If I quit smoking I'll start gaining weight.
- *Structural:* How am I going to survive at work when people are smoking everywhere in the building?

Marketers attempt to understand these and other costs from the target audience's perspective as they pose key resistance points to behaviour change. They then examine equally closely what the perceived benefits of a specific behaviour change are, and develop communication and marketing strategies that realistically address the cost issues and reinforce the benefits. Notice that cost issues are not skirted or ignored; to do so jeopardizes not only the credibility of the programme (they don't know what they're talking about!) but it is detrimental to establishing an empathy with the target group that allows them to draw the inference – 'they know what I'm going through!'

On the other side of the price equation are the 'benefits'. Again, these benefits cover the same types of categories as illustrated earlier for prices. The focus of marketers on benefits sometimes leads to segmentation strategies that are themselves based on the differing perceived benefits among the target group. For example, cigarette smokers might be segmented, not by socio-demographic factors, but by how they see the benefit of quitting: being a better role model for their children; having a healthy baby; not dying of cancer like their sibling; being able to exercise more easily; not feeling like cigarettes are controlling their life. The art of marketing lies as much in communicating effectively the benefits of behaviour change and making the 'price' worth it, as it does in production of the products to support the effort.

A focus on benefits also leads to another distinguishing characteristic of marketing programmes: their offering of incentives to motivate behaviour change. Again, there is often some resistance to the idea of 'bribing people to do something that they should do anyway' (i.e. not smoke, eat right). However, many theories of behaviour change suggest that it is the anticipation of rewards – and tangible ones at that – that increases the probability of an individual engaging in the desired behaviour (Bandura 1977). Incentives have been used successfully in a number of health promotion efforts including smoking cessation campaigns (Lefebvre *et al.* 1990) and weight loss programmes (Brownell *et al.* 1984; Nelson *et al.* 1987). One need review only consumer marketing programme – the types of incentives they use and the method of promoting the desired behaviour with the incentive – to begin to recognize the many ways in which incentives can be used in a positive way to influence trials of healthy behaviours just as trials of new consumer products are promoted. A reminder to oneself that these consumer marketers spend inordinate sums of money to develop and evaluate these promotional efforts also reinforces the important formative research being engaged in by these 'competitors' that can benefit our own social marketing programmes.

Place

Place characteristics, or communication and distribution channels, have already been discussed to some extent. As with other elements of the marketing mix, decisions about 'places' need to take into account the preferences and practices of the target population. Place decisions can have an immediate impact on the accessibility of messages, products, and services to the target group. Virtually all place decisions have associated costs as well. In the discussion of 'pricing', we noted the effect place can have in terms of consumer costs (i.e. geographic price). However, at least as important are place costs borne by an organization attempting to reach specific groups. Many of these costs are fiscal (e.g. buying media time, producing flyers and brochures), but others have to do with the temporal and personnel resources necessary to achieve efficiency and effectiveness within the channel (Kotler and Andreasen 1987).

Places, or channels, are almost limitless in type. In deciding which ones to employ in a social marketing programme, the function one seeks from a channel is important. If one is choosing to communicate information, mass media may be appropriate – but should it be by television, radio, outdoor signage, transit posters, or other means? The answer lies in the results of earlier channel analysis. However, if one is interested in opening a new type of clinic service, or distributing a new health promotion product, different types of channels – for instance, retail outlets, religious organizations, kiosks – are more appropriate. Here, channel analysis may help fashion a decision, but it is likely that pilot studies will also need to be undertaken to test the feasibility and acceptability of the channel before investing many resources in the project.

The function one wishes the channel to perform in relation to a particular message/product/service and specific audience is clearly a first decision. However, other tasks that confront social marketers are then to:

- Attract channel resources through direct appeals, inter-organizational agreements, co-option, financial payments, sponsorship arrangements, or development of new channels.
- Co-ordinate and control the channel system, including the development of working relationships with channel gatekeepers and middlemen, ensuring that the channel system reaches the appropriate target groups,

evaluating the efficacy and efficiency of the channel system and maintaining good working relationships with key gatekeepers.

- Maintain the flow of messages/products/services in an orderly manner and ensure the quality of the message/product/service is maintained. This latter point can be especially critical when intermediaries are involved as happens when volunteers are deployed for certain functions, influential citizens are involved in programme awareness functions, retailers are distributing products, and media representatives are producing messages.

Promotion

Although some people equate marketing with promotion, the concept of the marketing mix puts promotional strategies in their proper context: as they relate to the product, price, and place decisions made with respect to a specific target group (Lefebvre and Flora 1988). Promotion aspects of the marketing mix involve the communication aspects of social marketing and include such strategies as advertising (either paid or public service), personal selling or contacts, public relations events, point-of-purchase programmes, direct mail, telemarketing, and virtually every other opportunity the programme encounters (or can create) that puts it in front of a target group (e.g. T-shirts, balloons, newsletters, etc.). Before launching promotion after promotion however, Novelli (1984) recommends developing an overall communication strategy for a programme. Four elements need to be defined:

1   The *benefits* to the target group of responding to a message purchasing a product, or participating in a programme ('look better, feel great!', 'win a vacation for two!', 'feel good about yourself').
2   The *reasons why* the communication should be attended to and responded to by the target group ('doctors recommend . . .', 'people like you find that it works', 'more taste and less calories').
3   The *specific actions* the audience should undertake in response to the communication (i.e. 'call this number for more information', 'see your doctor', 'shop around the edges of supermarket').
4   The *tone* or *image* that should underlie all communications directed towards the public (i.e. fun and rewarding, serious and scientific, upscale and trendy).

The resulting communication strategy or concept platform (Lefebvre *et al.* 1988), should concisely state these four elements. Once decisions are made about the concept platform, the 'how to' communicate questions and creative execution of each promotion can be addressed as in Table 10.1.

Promotion strategies can be as inexpensive or pricey as one chooses. While it is not within the capacity of many health promotion programmes, to emulate the promotional budgets of large corporate advertisers, it is sometimes the less expensive – and often more creative – efforts that have the bigger pay off in terms of actual effectiveness. Costs of promotion need to be in relation to the actual impact they have. In the commercial world, the cost of advertising is typically calculated by the reach achieved (the number of people exposed to the advertisement) – usually expressed in costs per thousand, or CPM. The reach of a promotion is calculated by such methods as independent audits of listeners or viewers (in the case of radio or television) by companies who specialize in this type of service, circulation figures adjusted for multiple readers in print media (i.e. more than one person usually reads any single copy of a newspaper or magazine on average), and random telephone surveys. Thus a mass media campaign that costs $38,180 (US) and reaches 2 million people has a CPM of $0.02. However, one can raise the argument that reach, in and of itself, may not be the objective of a campaign; it may be more important to base promotion costs on actual participation rates in a pro-gramme promoted by the campaign. Thus in the example above of $38,180 spent (though donated) in mass media time, Elder *et al.* (1991) reported 802 residents enrolled in their 'Quit to Win' smoking cessation programme – for a promotion cost of $47.61 per enrollee. If one further refines the cost-effect to enrolled smokers who quit, then the media costs climb to $134.44 for each of the 284 self-reported quitters. These costs do not include 'direct' costs associated with salaries, material production, and related campaign expenses which were calculated by the authors to be $17.25 per quitter. The moral of this example is that promotional costs can be either quite inexpensive, or quite expensive, depending on the objective one sets for the effort. Clearly, a programme can reach many people rather inexpensively through the mass media, but it is not so evident that such costs are as efficient when partici-pation rates and behaviour, change are substituted in the denominator. Unfortunately, there have been few carefully documented cost accountings of health promotion programmes to allow for meaningful and generalizable conclusions to be drawn as to which types of promotional strategies are most cost-efficient for the type of objective one sets.

Process tracking

Process tracking systems are the most important element of the imple-mentation process once it has begun. These types of systems provide the integrative and control functions necessary for a programme manager to ensure (1) that the marketing plan is being implemented as designed, (2) that the programme is reaching its target audience, and (3) that an implementation record is maintained that can be used to modify and refine later programmes and campaigns.

In the Stanford Five City Project (Farquhar *et al.* 1990), the Minnesota Heart Health Program (Jacobs *et al.* 1986), and the Pawtucket Heart Health Program (McGraw *et al.* 1989), common needs were seen for developing tracking systems to manage and document their interventions. Each project developed a process tracking system to meet the unique needs and challenges of their intervention protocols. However, in a series of collaborative meetings, a hybrid tracking system was created that blended the major common features of each system in order to compare process tracking system data directly across the three projects (Flora *et al.* 1993).

The Community Education Monitoring System (CEMS) represents a consensus of these three cardiovascular disease prevention projects as to the major elements needed in a process tracking system – again, recognizing that each project had other elements not reflected in CEMS. As such, CEMS provides a useful heuristic in designing process tracking systems for different types of programmes and settings. The major elements of CEMS are outlined in Table 10.4. They are based on a common set of assumptions and strategies shared by the three projects including:

- *Interventions based on a number of perspectives* including social learning theory, diffusion of innovations research, social network theory, inoculation theory, social marketing, and community development models.
- *Multiple change objectives* such as increasing public awareness and knowledge of cardiovascular risk factors, changing risk behaviours, maintaining these changes, stimulating organizational changes, and encouraging community groups to adopt particular programme elements.
- *The use of a variety of communication channels* including electronic and print media, face-to-face and direct mail.
- *Multiple target audiences* including high risk individuals, children, adolescents, and healthy adults.

The CEMS model is presented to stimulate research and applications in health promotion programmes of all kinds. Whether it be a CEMS-derivative, or created for other needs and necessities, process tracking systems are integral to good marketing practice. While it is difficult to imagine commercial marketers not gathering information, for instance, on how many coupons they distributed, for what specific products, and how many were redeemed (the sophisticated ones will even tell you by whom and where), it is common-place to find health promotion organizations with only the most rudimentary and incomplete understanding of exactly what they have done and what immediate impact it had. This will have to change if we are to have well-managed and effective programmes that are sensitive to changes in the public's needs and priorities (Lefebvre and Flora 1988).

Marketing management

Implementation of a marketing orientation within an organization faces a number of potential barriers. Chief amongst these, if it is not already apparent to the reader, is that marketing programmes demand a great deal of planning and action that may be unacceptable – and actually disruptive – to the staff and organization (Lefebvre and Flora 1988). Marketing plans not only involve

Table 10.4 Major elements of the community education monitoring system

Date of entry
Product or programme identification code
Channel
1. Face-to-face
   a. Single session
   b. Multiple sessions
2. Mass media
   a. Television (PSA vs. news story vs. talk show)
   b. Radio (PSA vs. programme vs. talk show)
   c. Newspaper (advertisement vs. column vs. story)
3. Print materials
   a. Booklets
   b. Self-help kits
   c. Posters
   d. Brochures
   e. Flyers
4. Special events
   a. Health fair
   b. Contests
   c. Training
   d. Other special activities
5. Physical/social/political environment
   a. Smoking policies
   b. Restaurant menu-labelling
   c. Grocery store shelf-labelling
Objective of the specific intervention effort
1. Individual change
   a. Awareness
   b. Knowledge
   c. Behaviour
2. Organizational change
   a. Improved community relations
   b. Establishing networks
   c. Training health professionals
   d. Training lay volunteers
3. Environmental change
   a. Policy/regulation
Target of the intervention
1. Individuals
   a. Blood pressure
   b. Exercise
   c. Nutrition
   d. Smoking
   e. Weight control
   f. General heart health practices
2. Organizations
   a. Visibility
   b. Institutionalization
Community adoption and maintenance of interventions
1. Percentage of activity supported by project resources
2. Percentage of activity supported by community resources

Table 10.4 (continued)

Intervention accessibility
　1.　Available to general public
　2.　Available to employees/members only

Estimated reach of intervention activity
　1.　Number of print pieces distributed
　2.　Number of newspapers printed that day
　3.　Listener/viewer share (number of households) at specific time
　4.　Number of participants in activity
　5.　Number of people exposed on a quarterly basis to an organizational or
　　　environmental intervention

Source: Flora *et al.* (1993)

time, research, and turning the organization 'inside out' to assess consumer preferences, they also require careful attention to implementation timelines, co-ordination of diverse logistics and personnel (either paid or voluntary staff), and sufficient evaluation to ascertain the plan's effectiveness in achieving preset objectives and feedforward to the next set of activities. One or more of these tasks can cause an organization to discard the marketing orientation because 'it's too hard' or 'we don't have all those resources you talk about'.

Implementing a marketing orientation, and a marketing management structure, needs to start from the top. A commitment to the process of evolving to a true market-driven agency is the first step. From there, marketing audits (see Table 10.5) can help identify current strengths and weaknesses. Focus can then be placed on addressing as many, or as few, areas as need attention with timelines for completion, and resources allocated, as the agency's other demands allow. One does not have immediately to initiate, for example, a complete database management system to begin collecting process information, nor does one have to hire professional market researchers to get input from consumers. But, as with any marketing programme described in this chapter, the 'internal' marketing plan is just as important and needs to contain achievable objectives for both the short and long term.

The management of marketing operations within an organization involves the orchestration of organizational resources by senior management to meet consumer needs and the organization's objectives. It does not necessarily require a formal degree in marketing management to perform, yet it does require in-depth understanding of the social marketing elements and how they interrelate. It also requires good management skills and the development of an organizational culture that prizes what Dr Geoffrey Rose has been quoted as describing as 'Dirty hands and clean minds'. That is, the ability of staff to work in the field, staying directly in touch with their clients and getting things done while also being able to exercise the critical and strategic cognitive skills that make a good scientist. There may be no better definition of a social marketer.

Table 10.5 Outline of a marketing audit

Marketing environment

Markets
1. Who are the organization's major markets and publics?
2. What are the major market segments in each market?
3. What are the present and expected future size and the characteristics of each market or market segment?

Customers
1. How do the customers and public feel towards and see the organization?
2. How do customers make their purchase or adoption decisions?
3. What is the present and expected future state of consumer needs and satisfaction as they relate to the organization?

Competitors
1. Who are the organization's major competitors?
2. What trends can be foreseen in competition?

Macro-environment
1. What are the main relevant developments with respect to demography, economy, technology, government, and culture that will affect the organization's situation?

Marketing system

Objectives
1. What are the organization's long-term and short-term overall objectives and marketing objectives?
2. Are the objectives in a clear hierarchical order and in a form that permits planning and measurement of achievement?
3. Are the marketing objectives reasonable for the organization given its competitive position, resources, and opportunities?

Programme
1. What is the organization's core strategy for achieving its objectives, and is it likely to succeed?
2. Is the organization allocating enough resources (or too many) to accomplish the marketing tasks?
3. Are the marketing resources allocated optimally to the various markets, territories, and products/services of the organization?
4. Are the marketing resources allocated optimally to the major elements of the marketing mix (i.e. product development, service quality, personal contact, promotion, and distribution)?

Implementetion
1. Does the organization develop an annual marketing plan? Is the planning procedure effective?
2. Does the organization implement control procedures (monthly, quarterly) to ensure that its annual plan objectives are being met?
3. Does the organization carry out periodic studies to determine the contribution and effectiveness of various marketing activities?
4. Does the organization have an adequate marketing information system (i.e. process tracking system) to service the needs of managers for planning and controlling operations in various markets?

Table 10.5 (continued)

Organization
1. Does the organization have a high-level marketing officer to analyse, plan, and implement the marketing work of the organization?
2. Are the other persons directly involved in marketing activity able people? Is there a need for more training, incentives, supervision, or evaluation?
3. Are the marketing responsibilities optimally structured to serve the needs of different marketing activities, product/service markets, and territories?

Detailed marketing activity review

Products
1. What are the main messages/products/services of the organization?
2. Should any products in the product line be phased out?
3. Should any products be added to the product line?
4. What is the general state of health of each product and the product mix as a whole?

Price
1. To what extent are prices set based on costs to the organization, consumer demand, and/or competitive criteria?
2. What would the likely response of demand be to higher or lower prices?
3. How do consumers psychologically interpret current prices?
4. Does the organization use temporary price promotions (e.g. incentives) and how effective are they?

Place
1. Are there alternative methods of distributing messages, products, and services that would result in more services or less cost?
2. Does the organization render adequate service to its customers apart from its message/product/service line?

Promotion
1. Does the organization have a communications strategy (concept platform)?
2. Does the organization allocate an appropriate amount of resources to promotional activities?
3. Are promotional themes and copy effective among the target audiences?
4. Are media well chosen? Are costs accounted for and effective for the chosen media?
5. Are direct marketing opportunities utilized to complement other promotional activities and to maintain customer contact?

Source: Adapted from Kotler (1975)

Fashioning an organization that is market-orientated may require an elaboration of existing staff roles and functions. In the work of the Pawtucket Heart Health Program's Intervention Unit, eight key functions were identified, and organizational structure and staff responsibilities were modified accordingly. These functions included:

1   *Product development,* within which specific staff had responsibility for development, testing, implementation, evaluation, and refinement of

intervention messages, products, and services within their areas of risk behaviour change expertise (i.e. smoking cessation, blood pressure control, weight loss, blood cholesterol management, and physical activity). These staff assumed titles of 'product manager' for each intervention programme, and, as in the corporate sector, these product managers were delegated ultimate authority and responsibility for their product line, including the development of annual marketing plans for each product.

2 *Training*, in which specific staff with training expertise were designated as trainers for both paid and unpaid staff in various skills, including blood pressure measurement, blood cholesterol measurement, and dietary counselling, and group leaders for smoking cessation and weight loss programmes. These trainers were also responsible for supervision of volunteer staff in each of these areas, monitored service quality, and did annual recertification examinations of knowledge and skills for each staff person active in these programmes.

3 *Channel development* responsibilities for other staff not designated as product managers. Channels identified by the Intervention Unit for which one staff person had responsibility included worksites, religious organizations, mass media, and those channels through which the minority populations of Pawtucket could be reached most effectively (targeted radio and print media, religious organizations in those neighbourhoods, worksites with high ratios of minority employees, food retail outlets, and specific housing developments). These 'channel managers' developed and nurtured relationships with gatekeepers in their channel area, and worked with product managers in establishing distribution of messages, products, and services to meet organizational objectives of the project.

4 *Resource development* was most prominent in the project through recruitment of lay volunteers in the community. Again, specific staff – designated as the 'Volunteer Team' – made many contacts with community groups through which to recruit volunteers. They worked with product managers to identify staffing needs (e.g. weight loss group leaders), developed marketing plans to recruit and maintain volunteer staff, and managed the volunteer registry that enabled them to match emerging programme needs with expertise and talents of volunteers already involved in the project (see Roncarati *et al.* 1989 for more details about this process). Resource development also included assignment of staff to locate financial resources as well from local businesses, as when incentives were needed for major behaviour change campaigns or new product development.

5 *Promotion* for all products had in-house resource staff assigned to it including editorial and graphic services supported by desk-top publishing expertise in the Administrative Unit. All work went through this group to ensure that the project's concept platform and image were reinforced through the packaging and tone of the materials.

6 *Programme delivery* as a key function was defined by product managers who worked with their own volunteer staff to reach city residents

with behaviour change programmes. Participant registries were managed by staff and telephone and mail follow-up to people identified at risk for cardiovascular disease through screening, counselling, and referral programmes was an important element of the programme delivery process.

7   *Management* of the marketing programme was overseen by the Unit Co-ordinator, but occurred at a variety of levels in the organization. All staff had areas of management responsibility, whether it was products, channels, and/or resources. Annual two-day planning retreats and a mid-year one-day staff retreat to evaluate progress across the specific product marketing plans were important elements in co-ordinating staff efforts through the setting of annual objectives for the entire Unit which then drove the product planning process.

8   *Evaluation* of the intervention process was carried out through staff in the Formative and Process Evaluation section of the project's Evaluation Unit. The evaluation staff worked with product managers in testing new products and their efficacy in reaching target populations and promoting behaviour change amongst participants. This group also managed the programme's process evaluation system that monitored the Intervention Unit activities and is reflected in the earlier discussion of the CEMS. Readers interested in more details about the formative and process evaluation system may refer to McGraw *et al.* 1989.

These eight functions do not necessarily have to be translated into at least eight full-time staff positions in order for an organization to become effective in marketing. Rather, the organization should review its current staffing pattern and areas of responsibility with these points in mind. One staff person may have responsibilities that cut across several functions, and, indeed, in the Pawtucket Heart Health Program we approached each staff position as a mixture of each of these functions, with varying weights assigned to each one; for instance, volunteer team members were responsible for managing volunteer-related products and services, including marketing plans, were involved in promotion activities, and managed their own groups of volunteers. However, it is important that each of the areas receives an allotment of staff time for a fully functioning marketing operation.

Managing to market, versus managing for managing's sake, may also bring health promotion organizations to the point of evolving new management practices that reflect a very different world from the one we have been used to in the past. This new world, characterized by such trends as rapid and accelerating change, more consumer control over how they allocate their time, component lifestyles, an ageing population in developed countries, increasing globalization of many human endeavours, and changing work environments, requires new management strategies for organizations to survive, and even thrive, in it. Proposed management evolutions to meet these new demands and challenges note that dynamism, not control, is necessary for effective action and response. Flattened hierarchies, not more management layers, will ensure organizational responsiveness and closer touch with consumers. Fluidity in team building and development, as opposed to highly organized and sharply demarcated areas of responsibility, will encourage innovative approaches by staff to the new challenges of health promotion. Pushing responsibility and authority down in the organization, not centralizing them, will empower staff to make things happen and focus on consumers as the critical link – not what the boss thinks! Leadership by example, rather than by fiat, will further inspire greater efforts by staff. And finally, measuring what is important for success, not just what is convenient and measurable, will allow health promotion professionals to set their sights on the real objectives and goals necessary to fashion a healthier population (Peters 1987).

Concluding remarks

Social marketing is garnering much attention from public health professionals with an accompanying enthusiasm that it offers a new 'magic bullet' with which we can address social and health problems. While there are many success stories as to how social marketing principles led to significant and impressive results, it must also be recognized that these case studies lack the rigour of empirical investigations. Thus, while promising, one cannot – nor should not – suggest that social marketing is the health promoter's panacea. Many questions still remain.

There are numerous research questions that need to be addressed in social marketing. What is most unfortunate about this state of affairs is that it has changed very little since Bloom and Novelli (1981) surveyed the area. Some of the issues and questions they raised then have received scant attention since; amongst the more salient are:

- The difficulty in funding and completing consumer research studies in a timely fashion.
- The lack of behavioural data on which to base segmentation strategy, and the related challenge that few data are available as to which segmentation strategies are most appropriate for specific target behaviours.
- The formulation of messages, products, and services is hampered by the intangible quality of much of what health promotion is attempting to market and the scientific, social, and political context of many problems that require compromise, and at worst inaction, on important health concerns.
- In the area of pricing, the pressure is on social marketers only to reduce costs, due in part to the lack of information and models about how consumers view costs and benefits associated with health promotive behaviours.
- The difficulties associated with using intermediaries for much of our work, again due to a lack of understanding as to how to employ incentives appropriately to ensure co-operation and maintenance of quality.

- Communication strategies that are often driven by needs to communicate relatively large amounts of information but are restricted on such complete disclosures because of the nature of preferred media (i.e. television), the inaccessibility of paid advertising due to resource limitations, and pressures not to use certain types of appeals or 'tell the whole story'.

It is bringing together the practitioners of the art of social marketing with the scientists who can test and evaluate the approach that is the critical need at this time. Such a partnership requires that agencies who fund research look towards a more balanced portfolio in which the more 'pure' investigational studies (such as are found in much basic and clinical research) are complemented by the more 'dirty' work of understanding in the real world context how to translate new scientific knowledge into messages, products, and services that will improve the health and well-being of people everywhere. Social marketing may provide the type of strategic and practical tools with which Health For All can be achieved; it is incumbent on each of us to assure that it is applied appropriately and wisely.

References

Bandura, A. (1977) *Social Learning Theory*, Englewood Cliffs, NJ: Prentice-Hall.

Bloom, P. N. and Novelli, W. D. (1981) 'Problems and challenges of social marketing', *Journal of Marketing* 45: 79–88.

Brownell, K. D., Cohen, R. Y., Stunkard, A. J., Felix, M. R. J., and Cooley, N. (1984) 'Weight loss competitions at the worksite: impact on weight, morale, and cost-effectiveness', *American Journal of Public Health* 74: 1283–5.

Doremus Porter Novelli (1986) *Lessons Learned from the DuaLima Test Market*, Washington, DC: SOMARC/The Futures Group.

Elder, J. P., Campbell, N. R., Mielchen, S. D., Hovell, M. F., and Litrownik, A. J. (1991) 'Implementation and evaluation of a community-sponsored smoking cessation contest', *American Journal of Health Promotion* 5: 200–7.

Farquhar, J. W., Fortmann, S. P., Flora, J. A., Taylor, C. B., Haskell, W. L., Williams, P. T., Maccoby, N., and Wiid, P. D. (1990) 'Effects of communitywide education on cardiovascular disease risk factors: the Stanford Five-City Project', *Journal of the American Medical Association* 264: 359–65.

Fine, S. H. (1981) *The Marketing of Ideas and Social Issues*, New York: Praeger.

Flora, J. A., Lefebvre, R. C., Murray, D. M., Stone, E. J., Assaf, A., Mittelmark, M., and Finnegan, J. R. (1993) 'A community education monitoring system: methods from the Stanford Five-City Project, the Minnesota Heart Health Program, and the Pawtucket Heart Health Program', *Health Education Research: Theory and Practice* 8 (1): 81–95.

Jacobs, Jr., D. R., Luepker, R. V., Mittelmark, M. B., Folson, A. R., Pirie, P. L., Mascioli, S. R., Hannan, P. J., Pechacek, T. F., Bracht, N. F., Carlaw, R. W., Kline, F. G., and Blackburn, H. (1986) 'Community-wide prevention strategies: evaluation design of the Minnesota Heart Health Program', *Journal of Chronic Disease* 39: 775–88.

Kotler, P. (1975) *Marketing for Nonprofit Organizations*, Englewood Cliffs, NJ: Prentice-Hall.

Kotler, P. and Andreasen, A. R. (1987) *Strategic Marketing for Nonprofit Organizations*, 3rd edition, Englewood Cliffs, NJ: Prentice-Hall.

Kotler, P. and Bloom, P. N. (1984) *Marketing Professional Services*, Englewood Cliffs, NJ: Prentice-Hall.

Kotler, P. and Roberto, E. L. (1989) *Social Marketing: Strategies for Changing Public Behavior*, New York: The Free Press.

Kotler, P. and Zaltman, G. (1971) 'Social marketing: an approach to planned social change', *Journal of Marketing* 35: 3–12.

Lefebvre, R. C. (1990) 'Strategies to maintain and institutionalize successful programs: a marketing framework', in N. Bracht (ed.) *Health Promotion at the Community Level*, Newbury Park, CA: Sage.

Lefebvre, R. C. and Flora, J. A. (1988) 'Social marketing and public health intervention', *Health Education Quarterly* 15: 299–315.

Lefebvre, R. C., Lasater, T. M., Carleton, R. C., and Peterson, G. (1986) 'Theory and practice of health programming in the community: the Pawtucket Heart Health Program', *Preventive Medicine* 16: 80–95.

Lefebvre, R. C., Harden, E. A., and Zompa, B. (1988) 'The Pawtucket Heart Health Program: III. social marketing to promote community health', *Rhode Island Medical Journal* 71: 27–30.

Lefebvre, R. C., Cobb, G. D., Goreczny, A. J., and Carleton, R. A. (1990) 'Efficacy of an incentive-based community smoking cessation program', *Addictive Behaviors* 15: 403–11.

McGraw, S. A., McKinlay, S. M., McClements, L., Lasater, T. M., Assaf, A., and Carleton, R. A. (1989) 'Methods in program evaluation: the process evaluation system of the Pawtucket Heart Health Program', *Evaluation Review* 13: 459–83.

McGuire, W. J. (1984) 'Public communication: a strategy for inducing health-promoting behavior change', *Preventive Medicine* 18: 299–319.

Manoff, R. K. (1985) *Social Marketing*, New York: Praeger.

Nelson, D. J., Sennett, L., Lefebvre, R. C., Loiselie, L., McClements, L., and Carleton, R. A. (1987) 'A campaign strategy for weight loss at worksites', *Health Education Research: Theory and Practice* 2: 27–31.

Novelli, W. D. (1984) 'Developing marketing programs', in L. W. Frederickson, L. J. Solomon, and K. A. Brehony (eds) *Marketing Health Behavior: Principles, Techniques and Applications*, New York: Plenum.

Peters, T. (1987) *Thriving on Chaos: Handbook for a Management Revolution*, New York: Knopf.

Rice, R. E. and Atkin, C. K. (1989) 'Trends in communication campaign research', in R. E. Rice and C. K. Atkin (eds) *Public Communication Campaigns*, 2nd edition, Newbury Park, CA: Sage.

Rogers, E. M. (1983) *Diffusion of Innovations*, New York: The Free Press.

Roncarati, D. D., Lefebvre, R. C., and Carleton, R. A. (1989) 'Voluntary involvement in community health promotion: the Pawtucket Heart Health Program', *Health Promotion* 4: 11–18.

Weinstein, A. (1987) *Market Segmentation*, Chicago, IL: Probus.

Part III

Reflections and developments

11 Health promotion theory and its rational reconstruction

Lessons from the philosophy of science

Don Rawson

Confidence and crises in health promotion

As health promotion work has expanded in recent years so the accepted prescriptions for appraising health science and evaluating health interventions have proved to be inadequate. Theorists have either tended to search other disciplines for a scientific basis to their work (witness this volume) or else have concentrated on expounding the ideological basis of health promotion (compare, for example, the anthology in Rodmell and Watts 1986). Neither approach, however, has led to the creation of a corpus of knowledge particular to health promotion or to a coherent set of methods worthy of discipline status.

Is there a paradigm shift from health education to health promotion?

Since the 1970s the efforts of health educators have come under increasing criticism. (Contrast the vast array of critical evaluations from differing perspectives all summating into a disenchantment with the panacea health education had originally promised: Adams 1985; Bowman 1976; Dwore and Matarazzo 1981; Labonte and Penfold 1981; Neutens 1984; Tones 1983; Tones *et al.* 1990; Whitehead 1989; Williams and Aspin 1980.)

There has been at least a crisis of spirit as critics from a variety of perspectives have highlighted the relative ineffectiveness of health education campaigns which are focused on changing health lifestyles. Added to this are the overwhelmingly daunting problems of attempting to achieve major health reforms in the existing social and political order.

Whether or not the very foundations of health education have been shaken, the criticisms illustrate the cramped and teetering structure of a subject built on unsound philosophical grounds. Whether or not health education and health promotion can be regarded as possessing a scientific basis, the continuing growth of criticism suggests it will be necessary to become increasingly conversant with the kind of issues addressed by the philosophy of science: namely, elucidation of the essential nature of the subject, characterization of progress and growth, and questioning of the basis of its authority.

Champions of the self-styled new health promotion movement in public health have been vociferous in proclaiming a paradigm shift from the old health education to health promotion. Although there has been dissatisfaction with some health education work, is this the same as a transfer of allegiance to a new paradigm?

Thomas Kuhn's (1957, 1962) descriptions of scientific revolutions as paradigm shifts has been broadly welcomed as an explanation of the displacement and progression of ideas within disciplines. Kuhn argues that paradigm shifts take place as social movements in the scientific community, with researchers abandoning orthodox theories and methods (or paradigms) when a new paradigm is seen to assimilate or go beyond the older established one.

In just such a manner, it is said, the term health promotion appeared more or less abruptly during the 1980s and rapidly achieved a fashionable status. Many professionals who ten years ago were engaged in the development of health education now appear to align themselves with the new health promotion movement.

The distinction between health education and health promotion has, however, been both contentious and confused (Tones 1986). Recently, some consensus has begun to emerge, redefining health education almost exclusively in terms of individually focused campaigns designed to change health lifestyles (WHO 1984). As health promotion gains ground, health education is increasingly faced with a crisis of legitimacy. Where health education is identified solely with the attempt to change individual lifestyles it is also regarded as synonymous with victim blaming (Crawford 1977; Labonte and Penfold 1981).

Prior to the advent of health promotion, however, health educationalists had already begun to define the parameters of health education more widely to include consideration of structural features and advocacy of social reform (Anderson 1980; Crawford 1977; Draper *et al.* 1979; Thorpe 1982). In Britain at least, the proliferation and dissemination of hypothetical health education models during the 1980s facilitated a reconsideration of the appropriate aims and methods of health education. It may be that such collections of models are now more appropriately described as health promotion taxonomies, containing health education models.

Described in this way, the change to health promotion resembles a paradigm shift. Kuhn's analysis relies, though, on the scientists' ability to recognize truth (or at least the prospects of a going concern). As Kuhn (1970) expresses it, 'Scientific knowledge, like language, is intrinsically the common property of the group or else nothing at all'. Lakatos (1970), though, criticizes Kuhn's account as being little more than 'mob science', that is, scientific progress determined through consensus in the scientific élite.

The implication is that, although Kuhn suggests the new scientific paradigm has greater theoretical content than its predecessor (that is, it explains the world better), Kuhn's analysis excludes the possibility of a rational and normative means of appraising scientific growth.

In recent years Kuhn's work has suffered a declining influence amongst philosophers of science, partly because the historiographical basis is regarded as too simplistic. The idea of cycles between normal and revolutionary science has in particular been difficult to sustain. The epistemological basis to Kuhn's work has also received considerable criticism. Chalmers (1976) claims that Kuhn's popularity is undeserved and that he conflates three distinct views: subjectivist, consensual, and objectivist. Although Kuhn argues for elements of all three, Chalmers points out that ultimately Kuhn chooses the consensual criteria for appraising science.

Was the change to health promotion purely a social movement in the occupations of health education or has it entailed real changes in professional thinking and practice? Although many have adopted the health promotion rubric there is some doubt that it has been accompanied by changes in substance. In a nationwide study of the training and development needs of British health education officers, Rawson and Grigg (1988) were unable to locate any factors which reliably differentiated the work of those involved in health education as opposed to health promotion. Numerous health education organizations, moreover, are staffed by health promotion officers and likewise, some health promotion units are run by specialists with a health education title.

Another critical review of recent changes in public health policy similarly concludes, 'Health promotion to date has either comprised the strategies of health education under a new name or has consisted of much rhetoric and little action' (Research Unit in Health & Behavioural Change, University of Edinburgh 1989). In short, there appears to be more of a shift in title than a true shift of paradigms. In the occupations of health education the change of label to health promotion may none the less be welcomed as an opportunity to declare anew the purposes of an emerging profession.

Most writers now appear to have accepted that health education is redefined as a part of a broader health promotion perspective. It is to be hoped that the sudden professional exodus to health promotion does not in the end signal the complete abandonment of health education or replace one practice having an inadequate theoretical basis with another equally inadequate thesis bereft of epistemological foundations.

The philosophy of scientific method

As with all disciplines, the philosophy of scientific method is best characterized through the approach it takes to defining problems rather than by the current content of its subject matter.

Interestingly, Gellner (1974) contends that the philosophy of science has also been working through a crisis of legitimacy. Like politics generally, he argues, it fluctuates between poles of liberalism and authoritarianism. The first tries to protect science from the arbitrary limits imposed by authority which ultimately lead to scientific stagnation. The second attempts to protect science from stultification brought through the chaos of anarchy. Gellner goes on to identify two corresponding modes of resolving the crisis. One is to invoke something bigger than all of us, something, that is, objective. The alternative means of validation is to believe only in our own internal premises, resulting in something relative and subjective. Whatever scientists are, or do, supplies this agnostic and anthropocentric solution.

For Gellner, theories take on a political force with the movement from one pole to the other. In the struggle for scientific survival, it is necessary to discover how and why one theory comes to be regarded as more scientific or true than another. In the parlance of the philosophy of science a *universal demarcation criterion* is created (Popper 1959, 1963).

The philosophy of scientific method then directs us to appraise theories in the light of the generalized demarcation problem. This consists of asking how true science can be differentiated from pseudo- or non-science, and how rival theoretical accounts of the same subject matter can be reconciled. Translated to the field of health promotion the problem is to distinguish true or 'authentic' health promotion from other promotions of health (say, for example, commercial advertising which incorporates a pseudo 'health' message to motivate product buying). For public credibility to be maintained there is a pressing need to establish a clear demarcation criterion. Within the professional field there is no less urgent a problem of differentiating health educational from wider health promotional activity and of establishing the relative effectiveness of different approaches. If health promotion theory continues to develop it will become increasingly necessary to address the generalized demarcation problem.

The philosophy of scientific method approaches the demarcation problem through two complementary paths: by elucidating the epistemological basis of scientific method and by historiographical reconstructions of scientific progress. Theorists, though, have been slow to journey along either route in their discussions of health promotion.

The need for epistemology

Understanding human knowledge is more than a paradox. More than the vain pursuit of armchair philosophers, it is ultimately our only touchstone of truth. But to say that the shape of all knowledge is guided by our view of what knowledge is or should be is, of course, a mere metaphysical adage. And, like most well-worn issues, its significance declines over time. The original puzzle of understanding knowledge which so preoccupies philosophers can come to be seen as an impossible and largely irrelevant quandary. After all, it might be said, what point is there in procrastinating about such intangibles when there are real and practical issues to solve? More strongly, the same notion, that there are certain irreducible aspects of human existence, can be taken as a justification for activism, the ideology which opposes any kind of complacency, including theorizing (Popper 1957). Within health promotion some who advocate radical action are also intolerant of theory work. Equally, pragmatists who resist intellectual activity see philosophizing as irrelevant or misleading (e.g. Seymour 1984).

Even scientists sometimes show little patience with problems of epistemology. In trying to expand their body of systematic knowledge they focus only upon specific problems related to their discipline. Now scientists can, and some do, practise successful science without an explicit formulation of the epistemological assumptions underlying their methods. Claiming to hold no specific philosophy, however, is at best a pretence. Perhaps of greatest consequence, implicit epistemologies are more difficult to criticize, and therefore improve, than are explicit ideas. Epistemology is in this sense unavoidable. As Rosenberg (1988) aptly describes, 'Even the claim that philosophical reflection is irrelevant to advancing knowledge . . . is itself a philosophical claim'.

Some historiographical considerations

The models of health education debate

During the last decade health education (in Great Britain anyway) has been awash with debate about appropriate health education models. The subject frequently surfaces at conferences and has been carried along with the ebb and flow of journal correspondence. The professional field has expressed and continues to express concern with the appropriate selection of working models. (See, for example, the issue of the *Health Education Journal*, Vol. 49, 1990, devoted to theoretical debate.)

Health education models are hypothesized to be coherent approaches to health education practice, such as the 'self-empowerment model' or the 'social action model'. They are considered to embody different concepts of health and education, diverse methodologies and means of evaluation, and consequently different repertoires of knowledge and skills from practitioners. Most significantly, they have been generated, almost entirely, from within the practice field. In this sense, models of health education represent the most likely source for developing a body of knowledge particular to health promotion. They may be distinguished completely from explanatory models imported from other disciplines (e.g. the health belief model), though this has also been a major concern to some theorists in health promotion (see, for example, Catford and Parish 1989; Downie *et al.* 1990; Tones *et al.* 1990; Research Unit in Health & Behavioural Change, University of Edinburgh 1989).

From the models debate *within* health education, however, Rawson and Grigg (1988) identified seventeen published taxonomies or collections of health education models in Britain alone. Many of the taxonomies are only sketchily described in one- or two-page articles or have gone no further than brief presentations at professional conferences. One notable account has managed strongly to influence a generation of health education specialists whilst remaining largely absent from the usual channels of academic publication (Beattie 1980, 1984, 1991). The content of taxonomies ranges from simplistic linguistic juggling (e.g. Tannahill 1985) to complex structuralist arguments (e.g. Dorn 1983). Recent additions to the burgeoning catalogue of models include a health promotion model by Catford and Parish (1989), three historical 'approaches' to health education by Downie *et al.* (1990), interpretations of the Burrell and Morgan scheme (1985) by Caplan and Holland (1990) and Taylor (1990), plus a revision of the French and Adams taxonomy (1986) by French (1990).

The continuing proliferaton of models shows no sign of abating and brings the number of taxonomies to over a score. Strangely, most of the model makers seem to be unaware of the existence of each other's efforts. At least there is little cross-referencing with either critical appraisal or cumulative building of ideas. Generally, it appears that the taxonomies are produced from first principles, in order to explain some particular health education initiative or in order to set out the range of possible approaches to health education activity for different professional groups who have discovered a core health promotion role. The plurality of efforts leads inevitably to much redundancy and slow, if not retarded, theoretical growth. Whilst the expression of more models may testify to persistent underlying theoretical issues, there is also the real possibility of theoretical fragmentation and practical confusion with well over 100 resultant models to choose from.

Unfortunately there has been very little in the way of either analytical or empirical research to test the validity of the putative health education models. Collins (1982, 1984) explored the ramifications of different practice models across four professional groups using so-called illuminative methodologies. Nutbeam (1984) also investigated the health education models held by different professional groups, using a different but limited methodology. The samples were also respectively very small and eccentric, however, making generalization difficult.

In a more extensive empirical study Rawson and Grigg (1988) surveyed the health education models preferred by over 100 health education officers plus a similar number of their role partners and set these against actual records of health education activities. The methodology made innovative use of an interactive computer program (MODEFI or MOdels DEFinition Instrument). This locates individual or group preferences against a set of well-known taxonomies (Beattie 1980; Draper 1983; Ewles and Simnett 1985; Tones 1981). Factor analysis revealed that the nineteen separate models generated from the principal taxonomies represented could be subsumed in a spectrum of seven meta models. In all, the results showed that the occupational philosophy of health education officers could be characterized as a preference for working through intermediaries such as other health professionals and lay workers, rather than through direct appeals to at-risk groups. The role partners, however, saw health education work as influencing public health through more direct and less catalytic approaches. More than this, the health education specialists showed a marked concern with methodologies of facilitating rather than disseminating health education content.

Similar names are invoked by many of the model makers for their various models. French (1984) analyses several of the taxonomies and attempts to reduce the surfeit by identifying areas of linguistic overlap. French shows that many of the same themes are indeed reiterated, suggesting some theoretical unity and redundancy of effort. Closer analysis, however, also reveals that the same labels sometimes conceal quite distinct concepts. For example, Ewles and Simnett (1985) and Tones (1981) both describe an educational approach as a distinct model of health education. Ewles and Simnett say it aims to equip individuals with the knowledge and understanding for rational decision making about health issues. Appropriate health education is said to address the causes and effects of health and illness and may include an exploration of values and attitudes. They also specify, however, that the educational approach should inform but not influence. As they express it, 'Information about health is presented in as value-free a way as possible'.

Tones, in contrast, is critical of education based on the supposition that facts can be presented from a neutral position for people to make an untethered rational choice. Instead he advocates a sophisticated version of the educational model which recognizes the need to explore beliefs, clarify values, and give practice in decision making. Indeed, the concept of informed choice is central to any educational model but also implies inescapable assumptions about freedom of choice. As Tones (1981) cogently states, 'For many individuals the options are limited or non-existent'.

It is also relevant to note that, in countries where health education exists as an established academic subject, models' debates concerning the essential nature of health education have had little showing. In the United States, attention has largely focused on the appropriate role and function of health educators. This has tended to be both prescriptive and atheoretical, however, lacking process indications and making naive assumptions about the unity of purpose (Bowman 1976; Galli 1978). Neutens (1984) argues for further role delineation research as a means of establishing a unifying philosophy. Similarly, in the Netherlands, there has been a primary concern with role composition (Krijnen *et al.* 1982).

The relationship of models, taxonomies, and theories

Within the philosophy of science generally, models appear to be regarded unproblematically, and are usually described as preliminary or temporary devices to assist the scientists' thinking rather than as logically necessary components of theory building. Lakatos (1970), for example, says, 'A model is a set of initial conditions (possibly together with some of the observational theories) which one knows is bound to be replaced during further development of the [research] programme'. Nagel (1961) gives a stronger role to models for fleshing out the logical skeleton of a theories explanatory structure which he says is often in visualizable terms. That is, models make the theory concrete. Theories, in Nagel's view, cannot provide adequate explanation without models. In the social sciences a similar notion to Nagel's can be found in Blalock (1971) who argues that models enable a transition from the verbal form of theories to more precise research techniques. Mathematical formulations in particular, Blalock sees as helping 'recast' verbal theories as testable models. This insight has a special relevance for health promotion which continues to thrive in a mostly oral tradition. Major developments in practice tend to be told narratively at conferences rather than being documented in theoretical literature.

It is pertinent to ask whether health education models are necessary components of theoretical development or whether they should be regarded as temporary constructions in the development of health promotion theory.

French and Adams (1986) envisage a construction sequence from laying the foundations in ideology, through theory building, to the development of models. That is, models are regarded as the end product of health promotion philosophy. They function to support practice through identifying goals and shaping strategies.

For the most part, however, health promotion taxonomies can be seen to have developed in the opposite direction. At least, the greater abundance of models which have appeared have been unaccompanied by much detailed theory work or explicit ideology.

Models, moreover, are seldom followed through. At a descriptive level the models' wider and more extensive implications are excluded. The often-criticized medical model, for example, is seldom explored as a basis of appropriate intervention by medical professionals. As a normative (ideal) account the underlying theory receives only the crudest analysis. The educational model, for example, has little correspondence with the educational issues emphasized by educationalists (cf. Dearden 1972; Hirst 1983; Peters 1977).

Rather, health education models appear at first sight to be as much about forms of service delivery available to health education specialists as about health education principles. That is, the models may conflate role boundaries with health promotion principles. In describing the educational model, for example, are the models not describing the deployment of skills by practitioners from an educational background rather than unfolding an approach based on educational principles? Downie *et al.* (1990) are critical of the models debate on precisely these grounds. They see the putative models as misleading and oversimplified viewpoints detracting from interprofessional collaboration. Downie *et al.*, however, miss the epistemological point. They are mistaken to assume the models debate is only a reflection of professional rivalry. Rather, it is a manifestation of an emerging profession's struggle to develop core theoretical underpinnings from the practice base. What is required in health promotion, as in any other emerging occupation, is a new epistemology of practice (Schön 1983). That is, a means of distinguishing and codifying the essential operating characteristics of practice and of articulating the development of goals.

Iconic and analogic models in health promotion

Diesing (1971) lists eight separate usages of the term 'models' and cautions that the terms 'model' and 'theory' are often loosely employed and sometimes reversed in meaning. Warr (1980) provides a most useful summary of the function of models generally and notes that the term contains a confused collection of meanings. He also points out that various reviewers have been dismayed at the disparate variety of meanings and lack of theoretical integration. For Warr, however, models are separate from conceptual frameworks, paradigms, and theories. Although the language varies considerably, most contributors to thinking about the epistemological status of models typically differentiate two types of models, which Warr, somewhat prosaically refers to as Models 1 and 2. More lucidly, they are iconic or analogic representations. The first are simplified descriptions of some aspect of known reality, portraying a literal or isomorphic image of nature. The second are analogies or metaphors used to assist our understanding about nature and may have no direct counterpart in reality.

Although the term 'approaches' is preferred by Ewles and Simnett (1985), their taxonomy contains five detailed iconic models. In addition to descriptive accounts of each model they also supply examples of the application of each approach in practice along with the aim and appropriate health education activity for each model.

Model systems in health promotion which are predominantly iconic, such as the Ewles and Simnett taxonomy, have the advantage of being limited to that which is currently observable. By simplifying the reality of practice they also help reduce the complexities of health promotion to manageable proportions. This makes them readily believable and attractive to those who eschew intellectual work. Being tied to the here and now, however, means that they have limited generalizability and cannot be easily adapted to changes. In the world of health, of course, change is the one certainty.

Iconic models in the final analysis reduce to operational definitions. Health promotion comes to be defined as what health promoters do. As Tones (1981) warns, however, this is fraught with the same difficulties and circularity of reasoning as are other operational definitions (like intelligence being what intelligence tests measure). Effective and appropriate health promotion could instead be that which no one has yet developed. In the absence of any higher order theory showing how the various models are integrated to the same overall purpose there is also the constant danger of contradictory practice. Different health education models may cancel out the achievements of other approaches through mutually contradictory efforts. Theoretical growth at a practical level is thus essential to the development of coherent strategy.

Beattie's (1980, 1984, 1991) account of health education and health promotion offers in contrast a strongly analogic taxonomy. The work partly grew out of Bernstein's (1980) concepts of codes and control and makes use of the cross-classification scheme proposed by C. Wright Mills (1959). It thus stands on a firm theoretical footing. The resulting repertoire is drawn from the attempt to combine models of health with models of education. Two intersecting axes, which are claimed to be fundamental dimensions of health education, create a 'structural map' of the possible range of health promotion models.

Analogic taxonomies such as Beattie's, in contrast to iconic representations, can assimilate changes since the theoretical structure already contains the relationships and progressions between elements. They may even extend the possibilities of practice by indicating a form of health promotion which as yet has to be attempted.

The disadvantage of analogic systems is that they may be seen as remote from the detail of reality and so of limited help in dealing with the concrete issues encountered in practice. That is, the theoretical abstraction may require further translation to be of immediate benefit.

Caplan and Holland (1990), French and Adams (1986), and Tannahill (1985), amongst others, describe their sets of models as typologies. Typological systems, however, are more usually taken to refer to a dimensional classification, which means a continuously graded sequence of elements with labels attached to the extremes or poles (e.g. introvert–extravert). Although some of the collections of models are claimed to be dimensional (e.g. Beattie 1991; Caplan and Holland 1990; Nutbeam 1984), none actually treats the variety of models in this way. Mid-points on the dimensions are not considered, neither are progressions along the continua referred to in anything other than a cursory manner. Consequently, it would be more internally consistent if the intersecting axes of these systems were redrawn to recast the models as nominal categories.

There is, coincidentally, another sense in which taxonomies may be the more appropriate form of categorization. It is interesting to recall that much of evolutionary theory was propagated in the soil of taxonomic development. Darwin's work made essential use of the systematic collections of fossils and animal specimens catalogued by early naturalists who painstakingly assembled taxonomies of species. Regarded in this way, health promotion taxonomies may be best regarded as embryonic formulations necessarily preceding the maturation of theory.

The search for models has, however, been condemned by Kelvin (1980) who sees it as being empty. As he expresses it, 'To think of models is primitive. We should look for the phenomena for which we have to account'. Restated, there is a possible tautology in explaining the functioning of health promotion through modelling health education work. Can a part be used to explain the whole?

Suppe (1977) also criticizes the idea that models are essential explanations and cites quantum mechanics as an example of theory work not dependent upon models. Instead, Suppe contends that models may be heuristically fruitful but not necessary as integral components of theoretical development. For health promotion, however, model construction appears to be the only basis of core theoretical development thus far.

The models debate has unfortunately been limited mostly to discussion of models *within* taxonomies. What is required, however, is debate *between* taxonomies with an attempt to explicate the underlying theoretical principles. Further production of yet more taxonomies which only superficially describe health education and health promotion approaches will not of itself lead to theory development. Instead, health promotion theory should be directed at discovering what characterizes health promotion as opposed to any other subject matter. This should include an analysis of both content and methods. The philosophy of science may assist in this regard by extending the analysis of solutions given to the generalized demarcation problem.

In mainstream philosophy of science, the iconic–analogic distinction has a parallel in the epistemological status of theories. Controversies over the realist or instrumentalist nature of science have come to be redefined instead as debates over the generalized demarcation problem.

Essentials of health promotion

The nature of health and its attainment

The content of health promotion taxonomies is in part predicated upon alternative definitions of health. Health educationalists have long been outspoken in challenging the received notion of health as absence of illness and disease. Birn and Birn (1985) best characterize the prevailing bio-medical concept of health as a defect-apparatus. This means that disease and progressive failure of function are seen as inevitable features of life. Consequently, appropriate health promotion consists of timely screening and other interventions to reduce defects and minimize damage. Instead, Birn and Birn urge a complete move by health educators to a social-medical model emphasizing well-being.

From a wider cultural perspective, Burkitt (1983) has similarly challenged the fact that the Western medical model still dominates health education with an inappropriate basis for understanding health. The WHO concept of Health For All is unlikely to be obtained, moreover, as long as health is defined in terms of illness avoidance. Instead, Burkitt advocates a concept of positive health similar to that found in traditional Chinese medicine.

Downie *et al.* (1990) dispute the implied continuum from negative to positive health and suggest instead that the two concepts are independent. With this orthogonal relationship of concepts it would be possible to be in a state of illness and yet have a state of well-being. Equally, one might have a complete absence of illness but not experience well-being. Positive health, moreover, is said to be a broader concept, embracing well-being, fitness, and other related features (such as balance of physical, mental, and social elements). This analysis offers interesting possibilities for the development of health promotion to integrate with other forms of health intervention. At the very least it represents a move away from the dichotomized impasse between medical and health education ideologies.

Seedhouse (1986) takes a more pluralist view and argues that health is intrinsically composed of multiple meanings and definitions, being both a means and an end in itself. Consequently, he urges health promoters to adopt a fuzzy view of health as a potential, given definition by the wider personal and social context.

Whatever definition of health gains precedence, health is likely to remain an essentially contested concept for health promotion (Gallie 1956). How the issue is debated, more than the resolution of an agreed upon meaning, will in the end dictate whether or not health promotion achieves discipline status.

Another set of epistemic assumptions underlying different approaches to health promotion engenders levels of potential health attainment. That is, a set of expectations about what in principle can be achieved through health promotion. These range from superficial health (which merely keeps illness at bay) through to complete or absolute health (where health is a positive state). Seedhouse (1986) comes nearest to this understanding by distinguishing questions which address 'what is health?' from those which ask 'how can it be achieved?'

Both Seedhouse (1986) and Downie *et al.* (1990) make a strong case for health outcomes to be regarded as relative. The achievement of absolute health (as in the WHO's declaration of Health For All) is portrayed as Utopian. Not only are such goals considered to be unrealistic, but, they also imply fundamentally different strategies for health promotion methodology. Appropriate research and evaluation in health promotion would also need to focus on different health outcomes. Assessing relative health improvement requires different states of evidence than the measuring rod of absolute health.

As with all disciplines, health promotion can be best understood by the approaches it takes to solve such problems, rather than by the current nature of the subject matter. In any case, today's health topics will inevitably be replaced by other demands as the world of health continues to change. How well health promotion adapts to change and survives as a discipline will depend upon how efficient its methodologies are. In this sense the putative models or approaches epitomize the essential nature of the emerging discipline. They contain the special characteristics which distinguish health promotion from other subjects. Models debates then are disputes over the appropriate basis for the discipline. That is, they offer different solutions to the generalized demarcation problem in health promotion.

Possible solutions to the generalized demarcation problem in health promotion

The models question can be most usefully explored through a critical appraisal of the various solutions implied in the health promotion taxonomies. Revealing parallels may be drawn between solutions to the demarcation problem in the philosophy of science and the epistemic basis of health promotion theory. Three kinds of solution may be outlined:

1   that only one criterion is acceptable for promoting health (fundamentalist health promotion);
2   that no universal criterion is possible but some solution is possible (evolutionary health promotion);
3   that no criterion is possible, hence all versions are equally acceptable (eclectic health promotion).

Fundamentalist health promotion

Health promotion based on fundamentalist principles sections the world of health initiatives into the total range of possibilities and admits of only one universal criterion for deciding which course to adopt. Other approaches are seen as either irrelevant, misleading (drawing attention away from the 'true causes' of health problems), or, worse, as contradictory (simply adding to the problem). Freudenberg (1978), for example, contends that individually based health education programmes have signally failed to make any impact on public health. The only viable alternative, he insists, is collective action designed to alter the environment thereby facilitating lifestyle changes. Freudenberg also adds, however, that health professionals might resist this advocacy approach, not least because the politicization of their official role would expose them to the risk of censure from their employers.

The current vogue, however, is to make health promotion work community based (Hatch and Kickbusch 1984: Smithies and Adams 1990; Thomas 1983). Indeed, in Britain, a community development approach appears to be recognized as the most 'authentic' or ideal form of practice for health education specialists (Rawson and Grigg 1988).

Community development, however, can mean anything from attempts to change the lifestyle of communities, perhaps appropriately conceived of as a pluralistic version of individual health education (Puska *et al.* 1983), to the radical use of community empowerment as a vehicle for wider social and political reform (Freire 1972). Whilst community health promotion work offers a constructive possibility for improving public health, there is also a counterpart tendency to insert the term 'community' as a self-justifying prefix to any new health initiative.

Despite the radical politics implied by the health promotion examples, the underlying epistemology corresponds to the solution given by 'militant' positivism familiar to philosophers of science. In essence this led to a demand that all scientific statements be ultimately reducible to some verifiable observation. This form of scientific empiricism dominated the philosophy of science for nearly half of this century. The received view, as Suppe (1977) labels it, set limits on the basic framework for analysing problems in scientific method. This solution gave the sharpest cutting edge to the demarcation criteria but also perpetuated a narrow view of what constitutes scientific knowledge. In their haste to gain scientific respectability, social scientists, for example, tied themselves to the same sinking philosophical ship (Armistead 1974; Harré 1979).

The parallel for health promotion might be that acceptability comes to be synonymous with a demand for all health promotion statements to be ultimately reducible to social policy. Tones (1990) makes a similar point and urges that individualist health education approaches be regarded as complementary to structuralist (or non-individualist) health promotion rather than being disgarded as non-acceptable approaches.

Evolutionary health promotion

With this criterion health promotion might be seen as an outgrowth or logical progression of health education. The development of Tones' taxonomy (1981, 1983, 1985, 1986) best illustrates this solution. Health education models are depicted as progressive adaptations to the changing social climate and as a means of survival in the face of governmental health policies. Tones' work originally described a fourfold taxonomy of health education, but has since expanded to incorporate at least five distinct models and to redefine health education as a part of health promotion. Tones also attempts to delineate central and peripheral influences in the wider social and political context.

Several health education taxonomies invoke principles of hierarchical progression or other developmental sequences amongst models. Slavin and Chapman (1985), for example, postulate a developmental progression for both professionals and clients away from the inhibiting strictures set into the health establishment. Seedhouse (1986) also makes the point that health promotion should achieve some level of health in the health promoters. The reflexivity of health promotion is a further epistemological demand hitherto given little consideration in health promotion taxonomies. Perhaps like charity, health promotion should begin at home.

French and Adams (1986) advance a 'tri-phasic' map of health education models. The ordering also reflects the potential and significance for achieving changes in health. The taxonomy includes the corresponding aim, models of health and education along with underlying models of humanity and society for each of the three phases. The hierarchical progression reflects a sequential change or an evolution of health education strategies towards greater health effectiveness.

An evolutionary view of knowledge and scientific progress is mostly associated with Popper (1963) who argues that falsification could be used as a demarcation criterion between science and pseudo- or non-science. The falsificationist demands that all scientific theories should be capable of potential falsification. This means that all theories should be testable or refutable in principle. Popper sees science progressing through a cumulative process of conjectures and refutations in which weaker theories are eliminated and replaced by more powerful versions with increasing empirical verisimilitude (a closer correspondence with reality).

Developmental sequences in taxonomies of health education similarly imply a principle of *increasing health verisimilitude*. That is, succeeding or higher models in the sequence are considered to be more effective in realizing health benefits. Typically this has been associated with a greater emphasis on structural changes. Conversely, health education models further down the sequence are more likely to be associated with falsifications or failures to bring about health benefits. Any paradigm shift from health education to health promotion may be best understood in this light.

According to the Duhem-Quine thesis, however, theories can be rescued from falsification simply by a relevant adjustment to the background knowledge. The problem is to locate which components are refuted and which are to be retained. With health promotion it is similarly important to discover at what point health education initiatives cease to be effective or what aspect of different approaches may be modified to better suit the aims of health promotion.

Eclectic health promotion

This position is based on the principle that all approaches to health promotion are equally plausible, since no one criterion is possible. The selection of appropriate activity is therefore based either on pragmatic considerations or is arbitrary and random. The Ewles and Simnett (1985) taxonomy, for example, makes explicit the eclectic nature of health promotion work. As they expound, 'In our view there is no-one "right" approach to health education'. Whilst this may be viewed charitably as a liberal solution, in which choice is left to the sagacity of the practitioner, it amounts to an epistemologically arbitrary or anarchic solution. It may seem surprising to equate Ewles and Simnett's otherwise conservative work with epistemological anarchism. Of course their formulation was not intended that way. The epistemic basis of their work none the less implies such a solution by default, as does any pragmatist taxonomy offering no objective rationale for the selection of appropriate health promotion methodologies (cf. Catford and Parish 1989; Downie *et al.* 1990).

Beyond this, such approaches foresee neither contradictions nor professional dilemmas in choosing one model over another or electing any combination of models. The alternative interpretation is to see the health educator exercising choice as also exercising a form of élitism (which means a return to fundamentalist health promotion).

Within the philosophy of science, Feyerabend's thesis (1975) advocates an extreme form of relativism. A resolute anarchist and Dadaist, Feyerabend argues that all theories are equally right or wrong and therefore equally acceptable or rejectable. Originally a stout hearted Popperian, Feyerabend has since challenged all rational normative solutions to the generalized demarcation problem, contending that, if applied, they would have the effect of shackling scientific progress. Lakatos (1970), however, argues that unless we are to create a situation of real anarchism (where pseudoscience has equal status with true science) there is a need for a rational and conventional solution. But, Feyerabend insists, all rational alternatives are founded on unrealistic assumptions about epistemological commensurability of theories. Rather, he sees knowledge growing in an ocean of incompatible ideas. Epistemological anarchism, therefore, is offered as the only tenable solution.

Within health promotion, a number of theorists reach conclusions carrying the same epistemic implications. In filling out their 'choice-change-champion' framework, Catford and Parish (1989) present a highly eclectic battery of imported models to guide health promotion. Their selection ranges from social learning theory (Bandura 1977) with its emphasis on self-efficacy to social marketing (Manoff 1985). Whilst such models are arguably contradictory, the Catford and Parish framework treats them as totally discrete influences at different and apparently unrelated stages in the overall framework of health promotion. The theoretical influences, that is, are regarded as incommensurable. No linking mechanisms are hypothesized and no rationale is given for the selection of one imported theoretical model over any other.

Whilst we might hope that the assembled models represent a judicious selection in a creative proliferation of workable approaches, the overall framework appears to have no guiding principles. Such unabashed eclecticism leaves health promotion in a limbo of arbitrary influences. With no theoretical basis to call its own it may be easily assimilated by more powerful rivals or dismissed as an empty subject matter wholly dependent on other disciplines.

Despite his efforts in generating core theory work, French (1990) also contends that the theoretical content of health promotion is intrinsically eclectic. He is further unhopeful about the development of any overarching health promotion theory to integrate the diverse strands of influence.

Feyerabend, however, does not sustain a pessimistic outlook with epistemological diversity. In a doctrine of proliferation he suggests scientists should proceed with an 'anything goes' philosophy. This might be best regarded as a form of brainstorming in the scientific community. Although Feyerabend's methodological and epistemological pluralism has much force in promoting a creative scientific enterprise, he ultimately neglects the objective content of science. That is, theories may in fact be successful (or not) in predicting events or giving rise to powerful technologies. The need for a solution to the demarcation problem also becomes crucial when there are rival theories vying for limited resources or where there are direct implications for social engineering (Urbach 1974). Health promotion, of course, faces exactly these circumstances.

Unlike Kuhn, Feyerabend has had little impact on social scientists, but has been influential with philosophers of science. On epistemological grounds alone, Feyerabend's position represents a logically possible extreme form of relativism, which must be taken seriously by philosophers of science. It appears that much of health promotion should also be reconsidered in the light of this epistemology.

Health promotion and the theory–practice gap

Schön (1983) argues that a model of technical rationality dominates professional thinking. Practitioners can be seen to act instrumentally, applying the tools of science to solve problems. With the technical rationality of applied science, practical knowledge is entirely used as a means to an end. An assumption is made, moreover, that the ends are unambiguous and agreed upon.

Such a technical application of science in this way leads to a separation of research and practice. In turn this further polarizes the theory–practice gap, with practitioners becoming more doers than thinkers.

Since applied science is based on some scientific discipline it follows that problems are defined by the relevant scientific theory as much as the needs of practitioners. The importation of models from other disciplines in this way redefines health promotion, not as an emerging discipline growing out of the fruits of others, but as a practice ground for others. Contrary to what some advocates of the new health promotion movement think, the successful use of models imported into health promotion may not add to the discipline status of health promotion. Rather, it constitutes a victory of hegemony for the exporting discipline as it takes over further empirical ground (Laudan 1977).

Schön (1983) argues instead for the emergence of a new epistemology of practice in which practitioners reconstruct their own knowledge base from their tacit knowledge-in-action to become *reflective practitioners*. To this end he advocates incorporating into practice two sources of explicit knowledge building.

Reflection-in-action concerns knowledge which guides practice during the process of implementation. It embodies the 'tricks of the trade', or practitioner know-how.

Reflection-on-action takes a longer view and concerns the positioning of action relative to other possible courses. Both forms of reflection demand the emergence of concepts capable of encompassing practice operations. This may even necessitate the building of a new meta-language to describe the basis of appropriate knowledge. Like other practitioners, health promoters have their own language, though this is largely distinct from written accounts and is only overheard in day-to-day practice or occasionally at conferences.

It is important to caution, however, against repeating the theoretical cul-de-sac encountered by educational philosophy in the attempt to deduce theory from practice. Hirst (1983) reflects that it became concerned only with explanation and neglected to produce guiding principles. De Castell (1989) adds that educational philosophy is now generally regarded as over-intellectualized and of little practical use. It led to a divide between those who had time to reflect and write, and those who could take time only to talk about their practical world. This division of labour extended yet again the distinction between theory and practice.

To articulate and codify practical knowledge, as Schön would have it, scholarly discourse must take the form of theory construction through literate practice. De Castell warns, however, that institutional factors impose severe limits upon reflections about action. Practitioners are typically given neither the time nor the encouragement to engage in theory construction.

Without some form of objectification of practice, however, it is difficult to transmit the lessons of experience efficiently. Training is almost entirely limited to role modelling. Trapped in subjective relativism each new cohort of practitioners must reinvent the subject matter (including blind alleys and mistakes) as they necessarily strive to recreate the essential experience for acquiring competence. Of greatest consequence, the growth of knowledge is severely stunted through the lack of accumulated wisdom and restricted opportunities for shared criticism.

Schön's model of the reflective practitioner cannot, moreover, be grafted on to practice in yet another exercise of technical rationality. It does, though, provide an important challenge to our view of how disciplines emerge. This is significant for training and development work amongst health promotion specialists and offers an alternative to the constricting concepts of role delineation based upon task analysis (Rawson and Grigg 1988). Just as importantly, the prospect of a new epistemology of practice shows that health promotion need not be limited by the horizons of other disciplines. There is instead the opportunity to establish core theoretical work building on the development of practice.

For health promotion theory to be regarded as progressive it must be shown to accomplish all that rival approaches claim to plus it must uncover new possibilities for improving health or at least our understanding of what constitutes health (Lakatos 1970). This will be the most difficult aspect to establish but it would also generate the most powerful indicator for continued confidence in health promotion.

Conclusions

According to Shapere (1977), in scientific practice it is rational for scientists at various stages of development of a theory to continue pursuing and fostering it even though they may be explicitly aware that it is literally false. Indeed, it may be that all young theories go through such a primitive stage and it would be nonsense to attempt refutations. Theory may be put forward initially not as true, but as some idealization or as a model or even a useful fiction. In the development of a theory it becomes pertinent to ask at any particular stage whether it purports to provide a realistic explanation or else is offered as a conceptual device. In providing an adequate account of scientific practice Shapere also insists that we must accommodate the actual uses to which theory is put.

The same questions have to be addressed to health promotion. Even if no ready answers can be found, the asking will help better define the subject matter and create the discipline to discover the true potential of health promotion.

References

Adams, L. (1985) 'Health education: in whose interest?', *Radical Health Promotion* Spring: 11–14.

Anderson, D. (1980) 'Blind alleys in health education', in A. Seldon (ed.) *The Litmus Papers*, London: Centre for Policy Studies.

Armistead, N. (ed.) (1974) *Reconstructing Social Psychology*, Harmondsworth: Penguin.

Bandura, A. (1977) 'Self-efficacy: towards a unifying theory of behavioural change', *Psychological Review* 84(2): 191–215.

Beattie, A. (1980) *A Structural Repertoire of the Models of Health Education*, Exeter: Health Certificate Tutors Workshop.

—— (1984) 'Health education and the science teacher: an invitation to debate', *Education and Health* 2(1): 9–15.

—— (1991) 'Knowledge and control in health promotion: a test case for social policy and social theory', in J. Gabe, M. Calnan, and M. Bury (eds) *The Sociology of the Health Service*, London: Routledge.

Bernstein, B. (1980) 'On the classification and framing of knowledge', in M. Young (ed.) *Knowledge and Control*, London: Collier Macmillan.

Birn, H. and Birn, B. (1985) 'Education for wellness', *Community Dental Health* 2: 1–6.

Blalock, H. M. (ed.) (1971) *Causal Models in the Social Sciences*, Chicago: Aldine Atherton.

Bowman, R. A. (1976) 'Changes in the activities, functions and roles of public health educators', *Health Education Monographs* 4(3): 226–46.

Burkitt, A. (1983) 'Models of health', in J. Clarke (ed.) *Readings in Community Medicine*, Edinburgh: Churchill Livingstone.

Burrell, G. and Morgan, G. (1985) *Sociological Paradigms and Organizational Analysis*, Aldershot: Gower.

Caplan, R. and Holland, R. (1990) 'Rethinking health education theory', *Health Education Journal* 49(1): 10–12.

de Castell, S. (1989) 'On writing of theory and practice', *Journal of the Philosophy of Education* 23(1): 39–50.

Catford, J. and Parish, R. (1989) '"Heartbeat Wales": new horizons for health promotion in the community – the philosophy and practice of Heartbeat Wales', in D. Seedhouse and A. Cribb (eds) *Changing Ideas in Health Care*, Chichester: Wiley.

Chalmers, A. F. (1976) *What is This Thing Called Science?*, Milton Keynes: Open University Press.

Collins, L. (1982) *Concepts of Health Held by Members of Four Professional Groups*, National Conference on Research and Development in Health Education with Special Reference to Youth, University of Southampton, 10 September 1982.

—— (1984) 'Concepts of health education: a study of four professional groups', *Journal of Institute of Health Education* 23(3): 81–8.

Crawford, R. (1977) 'You are dangerous to your health: the ideology and politics of victim-blaming', *Journal of Health Services* 7: 663–80.

Dearden, R. F. (1972) 'Autonomy and education', in R. F. Dearden, P. H. Hurst, and R. S. Peters (eds) *Education and the Development of Reason*, London: Routledge & Kegan Paul.

Diesing, P. (1971) *Patterns of Discovery in the Social Sciences*, London: Routledge & Kegan Paul.

Dorn, N. (1983) *Alcohol, Youth and the State*, Bromley: Croom Helm.

Downie, R. S., Fyfe, C., and Tannahill, A. (1990) *Health Promotion: Models and Values*, Oxford: Oxford Medical Publications.

Draper, P. (1979) *Rethinking Community Medicine*, Unit for the Study of Health Policy, 11–15.

—— (1983) 'Tackling the disease of ignorance', *Journal of College of Health* 1: 23–5.

Draper, P., Griffiths, J., Dennis, J., and Popay, J. (1979) 'Three types of health education', *British Medical Journal* 16 August: 495–8.

Dwore, R. and Matarazzo, J. (1981) 'The behavioural sciences and health education', *Health Education* May/June: 4–7.

Ewles, L. and Simnett, I. (1985) *Promoting Health – A Practical Guide to Health Education*, Chichester: Wiley.

Feyerabend, P. (1975) *Against Method*, London: New Left Books.

Freire, P. (1972) *Pedagogy of the Oppressed*, Harmondsworth: Penguin.

French, J. (1984) *A Review of Contemporary Health Education Models and their Relevance in Postgraduate Education Courses in the U.K.*, unpublished MSc dissertation, Chelsea College, University of London.

—— (1990) 'Boundaries and horizons, the role of health education within health promotion', *Health Education Journal* 49(1): 7–10.

French, J. and Adams, L. (1986) 'From analysis to synthesis', *Health Education Journal* 45(2): 71–3.

Freudenberg, N. (1978) 'Shaping the future of health education from behavioural change to social action', *Health Education Monographs* 6 (4).

Galli, N. (1978) *Foundations and Principles of Health Education*, New York: Wiley.

Gallie, W. B. (1956) 'Essentially contested concepts', *Proceedings of Aristotelian Society* 56: 167–98.

Gellner, E. (1974) *Legitimation of Belief*, Cambridge: Cambridge University Press.

Harré, R. (1979) *Social Being: A Theory for Social Psychology*, Oxford: Blackwell.

Hatch, S. and Kickbusch, I. (1984) *Self-help and Health in Europe*, Copenhagen: WHO.

Hirst, P. (1983) 'Educational theory', in P. Hirst (ed.) *Educational Theory and its Foundational Disciplines*, London: Routledge & Kegan Paul.

Kelvin, P. (1980) 'The search for models is a delusion', in A. J. Chapman and D. M. Jones (eds) *Models of Man*, Leicester: British Psychological Society.

Krijnen, M., Schenk, R., and Garnick, W. (eds) (1982) *Health Education – A Major in Health Science: Philosophy and Exit Level Competencies*, Limburg State University, Maastricht.

Kuhn, T. S. (1957) *The Copernican Revolution*, Boston, MA: Harvard University Press.

—— (1962) *The Structure of Scientific Revolutions*, Chicago: University of Chicago Press.

—— (1970) *The Structure of Scientific Revolutions*, second edition, Chicago: University of Chicago Press.

Labonte, R. and Penfold, S. (1981) 'Canadian perspectives in health promotion', *Health Education* 19: 4–7.

Lakatos, I. (1970) 'Falsification and the methodology of scientific research programmes', in I. Lakatos and A. Musgrave (eds) *Criticism and the Growth of Knowledge*, Cambridge: Cambridge University Press.

Laudan, L. (1977) *Progress and its Problems*, Berkeley, CA: University of California Press.

Manoff, R. K. (1985) *Social Marketing: New Imperatives for Public Health*, New York: Praeger.

Mills, C. Wright (1959) *The Sociological Imagination*, Oxford: Oxford University Press.

Nagel, E. (1961) *The Structure of Science*, London: Routledge & Kegan Paul.

Neutens, J. J. (1984) 'Professional competencies of the health educators', in L. Rubinson and W. F. Alles (eds) *Health Education: Foundations for the Future*, St Louis, MO: Times Mirror/Mosby.

Nutbeam, D. (1984) 'Health education in the National Health Service: the differing perspectives of community physicians and health education officers', *Health Education Journal* 43(4): 115–19.

Peters, R. S. (1977) *Education and the Education of Teachers*, London: Routledge & Kegan Paul.

Popper, K. R. (1957) *The Poverty of Historicism*, London: Routledge & Kegan Paul.

—— (1959) *The Logic of Scientific Discovery*, London: Hutchinson.

—— (1963) *Conjectures and Refutations*, London: Routledge & Kegan Paul.

Puska, P., Salonen, J., Nissinen, A., and Tuomilehto, J. (1983) 'Change in risk factors for coronary heart disease during ten years of community intervention programme (North Karelia Project)', *British Medical Journal* 287: 1840.

Rawson, D. and Grigg, C. (1988) *Purpose & Practice in Health Education*, London: South Bank Polytechnic/HEA.

Research Unit in Health & Behavioural Change, University of Edinburgh (1989) *Changing the Public Health*, Chichester: Wiley.

Rodmell, S. and Watts, A. (eds) (1986) *The Politics of Health Education*, London: Routledge & Kegan Paul.

Rosenberg, A. (1988) *Philosophy of Social Science*, Oxford: Clarendon Press.

Schön, D. A. (1983) *The Reflective Practitioner: How Professionals Think in Action*, New York: Basic Books.

Seedhouse, D. (1986) *Health: Foundations for Achievement*, Chichester: Wiley.

Seedhouse, D. and Cribb, A. (eds) (1989) *Changing Ideas in Health Care*, Chichester: Wiley.

Seymour, H. (1984) 'Health education versus health promotion – a practitioner's view', *Health Education Journal* 43(2&3): 37–8.

Shapere, D. (1977) 'Scientific theories and their domains', in F. Suppe (ed.) *The Structure of Scientific Theories*, Urbana: University of Illinois Press.

Slavin, H. and Chapman, V. (1985) *The Application of Models of Health Education to Health Visitor Training and Practice*, 1st International Conference of Health Education in Nursing, Health Visiting and Midwifery, Harrogate, 23 May 1985.

Smithies, J. and Adams, L., with Webster, G. and Beattie, A. (1990) *Community Participation in Health Promotion*, HEA.

Suppe, F. (ed.) (1977) *The Structure of Scientific Theories*, 2nd edition, Urbana: University of Illinois Press.

Tannahill, A. (1985) 'What is health promotion?', *Health Education Journal* 44(4): 167–8.

Taylor, V. (1990) 'Health education – a theoretical mapping', *Health Education Journal* 49(1): 13–14.

Thomas, D. (1983) *The Making of Community Work*, London: Allen & Unwin.

Thorpe, P. (1982) 'Individual or collective responsibilities for health', *Nursing* May: 8–10.

Tones, B. K. (1981) 'Health education: prevention or subversion', *Royal Society of Health Journal* 101(3): 114–17.

—— (1983) 'Health education and health promotion: new directions', *Journal of Institute of Health Education* 21: 4.

—— (1985) 'Health promotion – a new panacea?', *Journal of Institute of Health Education* 23: 16–21.

—— (1986) 'Health education and the ideology of health promotion: a review of alternative approaches', *Health Education Research* 1(1): 3–12.

—— (1990) 'Why theorize? Ideology in health education', *Health Education Journal* 49(1): 2–6.

Tones, B. K., Tilford, S., and Robinson, J. K. (1990) *Health Education: Effectiveness and Efficiency*, London: Chapman & Hall.

Urbach, P. (1974) 'Progress and degeneration in the IQ debate', *British Journal of Philosophy of Science* 25: 99–135 & 235–59.

Warr, P. B. (1980) 'An introduction to models in psychological research', in A. J. Chapman and D. M. Jones (eds) *Models of Man*, Leicester: British Psychological Society.

Whitehead, M. (1989) *Swimming Upstream: Trends and Prospects in Education and Health*, London: King's Fund Institute.

Williams, G. and Aspin, D. (1980) 'The philosophy of health education related to schools', in J. Cowley, K. David, and S. T. Williams (eds) *Health Education in Schools*, London: Harper & Row.

WHO (1984) *Health Promotion: A Discussion Document on the Concepts and Principles*, Copenhagen: WHO.

12 Introducing ethics to health promotion

Alan Cribb and Peter Duncan

Introducing ethics

Our fundamental concern in this chapter is to explain and explore the relevance of ethics to the practice of health promotion. We will be considering ways in which the *content* of ethics (what ethicists talk about) and its *form* (the ways in which ethicists talk) can contribute to understanding and evaluating health promotion. We will, however, begin by making a few introductory remarks about ethics itself.

Ethics is the name of both an academic discipline and its subject matter. In very general terms, it is an enquiry into what is right or good. It is a disciplined attempt to (a) justify (or critique) particular values, or sets of values; and (b) to understand what kinds of conduct embody or promote these values. Put otherwise, it is about how we ought to live and to act. It ranges from very abstract theoretical questions about the bases and nature of ethical judgement to more applied concerns with important social questions about, for example, human welfare, social justice, and our duties to other animals or the environment

These concerns – with elaborating and justifying values, and analysing the kinds of conduct likely to produce these values – are closely connected. One way of understanding the history of ethics is as a range of projects attempting to justify forms of life and lines of conduct which embody or produce 'the valuable', whatever that might be. We want briefly to examine two such mainstream traditions in Western philosophy. Our summaries of these traditions (which are necessarily crude) will be followed later by an illustration of how they might be applied in the evaluation of health promotion practice.

Deontology (usually linked with the name of Immanuel Kant, the most famous German philosopher of the Enlightenment) is the ethical tradition based on the idea that we owe each other particular duties or obligations. There just are certain kinds of things we must do, or must not do – certain rules we must follow. For example, we have a duty to treat other people with respect, and not, for example, to lie to them. This duty cannot be reduced to further considerations; we cannot, for example, think that in a particular case we should put respect to one side because we want to keep a particularly painful truth from someone. Respecting persons is not merely an instrumental good – something that is valuable because it produces valuable consequences (and which might, therefore, be waived where it produces unhappiness) – it is simply our duty, whatever the circumstances in which we find ourselves.

The belief, by contrast, that circumstances do shape duties frames the second tradition we are introducing. This is *consequentialism*, a range of theories based around the idea that in considering the ethical acceptability of any action, we must focus first and foremost on the consequences it is likely to produce. One of the best-known consequentialist theories is *utilitarianism*; and arguably its most famous proponent is J. S. Mill, the nineteenth-century British philosopher. Mill's principle of utility treats an action as right or wrong to the extent that it produces more or less 'happiness'. Mill, and many other philosophers, have sought to refine this apparently bald theory in a number of ways. These refinements involve, for example, different conceptualizations of happiness, and other ways of characterizing that which we ought to optimize (e.g. 'preference satisfaction' rather than happiness). Another possible refinement is the idea of 'rule utilitarianism' – the idea that (rather than trying to assess things action by action) we should obey those rules that are likely to produce the greatest happiness if generally followed. (Here we can see the possibility of some of the gaps between deontology and consequentialism closing to some extent. Indeed, a fuller account of these two traditions would not only open up many rival currents within each tradition, but also the difficulties of definitively demarcating the two traditions.)

Both of these important traditions concerned with explaining ethical conduct suggest an important feature to do with the *form* of ethics. As an academic discipline, ethics is essentially analytic. It is oriented towards systematic argument and requires conceptual elucidation and justification of assumptions. This may give the impression of it being an abstract discipline, unconnected with the real world. But the field of 'applied ethics' connects the discipline of moral philosophy to areas of human concern and endeavour, including professional and occupational action.

The relevance of ethics to health care

One of our first jobs is to explain the rationale for applying ethics to health promotion or health care more generally. Perhaps this is not such a difficult task. Nowadays health care ethics is much more than just an academic discipline. It is very much a part of popular discourse. Indeed, these days we are almost as likely to demonize as to idealize health professionals. Dr Harold Shipman, the United Kingdom's first mass-murdering General Practitioner, is obviously an exceptional figure. Yet the terrible disruption of trust this must have caused in the local population he was supposed to be serving is a crude symbol for a more diffused and gradual leakage of public trust and confidence in those professionally engaged in health care; a leakage represented in debates over a myriad of 'lesser' controversies. Some of these controversies arise from exposures of what come to be judged as 'bad practice'; for example, failures of consent or of competence. Others stem from generalized, deeply-rooted fears about the directions in which health care is going. Do we really want to permit euthanasia, cloning, etc.? Our capacity to create, end, and change human life challenges our conceptions and understanding of what it is to be human. Moreover, even if we can understand and resolve this challenge, how can we be sure that such technological developments, if permitted, would be handled responsibly? Literally and metaphorically, health professionals are 'in the dock', subject to profound questioning and scepticism from a society once in thrall to their expertise.

Surely, though, health promotion is a case apart? What difficulty can there be in helping people stay healthy? We suggest that there is substantial difficulty; and that appealing to honourable goals and evidence of good intentions is not sufficient. (We do not, after all, consider it to be so in cases of bio-medical controversy.)

Why health promoters need ethics

Imagine two people, H and C. H is a health promoter seeking to promote C's health. To do so, H effects some change to C, either directly or to his environment (for example, she gives C information, puts fluoride in C's drinking water etc.). In any event, H's action affects C. But why should C trust H? H may argue that she is bringing a benefit to C; however, there are at least two difficulties with this argument. First, C may simply object to interference in his life, regardless of the intentions or consequences of H's action. Second, C may dispute that H's actions will, in fact, produce the intended (beneficial) outcomes; or disagree that the intended outcomes are actually beneficial. In short, there is no compelling reason why C should trust H on the basis of claims to 'benefit'. (If H transforms into a group of people and C into a community or population, the position becomes still more complicated.)

Why should we be any less sceptical about H's action than C? Why should we be less reluctant to cede trust and accept H's authority? One possible response is to suggest that H possesses a level of expertise which C lacks; that H is simply in a better position to judge what is best. But even if we accept that, in this case, technical judgement about 'effectiveness' or 'benefit' is possible (and very often in the field of health promotion it isn't), a difficulty remains. It is that the judgements required are not solely technical. The question, 'Will action x (water fluoridation, say) cause outcome y (reductions in caries, more dental health)?' might be considered a technical question subject to expert judgement. (Although even here there are disputes about the potential neutrality and legitimacy of scientific judgement.) But imagine the questions, 'Is it right for H to intervene in C's life by fluoridating his water supply?'; or 'Is more dental health of value to C?' These questions are definitely not susceptible to scientific expertise. They are questions of ethics and, like all such questions, cannot be resolved by reference to technical knowledge and expertise.

H's appeal to authority, then, cannot rest on technical or scientific expertise alone (or even at all); it has to be more broadly grounded and more carefully won. Fundamentally, the ethics of health promotion involves the careful examination of the authority or legitimacy of health promoters. It asks us to explain and justify our choice – if we make it – to side with H rather than C. If we fail to do so, we risk entailing the kind of arrogance sometimes associated with bio-medicine – an arrogance which is routinely condemned.

Ethics: from theory to practice

We have identified that C may have at least two worries about H, each apparently rather different to the other. The first is that it is just *wrong* for H to interfere in his life, even if it is for his own good. The second is that H's actions will not, anyway, produce *good* consequences. These worries correspond to the two broad traditions of ethics we introduced at the beginning of the chapter; deontology and consequentialism (which we will simplify respectively as 'rule-based' and 'consequence-based' approaches to ethics).

Are these two worries actually different in kind; or can they ultimately be reduced to the same sort of concern? We can use the positions assumed by the rule-based approach on the one hand, and the consequence-based approach on the other, to explore H's intervention with C. When and why might this intervention be wrong (or right) in terms of rules? And when and why might it be wrong (or right) in terms of consequences?

There are a cluster of 'rules' – many often unspoken in social conduct – which suggest H ought not to intervene. These include the general entitlement to be left alone; to be able to make one's own mistakes; to privacy. All these things can be summed up by our duty to respect others and in particular to respect their autonomy. Respect for autonomy is central to the cluster of social norms or 'rules' referred to above, that are widely accepted in liberal individualist societies. However, there is one important and fairly obvious set of exceptions to such norms: we do not believe that people should be left to live their own lives to the extent that in doing so they cause harm to others. (This is often referred to in ethics as the 'harm principle'.) Consideration of the 'harm principle' means that H would have to think long and hard before attempting to justify her health promotion interventions. She would have to balance a duty to respect autonomy with an examination of whether – and how – the 'harm principle' might apply in relation to her work. The principle does not necessarily rule health promotion out, but it does demand a careful examination of the case for intervening. The challenge, of course, is in interpreting its implications for practice. But leaving aside its application to practice for now, it is important to clarify its force. First, if we accept the 'harm principle', we cannot override it simply by claiming substantial benefits to C and others; we would need to show that leaving C alone will result in her causing harm to others. Second, H may pursue the alternative path of seeking to gain C's consent to the intervention. If she is successful, though, the intervention ceases to constitute 'interference' of the kind we have been concerned about. (But once again, while this further principle of 'informed consent' may have widespread currency, the challenge is how to interpret and apply it in practice.)

We turn now to thinking primarily about consequences rather than rules *per se*. Here we might still want to bear in mind certain principles (such as the 'harm principle') but do so because these are 'rules of thumb' providing helpful 'habits of thought' rather than sufficient and authoritative guides to action in themselves. Such principles now gain their value because, and insofar as, they generate good consequences. To put it crudely, society is made a better place because they exist; we can each live our lives, and pursue our own interests and projects, secure in the knowledge that others will give us the space to do so. Given that, in the main, we are each likely to be quite good judges of what suits us, and that other people may often be mistaken in this regard, this arrangement of non-interference is the surest means available to us of maximizing people's happiness. But – a consequentialist thinker might go on to argue – we should not make a fetish out of these general principles. The fact that many people accept the 'harm principle', that it *feels* strongly normative, does not make it sacrosanct. It is possible that while the principle is generally useful, it does not always and in every case generate the best results. What we need to do is to examine the effects of health promotion – in general and in particular cases – and ask whether or not health promotion interventions produce sufficiently worthwhile societal outcomes, all things considered, for them to be justified. If this is the case, then we are ethically right to allow them (indeed we may decide we are obliged to put them in place), even if they do entail a measure of interference. (In such cases, if we are working with individuals, this does not of course preclude application of the principle of 'informed consent' – although this is likely to become extremely problematic if we are working with communities or populations. How precisely do we obtain informed consent from a large population?)

We will now move on from this rather abstract debate. In the rest of this chapter we will assume that both rules-based and consequence-based accounts of ethics have something to offer health promotion. However, it is important to summarize our discussions so far. In brief, we have argued that there can be no presumption in favour of health promotion. (For all sorts of reasons, simply to assert that 'it's a good thing' is plainly insufficient.) Health promoters must be able to justify their actions and, in this process, should have regard to whether or not they breach the 'harm principle'; and if so, why their work might justify such a breach. At least part of any task of justification will entail a close examination of the multiple effects of their actions: some analysis of what are 'good' and 'bad' consequences; and how these different kinds of consequences are to be identified and balanced together. The task of justification is likely to be demanding and complex.

Debating the ethics of health promotion

So far we have attempted to do two things. First, to introduce some of the basic *content* of ethics, and of ethics applied to health promotion; and second to introduce its *form*. In talking of form, we have tried to indicate that ethics – including, of course, applied ethics – is at its heart about dispute and debate. This suggests that there is no correct 'ethical formula' for decision making, no single set of 'right answers'. We agree with this, but we also wish to stress the value of gaining familiarity with the different voices in ethical debate, and of learning what lies behind particular disputes and disagreements. When we can, as the saying goes, 'see things from both sides' (or even 'from many sides'), we are better placed to explain and defend our own ethical stances.

In what follows we will continue to open up the debates in health promotion ethics, using examples of influential work in the field to do so. We should stress immediately that we cannot do proper justice to any of this work here. We are obviously limited to drawing out a very few descriptive comments and summary notes on the work to which we draw attention; and, as we have noted, the essence of applied ethics is in its arguments rather than its conclusions. However, we believe that each example of work to which we refer says fundamental things about the ethics of health promotion. We briefly bring these together and reinforce their connections to practice in our conclusion. But we hope that anyone with an interest in the field will go on to read these texts themselves.

1 Daniel Wikler and the ends and means of health promotion

One of the most closely argued and penetrating discussions on health promotion ethics is also one of the oldest. In 'Persuasion and Coercion for Health', the American philosopher Daniel Wikler debates possible justifications for government-sponsored forms of 'lifestyle' health promotion (Wikler 1978). His paper further unpacks the issue of 'interference' that has dominated our discussions and sets the relationship between health promoters (our H) and their 'clients' (our C) in a broader context. Does it make a difference to our consideration of activity if H is the government (or health promoters working on its behalf); and if C is a community of people or a population rather than an individual client? While we may intuitively feel these factors make a difference to our considerations, Wikler considers this question much more systematically. Part of our intuition is that while we may strongly feel that it is wrong for equal citizens to interfere in the lives of each other, we do not necessarily feel so in respect of the relationship between a *government* and its citizens. As Wikler points out, most of us routinely accept that the state is entitled to regulate to try and protect health, even though this clearly involves 'interfering' in people's lives. What is important, he argues, is to look carefully at why and how the government might be entitled to intervene to promote health; what are its 'ends' in doing so and what are its 'means'?

Wikler concentrates his analysis on government intervention in 'unhealthy lifestyles' (although he does refer to other examples), such as smoking, overeating, lack of physical exercise, and so on. He considers three possible ends or goals for government-sponsored health promotion for 'lifestyle reform':

1   The government may simply be interested in promoting health as an end in itself.
2   It may be interested in preventing some people in society from the unfairness of having to pay for the costs of the unhealthy choices of others (the rising bill of hospital and insurance services).
3   It may be interested in promoting other social benefits (or 'utility') to which better population health contributes, such as national economic well-being.

Considered separately, each of these three possible goals or ends may not provide a justification for much health promotion. Taken together, however – and, crucially, bearing in mind the means to achieve them – they become more persuasive. An individual citizen might dismiss the first reason as unjustified 'paternalism' – 'choosing' to be healthy or unhealthy is up to her or him. However, the second and third reasons provide a crucial social dimension. He or she cannot so easily dismiss arguments from 'fairness' and 'social utility'. Our lives are caught up in a complex social nexus. Another way of making this same point is to highlight the ambiguity and contestability of the 'harm principle' – it is very difficult to draw a sharp line between those of my choices which risk harming others and those which do not.

Nonetheless, as Wikler persuasively argues, so much of what we value about life in largely liberal societies depends upon setting a high weighting on individual privacy and choice before we try to 'force' social ends, however laudable, on people. Furthermore we would need to be convinced that the desired social ends would be of substantial value; we would also have to be confident that health promotion measures (our 'lifestyle reform') would actually bring them about. Here, however, the question of 'means' becomes important. There is a wide range of possible interventions open to health promoters in their attempt to achieve 'ends'; and these can be more or less intrusive and coercive:

> Health promotion programs that are only very mildly coercive, such as moderate increases in cigarette taxes, require very little justification; non-coercive measures such as health education require none at all. And the case for more intrusive measures would be stronger if greater and more certain benefits could be promised.
>
> (Wikler 1978: 117)

In other words, it may be possible to construct some goals or 'ends' of health promotion which have sufficient social importance to justify 'intrusion' to at least some degree, provided there is a level of confidence that this 'intrusion' would be likely to result in this 'end'. (The problem lies partly, of course, in establishing agreement on the 'ends'; and evidence of the relationship between intervention and goal.)

2 Health education and persuasion for health: a view from Alastair Campbell

We want now to examine an argument extending Wikler's suggestion above that there are more or less intrusive and coercive methods available to health promoters. Some of these (on the 'less' end of the scale) may not actually involve 'interfering' in people's lives – at least not in a way that has much ethical significance. Thus our concern about a health promotion activity or intervention may be significantly lessened or even completely misplaced. What, for example, could be wrong with health *education*?

This is a theme developed by Alastair Campbell (1990). He accepts that certain forms of educational 'intervention' are not intrusive and pose no threat to individual autonomy. If H 'offers' C a carefully tailored, reasoned, and balanced account of the best available evidence about the relationship between 'x' (health-related action) and 'y' (health status) – so that C can decide whether or not to 'listen and take note' – then C can hardly claim his autonomy is being compromised. Indeed, it may seem that perhaps the only way to support and respect C's personal autonomy is to provide education of this sort. (Would we be respecting autonomy if we failed to work with, say, C the smoker to develop a balanced account of the health risks – and benefits – cigarettes pose to him?)[1] Yet this is precisely Campbell's concern! He is not questioning whether this sort of 'pure' health education is ethically justifiable; he is trying to establish whether or not this is the *only* sort of health education which is ethically justifiable. What about educational campaigns that are 'attention grabbing', which use powerful images, or glamour, or persuasive rhetoric and slogans, etc.? Aren't these forms of persuasion ethically dubious? Aren't health promoters, then, guilty of unethical conduct – to the extent that at least sometimes they rely on, or borrow from, these more persuasive techniques?

This is a crucial issue for health promoters because all health promotion involves 'trading' in information (albeit typically in conjunction with other activities). What are the limits of 'ethical trading' in information? Campbell is concerned that health promoters should not draw the limits so narrowly that only very high-minded, and perhaps one-to-one, appeals to 'cold' rationality will qualify as acceptable. On the other hand, it is clear that there are some communication styles, and some 'messages', that are unacceptable. If this were not the case, there would be nothing wrong in principle with television campaigns frightening parents with images and scare stories of heavy infant mortality caused by the consumption of sweets and chocolates. As it is, most of us would surely feel that such approaches were unacceptable. And we would feel this way not simply because at a technical level they might be ineffective or counter-productive; but perhaps much more importantly because it seems to us simply wrong, in an ethical sense, to lie to and mislead people, and equally wrong to deliberately frighten and alarm others without very good cause indeed. Where, then, should we draw the limits?

Campbell argues that we cannot afford to be simply 'for' education and 'against' persuasion. After all, many of the fundamental goals of health promotion require political change of one kind or another; and persuasion is a fundamental tool of politics. To disbar health promoters from the use of this tool would seem to disbar them from a place in the real world. What is needed instead, he argues, is a distinction between legitimate and illegitimate forms of persuasion. For example, measures that seek to 'indoctrinate' – that is, that seek 'to impart beliefs regardless of the evidence' (Campbell, 1990: 21) – would be illegitimate. We need, then, to ask at least two kinds of questions of an activity to work out whether it is legitimate persuasion. First, are its 'recipients' clear that the health promoters are trying to persuade them of something?. Second, are the 'persuaders' careful to avoid concealing or distorting the relevant facts? If we can answer both of these questions in the affirmative and if we are dealing with competent adults, then, Campbell argues, there is no reason why health promoters should shun persuasive techniques.

It is important to see that the distinction Campbell draws is not a sharp one; it will always be subject to a degree of debate and interpretation. The key point he defends is that the line between legitimate and illegitimate 'trading' in information should not be drawn at 'pure education'. If the conditions contained in the above questions are met, it is possible to respect an individual's autonomy just as much by seeking to persuade, as by seeking to educate, them.

3 Is 'health' good for you? Robin Downie, Carol Tannahill, and Andrew Tannahill vs. David Seedhouse

Up to this point, we have rehearsed some of the ways in which we might be more inclined to offer approval of health promoters in an ethical sense, rather than disapproval. Although there is a general presumption against H interfering in the life of C, the case may be different if H were acting on behalf of some accountable body such as the government; or if the 'intrusion' were not only comparatively moderate but also transparent; or if the social benefits of intervening were comparatively significant. Each case would need to be considered on its own merits, but the overall importance of accountability and transparency is fixed. After all, C as well as H must have some say about the justifiability of any intervention. If H does not make her goals and methods transparent, then C is effectively being treated as an object. We think that most health promoters would instinctively agree with this concern to treat the perspectives and values of C (the client) equally as seriously as those of H (the health promoter). Indeed, Downie *et al.* (1996)

argue that there is a tendency amongst some health promoters to carry this position of 'equal seriousness' to unwarranted lengths.

Downie *et al.* challenge the view that health promotion is a relativist activity; that what ought wholly to guide work is a concern for complete compatibility between whatever is being promoted and the values of the client or clients. This is the kind of view apparently embodied in this quote from a leading textbook of the field: 'In our view, there is no one "right" aim for health promotion, and no one "right" approach or set of activities' (Ewles and Simnett, 1995: 37).

In response to this view, Downie *et al.* write:

> The health promoter is presumably committed to believing that health is at least one important value . . . if every set of values is as good as every other, then health promoters might as well pack up and go home. It is surely the belief that there are better and worse ways of living one's life that make the whole practice of health education, promotion, social work, nursing and medicine worthwhile.
>
> (Downie *et al.* 1996: 171)

The authors' argument is too extensive to consider here, but this quote begins to draw out a number of the fundamental issues they raise. Whatever other arguments can be advanced to justify the 'interference' of health promotion, at root these justifications must stem from a commitment to a set of values, including the value of health. The health promotion movement might, for example, place a lot of weight on the importance of autonomy and the closely connected notion of empowerment. However, Downie *et al.* argue, what we are doing is *health* promotion, not *autonomy* promotion or *empowerment* promotion. They attempt, therefore, to seek to clarify the meaning and ethical importance of 'health'. They argue that health is an important value in its own right and should not just be treated as a means to achieving other ends. It is not merely something that is useful but also something 'to be approved of' (ibid.: 176). In short, this means that the fact that something is bad for your health gives someone (our C, say) a good *prima facie* reason to avoid it; and gives someone else (H, for example) *prima facie* grounds for encouraging C to do so. Of course, these value judgements might be overridden by other value judgements. But the point is that 'health' must count for something ethically; nor can any old preference, opinion, or whim count against it. To repeat the core point above; 'there are better and worse ways of living one's life'. For Downie *et al.* health is an important part of a good or worthwhile life.

David Seedhouse (1997) takes issue with some of the arguments advanced by Downie *et al.* He seeks to find some middle ground between the relativism espoused by some practitioners and theorists (such as Ewles and Simnett 1995); and what might be described as the 'idealism' of Downie *et al.* He agrees that simple relativism about values is untenable but he is equally suspicious of any suggestion that health promoters might 'know better' about values than their clients. If someone chooses to live a life of much smoking and drinking, relishing the lifestyle, relishing the risk, accepting the consequences, and generally unattracted to the norms of 'respectability', then should a health promoter find this person wanting? On what basis could a health promoter prefer her (or his) values to those of this potential client, and with what authority? Seedhouse argues that it is not part of the health promoter's job to promote her (or his) conception of a good or worthwhile life; he criticizes Downie *et al.* for making the fundamental mistake, as he sees it, of mixing up 'health' and 'good lives'.

Whether or not Seedhouse's argument is a fair criticism of Downie *et al.*, it is an important one for the practice of health promotion. How can health promoters be sure that they are not 'smuggling' a whole range of irrelevant values into their work under the guise of 'health'? For example, there is an obvious risk of moralism creeping into sexual health promotion; but there are less obvious, although equal, risks of certain conventional norms simply being assumed in other, less controversial, areas. Seedhouse suggests at least two responses to this 'smuggling' dilemma. First and foremost he argues that health promoters must settle upon a clear, and defensible, account of the nature of health; what it is and what it is not (in this and previous work, he sets out and defends his own 'foundations' account). Only such an account, he argues, can enable health promoters to differentiate the goal of promoting people's health from the much more generic, and hence much less defensible, goal of 'improving their lives'. Second, he argues that health promotion policy and practice cannot be purely 'evidence based'; by its nature it must rest on specific sets of value commitments, which – to emphasize the point – he calls 'prejudices'. Everyone involved in formulating or implementing health promotion policy will bring their own value prejudices – or 'pre-judgements' – to bear in the way they conceive the 'problems' and 'solutions' of health promotion. This fact, however, should not allow us to descend into relativism, or allow us to feel complacent about the inevitability of moralism. Rather, we should strive towards what he calls 'reasoned prejudices' – that is to say, towards making our underlying value judgements as transparent as possible and explaining and defending them to others.

On this final point all the contributors to work on health promotion ethics are likely to agree. We cannot expect that 'reason' will usher in some wonderful consensus about health promotion values and ethics. We can, though, expect health promoters to be accountable for their values; setting out the content and the contours of the ethical debates will allow everyone involved to make a more reasonable appraisal of the issues from case to case.

Can these arguments help in practice?

There may be a tendency to believe that the arguments advanced by Wikler, Campbell, Downie *et al.* and Seedhouse are remote from the hard, everyday world of health promotion's practice; that in the messy confusion of this world the clarity of their arguments will dissipate. We want to suggest the contrary position. Collectively, these writers in fact provide the opportunity systematically to raise questions about the ethical nature of health promotion practice, and the values embodied in this field of activity.

The first, and fundamental, question is: what is the 'health' we are trying to promote? Only in an extremely limited sense is this a technical question. Much more importantly, it is a question of values. We need to be clear about the extent to which the 'health' we as health promoters are trying to promote aligns with conceptions of the value held by those we are supposed to be serving.

Further questions naturally flow from addressing this fundamental one. If alignment between our values as health promoters and those of our clients is not complete, what ethical justification exists for 'intervening' to promote our own values? If we believe a justification can be found, there is the further question – given the array of potential methods in the armoury of health promotion – of deciding what level of intervention is ethically acceptable.

The writers and the broader ethical theory that we have mentioned raise these questions, either explicitly or implicitly. In analysing them, some 'answers' have emerged. Health promotion is located in social and political contexts. It may be, therefore, that particular social goals (sponsored by an accountable government) justify the promotion of particular 'versions' of health in a way that is not compatible with the preferences of certain individuals. If this is so, then certain levels of persuasion or 'weak' coercion may be justified, especially given that these are endemic in public life. Of course, in the midst of public health threats, where the stakes are very high, consequentialist arguments will push us in the direction of stronger forms of interference and coercion.

But it is important to remember that there is an alternative set of 'answers'. We may believe that particular goals are not sufficiently compelling to override the wishes and preferences of individuals. As a result, we may be alarmed by any suggestion that anything other than the blandest and least intrusive kind of information-giving will constitute legitimate health promotion work.

We began our application of ethics to health promotion by asking, 'Why should H, the health promoter, be allowed interference in the life of C, the prospective client?' The fact that there are alternative sets of potential 'answers' to this question is not a problem. These competing answers represent the questioning and discussion which characterize the application of ethics to health promotion. And engaging in this questioning and discussion constitutes an important part of 'good practice' in a field where 'expertise' and 'professional judgement' can never be enough by themselves to justify action.

Health promoters need to familiarize themselves with these debates in general terms. But, much more crucially, they need to be ready to reflect upon, and enact, these debates in the messy realities of their working lives – from setting to setting and from case to case.

Note

1   We need to note that Campbell is not particularly concerned about how and where 'health education' is placed on the map of 'health promotion', i.e. he is not primarily concerned with definition and delineation of these terms. He seems to accept that the former is part of the latter and for the purposes of considering the argument presented here, we do the same.

References

Campbell, A. (1990) 'Education or indoctrination? The issue of autonomy in health education', in S. Doxiadis (ed.), *Ethics in Health Education*, Chichester: Wiley.

Downie, R. S., Tannahill, C. and Tannahill, A. (1996) *Health Promotion: Models and Values*. 2nd edn. Oxford: Oxford University Press.

Ewles, L. and Simnett, I. (1995) *Promoting Health: A Practical Guide,* 3rd edn. Scutari.

Seedhouse, D. (1997) *Health Promotion: Philosophy, Prejudice and Practice,* Chichester: Wiley.

Wikler, D. (1978) 'Persuasion and coercion for health: ethical issues in government efforts to change lifestyles', *Millbank Memorial Fund Quarterly/ Health and Society*, 56 (3): 303–38.

13 The new genetics and health promotion

Sarah Cunningham-Burley
and Amanda Amos

Introduction

The new genetics refers to the body of knowledge and techniques developed since the discovery of recombinant DNA in the 1970s. It involves research into the genetic components of a range of disease, illness, and behaviour and its application in the clinic in the form of genetic testing, screening, and subsequent treatments. Prior to these developments, the application of genetics to medicine remained within the realm of clinical genetics, with a focus on rare genetic disorders. Population and preventive medicine eschewed genetics in the wake of the eugenics movement earlier in the twentieth century. Until recently, genetics, in the context of health and medicine, had little to offer beyond those families known to be at risk of hereditary disease.

The situation now is somewhat different. New technologies have led to the identification of genes or markers of genes for a range of disorders. In 1983 a marker for Huntington's disease was mapped and in 1993 a specific genetic mutation was identified (Gusella *et al.* 1983; Huntington's Disease Collaborative Research Group 1993). Huntington's disease is an autosomal dominant disorder of high penetrance; where a person will be affected by inheriting a single copy of the faulty gene (BMA 1998). The disease is of late onset, serious and eventually fatal (Harper 1997). The gene for cystic fibrosis was cloned in 1989, paving the way for testing for carrier status as well as for the condition itself. Cystic fibrosis is an autosomal recessive disorder, which means that an affected person must inherit two copies of the genetic mutation, one from each parent, in order to develop the disease. Carriers remain free of the disease. The disease is also variable in its severity but is commonly associated with lung and digestive disorders and a shortened lifespan. Yates (1996) noted that in 1995 alone some 60 disease genes were isolated, and for example mutations have been identified for susceptibility to breast cancer.

Such discoveries, contingent on the ability to produce and manipulate DNA in the laboratory, quickly led to the development of genetic tests for a range of diseases, such as those outlined above. These developments also bring different understandings of disease (Savill 1997), while knowledge of the genotypes associated with specific diseases is leading to reclassifications of some diseases, such as diabetes (Bell 1998). New interventions are developing, for example through gene therapy or other experimental treatments, and it is anticipated that pharmocogenetics will lead to increased sophistication in drug therapy, tailored more specifically to an individual's genotype (BMA 1998; Hollingsworth and Barker 1999; Frears *et al.* 2000).

The new genetics, then, is moving from 'clinic to community', or from those in families known to be at high risk of inherited disease to wider populations as well as to mainstream health care. However, there are mixed views on the extent of the influence of the new genetics on matters of health, illness, and well-being. Beskow *et al.* (2001: 2) suggest that 'This information explosion is expected to bring nothing short of a revolution in medicine and public health'. However, others are more cautious, and see neither a paradigm shift nor great advances (Jones 2000; Lippman 1992). Recent research on general practitioners suggests that they do not feel that the new genetics will influence their management of chronic diseases (Kumar and Gantley 1999). On the one hand, the new genetics is ubiquitous in medicine, as the genetic turn greatly affects the direction of medical research, much of which is now genetic (Savill 1997). On the other hand, the influence of the new genetics in terms of medical application is rather more limited, and there has been no rapid improvement in health as a result (Jones 2000). The heralded cures for disease are still awaited.

The subject of the new genetics is hotly debated in a range of media and by a range of groups, including those directly engaged with genetic science and medicine. Developments excite considerable media coverage, sometimes prematurely heralding scientific 'breakthroughs', but also exploring, especially through documentaries, many of the complex issues which the new genetics raises for individuals and society. Much of this broader public debate is dominated by scientists, including protagonists and critics as well as science popularisers (Mulkay 1976; Nelkin 1994; Nelkin and Lindee 1995). The discipline of public health is beginning to play a part in these wider debates as well as in direct engagement with genetic research, especially through genetic epidemiology, and genetics in public health practice, particularly through genetic screening (Zimmern *et al.* 2000; Khoury *et al.* 2000; Beskow *et al.* 2001).

However, health promotion has yet to engage seriously with the issues raised by the new genetics, at the level of research, theory, and practice. Although the new genetics may not yet influence health promotion practice, other than tangentially through issues relating to genetic screening for disease or disease susceptibility, it certainly raises issues that are fundamental to the core values and practices of health promotion. Health promotion must begin to tackle these issues for two main reasons. First, health promotion must find its own place within the range of developments and changes that the new genetics embraces and propels. Second, it must provide a sophisticated analysis of some of the specific and general issues embedded in current trends and directions in order to be able to influence its shape.

The first section of this chapter will outline developments in the new genetics, as well as considering the social production and implications of such developments. The second section will consider what issues these developments raise for health promotion, focusing specifically on models of disease and prevention; the social context of individual choice and issues for families and society; public involvement and the democratic deficit in relation to science. The third section will discuss how public health and health promotion are and should engage with the new genetics, finally outlining suggestions for health promotion's influence in this complex area.

The development of the new genetics

The Human Genome Project (HGP), which involved the mapping and sequencing of every gene in a typical human being, has now been completed. The Human Genome Project was perhaps the most flamboyant expression of the promise and pace of developments in molecular genetics. Its high profile as an international endeavour combining public and private funds has helped propel genetic science into the public domain. Many of the protagonists of the HGP heralded it as providing the key to understanding human disease and behaviour, or providing the book of life or the 'holy grail' (Gilbert 1992). Petersen, among others, notes that the HGP 'was seen to hold immense promise in illness prevention, and to have the potential to transform preventive medicine and public health practice' (Petersen 1998: 59). Although others in the scientific community offered words of scepticism about the scientific value of the endeavour (Kevles and Hood 1992; Tauber and Sarkar 1992), the imperative to accelerate genetic research on a grand scale has remained. Science does not develop in a social vacuum, and it is important to consider the factors that shape its development, for science is a social activity (Barnes *et al.* 1996). There are issues of power involved in the development of science and technology and there is a complex interplay between economic, political, and cultural values and concerns (Kevles and Hood 1992). Understanding the social shaping of science means taking seriously the way in which social, political, and economic processes influence the way in which science and technology are developed in any given society. Among other things, genetic science in general, and the Human Genome Project in particular, came to align itself with matters of health and illness. Rose (1994) identifies this as a powerful discourse – genetics, through medicine, can alleviate suffering and eliminate disease. The HGP seemed to successfully place genetic research at the centre of cultural, economic, and health-related arenas. It also embraced powerful new alliances between academia, the state, and the biotechnology industry (Lewontin 1991; Keller 1992).

However, genetics did not always play such a prominent position in science, medicine, or popular culture. Its association with the eugenics movement in the first half of the twentieth century left a legacy of suspicion and concern after the atrocities of Nazi Germany. The eugenics movement embraced a range of scientists, social scientists, and social reformers, and was widespread in democratic as well as totalitarian regimes (Kerr *et al.* 1998a; Kevles 1995; Paul 1992). Subsequently, human genetics had to realign itself in order to gain credibility as an objective enterprise, eschewing either positive (enhancing the numbers in the population with desirable traits) or negative (eliminating those with undesirable traits) eugenics. Although state-sponsored eugenics ended, some sterilization laws were only repealed in the 1970s, and a reconfigured 'reform eugenics' emerged in the 1950s (Kevles 1995). Human genetics could once more become a socially useful discipline by aligning itself with clinical medicine and by studying well-defined disease traits. Its focus became preventive and therapeutic medicine, targeting families rather than whole populations.

This reconfiguring and realignment might help explain public health and health promotion concerns about overt involvement in the development of genetic services. Both disciplines are concerned with population health, and interventions at this level are perhaps harder to separate from eugenic concerns than individual interventions. It is only now, once the new genetics is becoming truly embedded in medical research, clinical practice, and popular culture that strategies for populations or specific social groups can develop. Wider transformations impel such developments – rapid developments in genetic science since the invention of the polymerase chain reaction in the 1970s that allowed the manipulation of DNA in the laboratory; the revival of genetic explanations in the 1970s heralding a move away from sociological and psychological explanations that had been dominant in the previous decade in particular; the popularization of genetics; and the rise of the biotechnology industry as a leading force in global capitalism.

Specific professional and economic interests serve to shape the developments in genetic sciences. Nelkin has identified three specific promotional messages that scientists have used to justify and enhance their claims, giving space for social acceptability. These are the definition of 'the gene' as the essence of identity; the promise to predict and therefore control disease and behaviour; and that the genome is the text defining the natural order (1995: 26). Such strategies help to promote a specific form of science and also protect the cognitive authority of science. In the late twentieth and early twenty-first century, this becomes all the more important, given the well-documented scepticism and lack of trust in science and experts in the 'risk society' (Beck 1992; Giddens 1991). Kerr *et al.* (1997) have identified how flexible appeals to the objectivity of good science as distinct from bad eugenics, alongside responsibilities for beneficial applications, help to maintain the position of geneticists and genetics science in the context of human health.

Although there is considerable hype about the promise of the new genetics, the extent of actual applications regarding human health and health care has been rather more limited. However, as noted in the introduction, the identification of genes or markers for genes has led to the development of genetic testing and screening for a range of diseases. Bell notes that current developments in genetics are shifting away from prevention of disease to its early detection and treatment (1998).

Genetic testing refers to testing individuals who are known to be at risk of a particular genetic disorder because of their family history (BMA 1998). Much of the early promise of genetic research that led to the identification of genes has only been realized in the clinic through genetic testing. Genetic testing identifies the presence or absence of a specific gene or mutation associated with a disease. Harper (1997: 31) notes that DNA-based testing differs from all other kinds of tests because of 'its constancy and its separation from the actual occurrence of disease'. However, testing is far from straightforward either technically or in terms of weighing benefits from harm. Most diseases are multifactorial in origin, and even where there is a genetic component, this is often polygenic, the result of many genes perhaps operating in interaction with one another or with the environment.

Even in single gene disorders, genetic testing is problematic. With Huntington's disease, a late onset genetic disorder, testing cannot predict exactly when the disease will occur, only that it will do so. However, do people really want to have this information, especially given that there is no treatment for the condition? The reasons why people may want this information include the ability to make reproductive choices, thus avoiding passing the gene on to their children; the desire to obtain an early diagnosis and thus plan their future including their care needs; or to establish that they are free of the disease. However, evidence suggests that many who know themselves to be at risk of HD do not wish to be tested, and living with uncertainty is part of their identity (Craufurd *et al.* 1989).

Using cystic fibrosis (CF) as another example, testing is complicated by the fact that over 600 mutations of the CF gene have been discovered. Although testing can be offered for the most common mutations, these still only account for about 85 per cent of the total incidence (BMA 1998). Testing may result in false reassurance to individuals who have been tested. Further complications emerge in relation to CF, where the disease spectrum is large and the association between genotype and phenotype is quite varied and complex (Alper 1996).

Moving this analysis on to more complex disorders, then testing becomes a less certain venture. A range of social and individual issues also ensue – who has the right to information? Should insurance companies and employers know? What about other family members? Does the prospect of testing raise anxiety and does this continue even after a negative result? What if available treatments are limited and other surveillance strategies offer no guarantee that disease will be picked up early and treated? Genetic testing can be presymptomatic as well as diagnostic, so people will be identified as having a disease often long before symptoms develop. In the case of diagnostic tests, these may result in earlier treatment, such as for cystic fibrosis, or in the case of prenatal diagnosis, the identification of affected foetuses (BMA 1998; Harper 1997).

Genetic screening refers to testing particular populations for a genetic disorder or for carrier status in the case of recessive conditions (BMA 1998). Some geneticists have expressed specific concerns about population screening and ambivalence about its impact or effects (Harper 1992; Clarke 1995; Stone and Stewart 1996). Population screening may raise people's concerns about risk (Harper 1997), as genetic testing moves from the genetics clinics, working with families known to be at risk, to the wider community. There are different kinds of genetic screening. Screening for carrier status for recessive conditions may help identify those few who may be at risk of passing on a genetic condition to their children; but it may also create problems for those who are simply carriers, as experienced by the sickle cell screening programmes in the USA in the past. Prenatal screening may identify those at risk of having a child affected by a genetic condition, but it may also raise anxiety in all pregnant women, requiring them to engage in decisions that affect how they feel about their pregnancy (Rapp 2000). As Shakespeare has pointed out, the existence of such screening programmes also affects the population of disabled people themselves (Shakespeare 1995). Newborn screening programmes may be offered where early treatment would be beneficial, or where the family as a whole may benefit from an early diagnosis of a genetic condition in their child. Genetic screening may be offered in the future for susceptibility to common diseases that are multifactorial in origin. Here there may be benefits in terms of interventions that prevent the onset of disease, whether these involve preventive drug therapy or lifestyle modifications. However, the potential disbenefits may also be large as ever more people are identified as being at risk of one disease or another. The commercial imperative to develop such tests that would embrace large populations through screening programmes should also not be ignored (Harper and Clarke 1997: 76).

Other developments include pre-implantation genetic diagnosis, where embryos fertilized in vitro can be tested for genetic disease and only 'healthy' embryos implanted in the womb. This is a high-tech procedure making considerable emotional, physical and financial demands on the woman going through it. Like many other areas in genetics, it is highly controversial, especially as such manipulation extends the frontiers of what is acceptable – should embryos be selected in order to provide suitable tissue for donation to a sibling? Should there be selection on the grounds of sex or other traits?

Gene therapy involves the manipulation of somatic cells, i.e. those not involved in reproduction (germ line gene therapy is not allowed currently and involves manipulation of the germ line, thus affecting future generations). Usually some kind of vector, such as a virus, is used to carry a new copy of a gene into affected cells in order to alter the course of disease. So far, trials have had limited or no success, and it seems unlikely that gene therapy will provide a rapid solution to the problem of human disease. However, wider developments in pharmaceuticals, resulting from developments in genetics, pharmacogenomics, are likely to be more rapid. Drug therapy is likely to become more tailored to individuals, taking into account their specific responses to medication, which their specific genotype will indicate (Zimmern and Cook 2000).

Other developments associated with genetics include treatments developed as a result of genetically engineered animals (for example, through specific proteins expressed in milk, or xenotransplantation). Research is also beginning to be carried out on large populations through proposed DNA databases, in order that epidemiological studies can investigate the interrelationship between genes and disease or susceptibility to disease, estimate population prevalence of genes, and examine gene–environment interaction (Lowrance 2001). Again, these are not uncontroversial as the experience in Iceland indicates (Rose 2001). Consultation exercises have been carried out by funding bodies such as the Medical Research Council, and it remains to be seen how successful these endeavours will be in eliciting public support and active participation in research.

As noted earlier, scientists and others disagree about the extent to which the new genetics will truly revolutionize medicine and science. However, most seem to agree that the rapid acceleration of developments is unique; the specific constellation of alliances between industry, state, and academia is also new. All commentators agree that the new genetics brings ethical and social issues to the fore too, indeed many articles on the new genetics contain at least passing reference to social and ethical implications (see Cunningham-Burley and Kerr 1999a, 1999b). Again, not all say that these issues are new or unique to the new genetics. However, concerns exist around issues for individuals, families, and society. They relate to informed consent, disclosure, anxiety, right to know, the increase in at-risk populations, the risk of discrimination and stigmatization, the possibility of a genetic underclass unable to access services including insurance, and concerns about welfare cuts and health care expenditure.

It is important to analyse how debates about social and ethical issues are framed. Recent research suggests that much attention is given to the implications of the new genetics, with a focus on its applications (most often testing or screening) and their likely effects. Although such a focus is important, public health genetics and clinical genetics have also both been involved in evaluating, screening, and testing programmes and in drawing up protocols for appropriate interventions (Beskow *et al.* 2001; Khoury *et al.* 2000). Much of this debate has been around issues relating to informed consent, choice, and non-directive counselling (Hallowell 1999a, 1999b; Petersen 1999), but also the wider concerns of whether genetic screening meets the traditional criteria of screening, especially where no subsequent effective intervention can ensue. The next section of this chapter goes on to consider some of the issues raised by the new genetics that are particularly relevant to health promotion.

Emerging issues for health promotion

This section focuses specifically on models of disease and prevention; the social context of individual choice including issues for individuals, families and society; and lastly public involvement and the democratic deficit in relation to science. Issues arising in the context of new genetics cut at the heart of health promotion but in contradictory and ambivalent ways. Perhaps these mirror some of the ambivalences within health promotion itself, especially in terms of its relation to medicine, its adoption or eschewing of a disease model, an emphasis on lifestyle and personal responsibility, as well as a concern for population health. The new genetics and health promotion may bring to the fore contradictions inherent in late modern societies, where reification of the individual, able to make life choices and 'colonise their futures' (Giddens 1991) exists alongside continuing discrimination and exclusions (Bauman 1997) as well as environmental risks of society's own making (Beck 1992). Nelkin and Lindee (1995: 191) note that popular culture embraces a discourse of genetic responsibility that constitutes a 'set of ideals about a perfect health culture', again mirroring rather than challenging some of the assumptions and values within health promotion.

A conflict between the needs and desires of individuals, their families, and the wider society of which they are part may be starkly reproduced when we think about genetic information, its production, and impact. As Kerr and Cunningham-Burley have argued, the science and technology of the new genetics is both post-modernist and modernist in its tendencies. The former is embodied in the alliances between global capitalism and a range of clinical and scientific disciplines and in the risk estimates offered to individuals so that they can plan their lives (Kerr and Cunningham-Burley 2000: 284). It is modernist in its traditional tendency to map, categorize, and control. Even pre-modern notions are rebuilt, through renewed emphasis on kinship, biological ties, and ideas about destiny and fatalism. All of these tendencies lead to a reconsideration of old dilemmas: the balance between nature and nurture, between population and individual health, and between behavioural change and fatalism in the light of genetic knowledge.

Models of disease and prevention

The new public health and health promotion are concerned with identifying and changing the social determinants of ill-health and ameliorating the social conditions that may limit an individual in living healthily. The social model of health, which operates with broad definitions of health, emphasizing health and well-being over disease and illness, underlies much thinking and practice in both disciplines. However, developments in the new genetics and their adoption or reflection within wider popular culture (Nelkin and Lindee 1995) challenge such an emphasis. Biological explanations for a range of diseases and traits are reasserted, and prevention itself may become narrowly focused in terms of specific diseases or susceptibilities identified at the genetic level. The new genetics may give the dominant medical model renewed vigour, as well as providing medical technology and pharmaceutical companies with a future full of new pharmaceuticals and tests to widen their markets and extend interventions.

Medicalization is a common term used to capture the way in which medicine can expand its claims over more and more areas of our lives. Health promotion has often sought to challenge such claims by locating health in the social rather than medical realm, and enabling individuals to take some control of their lives. 'Geneticization' is a term originally coined by Lippman in order to capture the growing tendency to distinguish people from each other on the basis of genetics; to define many disorders, variations, traits and behaviours as wholly or in part genetic in origin (Lippman 1993). In other words, geneticization involves the privileging of genetic research and explanations over an ever-broadening range of conditions and disorders it is likely to lead to a more genetically determinist view of the nature and the determinants of health, disease and social problems but also of their solutions. Geneticization may lead to the neglect of other causes of ill health both in terms of research as well as interventions, especially at the environmental or social level. 'Geneticization exaggerates personal responsibility for health, denigrates the collective solution to health problems that may be the only hope for those with few resources, and favours corporate profits over the collective and equitable provision of health care around the world' (Clarke 1995: 36). Lippman (1993) notes that geneticization is an ideology as well as a set of practices, and as such it can structure how we all think about health and illness as well as drive directions in research and clinical practice. It is clear from the history of medicine, and even public health and health promotion, that biological and individual explanations – and consequently solutions to health problems – are often favoured over environmental, social, and structural analyses. The new genetics is unlikely to challenge this.

New genetics aims to name, classify, and control (Petersen 1998; Kerr and Cunningham-Burley 2000), and will involve ever narrower definitions of disease requiring ever more complex technological solutions. Although currently aligned with clinical medicine and the prevention of disease, research into behaviour and other traits (such as intelligence) is gathering pace. The boundary between disease and behaviour has frequently been challenged in the past, and it may now become increasingly blurred, possibly allowing further geneticization and medicalization of aspects of everyday life. The new genetics is already having an impact on the criminal justice system and immigration services.

There are concerns over the extension, through genetic screening, of 'at-risk' status to larger and larger numbers of the populations. This increase in surveillance may result in heightened anxiety among individuals and their families, threaten privacy and autonomy, reinforce victim blaming, and create a situation where everyone is at risk and no one is 'healthy'. Genetic determinism is also part of the process of geneticization, and an issue for public health and health promotion (Petersen 1998). Although many scientists seem keen to argue for a balanced appreciation of the relationship between nature and nurture, this frequently masks a priority to the former (Cunningham-Burley and Kerr 1999b). The environment is rather undertheorized or underresearched, and the genetic turn may detract further from environmental concerns (Willis 1998; Petersen 1998). There are of course critics who argue strongly against genetic determinism and reductionism (Rose 1994; Tauber and Sarkar 1992); however, deterministic language pervades popular culture and may begin to influence the way in which we perceive ourselves and our health (Nelkin and Lindee 1995).

Where genetic differences are reified and used to distinguish between groups, a situation of increased discrimination and lack of tolerance of difference may result. However, some argue that the fact that everyone will have some deleterious genes will militate against such stigma. Yet, when the situation of disabled people in our society is considered, there seems little ground for optimism. The social model of disability (Oliver 1990) contrasts most starkly with the medical or genetic model of disability. This clash of perspectives is reflected in the quite different accounts of the new genetics from those writing from the point of view of disabled people or from those adopting a social model of disability (Shakespeare 1999; Asch 1999). Shakespeare (1995) has argued that the taken for granted assumptions about quality of life of disabled people should be revealed and contested: the new genetics undermines the authenticity of disabled people's lives and reinforces medical hegemony. Asch (1999: 1650) writes that 'Medicine and public health view disability as extremely different from and worse' than other 'forms of human variation'. In the context of welfare cuts and concerns about health service expenditure, prenatal testing for certain genetic impairments may carry a message that suggests that such lives are not worth living or simply too expensive for society to manage. This is far removed from an account which proposed that, for example, Down's syndrome is just 'one way, among others, of being human' (Clarke 1994: 19).

Genetics may, then, strengthen the biomedical paradigm to the detriment of the new public health and health promotion's agenda to seek collectivist solutions through social and political change (Willis 1998). The trend to individualize and privatize responsibility for health is taken up further in the following discussion of individual choice (see also Bunton and Petersen 2002).

The social context of individual choice

The association between genetics and eugenics in the past has resulted in very specific strategies to avoid any charge of association with eugenics today. As noted in the section above on the development of the new genetics, attempts are made by scientists and others to separate the new genetics from the 'old eugenics' (Kerr *et al.* 1998a). Paul (1992) in her historical analyses suggests that defenders of the new genetics distance it from eugenics by stating that they do not have eugenic goals; and that eugenics involved coercive practices rather than voluntary action, and societal good rather than individual rights. The discourse of individual choice, upheld in democratic societies and through so-called non-directive genetic counselling, is often portrayed as mitigating against eugenic abuse, which involves coercion. While most agree that state-sponsored eugenics is unlikely to reappear in Western democratic societies, some critics suggest that there is no ground for complacency. For example, Duster (1990) has argued that the 'back door' of disease prevention is now a reality even though the front door to eugenics appears to be closed.

Fears about eugenic abuse are often dismissed as irrational or sensationalist. This tends to divert attention away from discussions and analyses of the social and cultural processes which may operate to constrain individual choice. It has already been noted above that science does not operate in a vacuum, but both reflects and influences wider social, political, economic and cultural values. In the same way, appeals to individual choice as acting as a brake on eugenic abuse do not take seriously the social context within which choices are made. At a societal level, it may be that 'healthism', the promotion of health as a right and value, actually constrains choice, where to choose *not* to know one's risk status, or that of one's unborn child, may be deemed irresponsible. Disease or being diseased may be seen as undesirable, even where quality of life may be maintained and even when more and more traits might be reclassified as disease. Wider concerns about welfare expenditure may also limit choice both directly at the level of an individual, where lack of appropriate social or medical care may affect choices, and more indirectly in terms of what services are offered in the first place and how they are evaluated for costs and benefits.

The mere fact of offering particular tests alters the choices made and raises questions about who decides what is appropriate intervention for what diseases. As Rose notes, there is a taken for granted eugenics where someone decides which of the impaired foetuses have to have maternal decisions made about their survival (1994). She notes that a consumer eugenics has replaced state eugenics. Others have argued that ante-natal screening policies implicitly assume a negative view about the impairment being screened for. For example, Alderson (2001: 370) writes:

> Cost-effective justice, autonomy and prevention of harm can be diverted into supporting arguments that are hostile to people with Down's syndrome. Choice is oppressive when all the options are unwanted and responsibility for public health policies to reduce the incidence of Down's syndrome is borne by individual mothers.

Similarly, Asch (1999) notes that there are tensions between the goals of enhancing reproductive choice and preventing the births of children who would have disabilities. The language of individual rights thus masks cultural imperatives to make particular choices, and to hold individuals responsible for their own health and for the genetic health of their offspring. 'When considered in this way, the line between individual, voluntary choice and socially enforced coercion becomes blurred' (Kerr *et al.* 1998a: 192). Genetic counselling also may involve implicit or explicit values that favour particular actions or decisions; many consider that counselling can never be truly non-directive in the same way that individual choice can never been unfettered by social constraints (Petersen 1999; Hallowell 1999a).

Public involvement and understanding

Like individual choice, public involvement and understanding are also heralded as a way of preventing eugenic abuse (Nuffield Council on Bioethics 1993; Harper 1992). A 'deficit model' of public understanding of science underpinned many early calls for increased public understanding in order to safeguard against eugenics. This model implies that the public is ignorant of science, a claim supported by survey evidence which assesses people's knowledge of scientific facts (Durant *et al.* 1996). It also suggests that knowledge of such scientific facts is all that is required to enable informed public debate and involvement. This effectively eschews the more interesting questions about what type of knowledge is required for what purpose, as well as what types of public involvement for what purpose (Turney 1995). In an age of heightened scepticism about science in general and genetics in particular, managing public understanding in a way that reinforces scientific hegemony may be a strategy to bolster scientific authority.

The deficit model of public understanding has now been soundly criticized (Kerr *et al.* 1998b; Turney 1995; Macintyre 1995):

> Standardized questionnaires derived from textbook accounts of genetics inevitably document gaps in lay knowledge of scientific information. By contrast, research methods that put lay knowledge at centre stage are able to reveal the extent of expertise amongst the general public.
> (Cunningham-Burley and Boulton 2000: 183)

Much evidence suggests that people make sense of genetic knowledge in different ways, depending on their social location or the specific relevance of that information to them (Lambert and Rose 1996; Parsons and Atkinson 1992). Rather than being ignorant of scientific fact, people may bring a range of different expertise to debates about the new genetics (Kerr *et al.* 1998b, 1998c). This includes technical knowledge, but also institutional knowledge about the wider structures of science and medicine, methodological knowledge about science and how proof and certainty are difficult to assure, and cultural knowledge which refers to the wider social and cultural context that affects genetics, associated applications, and social responses. Similarly, people make sense of risk in different ways, often embedding risk estimates into the everyday contexts of their lives in ways meaningful to them (Parsons and Atkinson 1993). Again this does not reflect ignorance or an inability to grapple with complex test results, but rather reflects their own concerns about decision making and life choices.

Public involvement in debates and decisions about genetics is encouraged but is frequently limited to consultation, where the public are often cast in the role of consumer or future consumer of genetic services. Models of public involvement that embrace concepts of citizenship are less frequently used and are themselves limited in effect (Glasner and Dunkerley 1999; Irwin 1995). Irwin (2001) has pointed out that there is a new mood for dialogue that has replaced the deficit theory outlined above. However, he notes that moving from general statements of intent to actual applications of dialogue between scientists, policy makers, and citizens presents the next challenge. 'The relationship between science and democracy should not be about the search for universal solutions and institutional fixes, but rather the development of an open and critical discussion between researchers, policy makers, and citizens' (ibid.: 16).

The transfer of power, necessary to make up the democratic deficit in science, has not taken place, even though attempts have been made to engage with the public, promote debate in a range of arenas, and run consultation exercises especially around high-profile or controversial developments such as behavioural genetics and DNA databases. Such debates need to be 'vigorous and informed', including discussion 'about the role of power and the relative social locations of key actors in the determination of the knowledge and its application' (Duster 1990: 128). Numerous barriers must be overcome in order to achieve effective public engagement, including self-deprecation on the part of citizens themselves (Kerr *et al.* 1998b).

Health promotion and the new genetics

Where does health promotion fit in relation to these three emerging issues: (i) geneticization and biomedical models of disease; (ii) eugenics and the limitations of individual choice; (iii) public understanding and public engagement? And is there a role for health promotion within the developments associated with the new genetics in terms of promoting health and preventing disease?

Gabbay (1999) has argued that public health has to face a number of dilemmas. On the one hand, public health focuses on the social determinants of disease; on the other hand it remains firmly within the biomedical discourse, generating understanding of disease aetiology and health intervention effectiveness. The same dilemmas persist when considering public health's role in relation to genetic science. On the one hand there was some initial reluctance to engage with genetics, especially because of concerns about population screening. There are also critical voices outlining some of the concerns considered above (Bunton and Petersen 2002). Willis notes that 'the danger is that the new public health is being overtaken by outside social, political and economic forces so that the more traditional messages of public health are in danger of being lost' (1998: 135). On the other hand, public health genetics is a growing speciality, using its expertise to assess effectiveness and to design screening protocols. Zimmern *et al.* (2001: 1005) note:

> In time, health promotion programmes may take into account individual susceptibility to disease and provide more individualised approaches to behavioural change. Public health professionals will need to explore how genetic factors influence health and disease in populations and target interventions, such as screening programmes, at genetically defined sub-populations to improve their efficiency.

Beskow *et al.* (2001) write that genomics should be fundamental to public health, disease prevention, and health promotion programmes where at last those most susceptible to disease can be targeted.

Professional interests are at stake for public health, and the relationship between new genetics and public health is contested ground (Cunningham-Burley and Kerr 1999). Gabbay (1999: 264) asks:

> Should it try and rely on a new biomedical paradigm, which would have the advantage of helping epidemiology hold its own in the face of molecular biology and the new genetics? Or should it consciously draw much more than it does on social and behavioural sciences, thus risking being dismissed as a 'soft' science by the medical elite, which hold so much sway over the public health research world?

Larger economic and scientific interests have their part to play in the likely resolution of this dilemma.

Health promotion can be characterized as facing the same difficulties, and it needs to reflect on its role in relation to the new genetics. First, in considering models of disease, health promotion needs to retain a focus on the wider social determinants of health and on the social structures that limit individuals' capacity to make healthy choices. This requires continual research at both societal and individual levels, as well as involvement in interventions aimed at ameliorating socially caused inequalities in health. While the new genetics may have a preventive component, at present this mainly involves the selective termination of affected foetuses, which is an individual issue with wider social effects. Challenging the biomedical paradigm should be at the forefront of health promotion research, theory, and practice. However, health promotion can also provide a critical analysis of the wider endeavour of genetic science itself, thus bringing into the public domain understandings of power relationships and their influence on genetic science and its applications.

Second, health promotion can support individuals, their families, and wider society by challenging naïve typifications of the notion of individual choice and outlining the limits to such individual choice. Wider concerns about discrimination of disabled people as well as the overall impact of promoting 'genetic health' should be addressed. More specifically, individuals should be supported to make informed choices, where sufficient information is given about the range of options, including the quality of life of those with the genetic condition under scrutiny, as well as support for the range of options, including adequate social and medical care, for those who have a genetic condition. Health promotion can also contribute to understanding behaviour and behavioural change, especially as genetics moves to considering predisposition to disease. As Marteau and Lerman note, 'Providing people with personalised information on risk is not new. The question is whether responses will be any different if the information is based on DNA' (2001: 1057). They note that genetic risk could both increase and decrease motivation to change behaviour and the ability to do so.

Third, health promotion can contribute to more effective public engagement. As noted above, self-deprecation may be a barrier to effective public engagement (Kerr *et al.* 1998b). Health promotion can work to empower individuals, social groups, and communities. Health promotion can embrace grassroots activity, alongside political lobbying, in order to challenge both the deficit model of public understanding and the democratic deficit in involving citizens in science policy and practice.

Health promotion should not ignore the new genetics, but neither should it embrace it. Providing a critical contribution at every level will help promote a civil society that is not shaped by technological imperatives and medical fixes to social problems, nor one where the balance between individual and collective responsibilities for health tips too far towards the individual.

References

Alderson, Priscilla (2001) 'Prenatal screening, ethics and Down's syndrome: a literature review', *Nursing Ethics* 8 (4): 360–74.

Alper, Joseph (1996) 'Genetic complexity in single gene diseases', *British Medical Journal* 312: 196–7.

Asch, Adrienne (1999) 'Prenatal diagnosis and selective abortion: a challenge to practice and policy', *American Journal of Public Health* 89: 1649–57.

Barnes, Barry, Bloor, David, and Henry, John (1996) *Scientific Knowledge. A Sociological Analysis*, London: Athlone Press.

Bauman, Z. (1997) *Postmodernity and its Discontents*, Cambridge: Polity.

Beck, Ulrich (1992) *Risk Society: Towards a New Modernity*, London: Sage.

Bell, John (1998) 'The new genetics: the new genetics in clinical practice', *British Medical Journal*, 36: 618–20.

Beskow, Laura M., Khoury, Muin J., Baker, Timothy G., and Thrasher, James F. (2001) 'The integration of genomics into public health research, policy, and practice in the United States', *Community Genetics*, 25 July.

British Medical Association (1998) *Human Genetics. Choice and Responsibility*, Oxford: Oxford University Press.

Bunton, R. and Petersen, A. (2002) 'Genetics, governance and ethics', *Critical Public Health*, Special Issue.

Clarke, Angus (1995) 'Population screening for genetic susceptibility to disease', *British Medical Journal*, 311: 35–8.

Clarke, Angus (1994) 'Genetic Screening: a response to Nuffield', *Bulletin of Medical Ethics*, 97, 13–21. (www.cdc.gov/genetics/info/reports/wheelhtm)

Craufurd, D., Dodge, A., Kerzain-Storrar, L., and Harris, R. (1989) 'Uptake of presymptomatic predictive testing for Huntington's disease', *Lancet* ii: 603–5.

Cunningham-Burley, Sarah and Boulton, Mary (2000) 'The social context of the new genetics' in G. Albrecht, R. Fitzpatrick, and S. Scrimshaw (eds) *Handbook of Social Studies in Health and Medicine*, London: Sage, pp. 173–87.

Cunningham-Burley, Sarah and Kerr, Anne (1999a) 'Defining the "social": Professional discourses on the social implications of the new genetics', *Sociology of Health and Illness* 21 (5): 647–68.

—— (eds) (1999b) 'Risk and the new genetics', *Health, Risk and Society*, 1 (3): 249–357.

Durant, John, Hansen, A., Bauer Martin (1996) 'Public understanding of the new genetics', in T. Marteau and M. Richards (eds) *The Troubled Helix: Social and Psychological Implications of the New Human Genetics*, Cambridge: Cambridge University Press.

Duster, Troy (1990) *Backdoor to Eugenics*, New York/London: Routledge.

Frears, Robin, Roberts, Derek, and Poste, George (2000) 'Rational or rationed medicine? The promise of genetics for improved clinical practice', *British Medical Journal* 320: 933–5.

Gabbay, G. (1999) 'The socially constructed dilemmas of academic public health', in S. Griffiths and D. J. Hunter (eds) *Perspectives in Public Health*, Abingdon: Radcliffe Medical Press.

Giddens, Anthony (1991) *Modernity and Self-identity. Self and Society in the Late Modern Age*, Cambridge: Polity Press.

Gilbert, W. (1992) 'A vision of the holy grail', in D. Kelves and L. Hood (eds) *The Code of Codes*, Cambridge, MA: Harvard University Press.

Glasner, Peter and Dunkerley, David (1999) 'New genetics, public involvement and citizens' juries', *Health, Risk and Society* 1 (3): 313–24.

Gusella, J. F., Wexler, N. S., Conneally, P. M. *et al.* (1983) 'A polymorphic DNA marker genetically linked to Huntington's Disease', *Nature* 306: 234–8.

Hallowell, Nina (1999a) 'Advising on the management of genetic risk: offering choice or prescribing action?' *Health, Risk and Society* 1 (3): 267–80.

—— (1999b) 'Doing the right thing: genetic risk and responsibility', *Sociology of Health and Illness* 21 (5): 597–621.

Harper, Peter (1992) 'Genetics and public health', *British Medical Journal* 340: 721.

—— (1997) 'Presymptomatic testing for late-onset genetic disorders: lessons from Huntington's Disease', in P. Harper and A. Clarke (eds) *Genetics, Society and Clinical Practice*, Oxford: Bios Scientific Publishers.

Harper, Peter and Clarke, Angus (1997) (eds) *Genetics, Society and Clinical Practice*, Oxford: Bios Scientific Publishers.

Hollingsworth, Simon and Barker, Stephen (1999) 'New technologies: Gene therapy. Into the future of surgery', *Lancet* 353 (suppl. I): 19–20.

Huntington's Disease Collaborative Research Group (1993) 'A novel gene containing a trinucleotide repear that is expanded and unstable on Huntington's disease chromosomes', *Cell*, 72: 971–83.

Irwin, Alan (1995) *Citizen Science. A Study of People, Expertise and Sustainable Development*, London: Routledge.

—— (2001) 'Constructing the scientific citizen: science and democracy in the biosciences', *Public Understanding of Science* 10: 1–18.

Jones, Steve (2000) *Genetics in Medicine: Real Promises, Unreal Expectations*, New York: Milbank Memorial Fund.

Keller, Evelyn Fox (1992) 'Nature, nurture, and the Human Genome Project', in Kevles and Hood *The Code of Codes*, Cambridge, MA: Harvard UP.

Kerr, Anne and Cunningham-Burley, Sarah (2000) 'On ambivalence and risk: reflexive modernity and the new human genetics', *Sociology* 43 (2): 283–304.

Kerr, Anne, Cunningham-Burley, Sarah, and Amos, Amanda (1997) 'The new genetics: professionals' discursive boundaries', *Sociological Review* 45 (2): 279–303.

Kerr, Anne, Cunningham-Burley, Sarah, and Amos, Amanda (1998a) 'Eugenics and the new genetics in Britain: examining contemporary professionals' accounts', *Science, Technology and Human Values*, 23 (2): 175–98.

Kerr, Anne, Cunningham-Burley, Sarah, and Amos, Amanda (1998b) 'The new genetics and health: mobilising lay expertise', *Public Understanding of Science* 7: 41–60.

Kerr, Anne, Cunningham-Burley, Sarah and Amos, Amanda (1998c) 'Drawing the line: an analysis of lay people's discussions about the new genetics', *Public Understanding of Science* 7: 113–33.

Kevles, Daniel, J. and Hood, L. (eds) (1992) *The Code of Codes. Scientific and Social Issues in the Human Genome Project*. Cambridge, MA: Harvard University Press.

Kevles, Daniel J. (1995) *In the Name of Eugenics. Genetics and the Uses of Human Heredity*, Cambridge, MA: Harvard University Press.

Khoury M., Beaty, T., and Cohen, B. (1993) *Fundamentals of Genetic Epidemiology*, Oxford: Oxford University Press.

Khoury, M., Burke, W., and Thomson, E. J. (2000) *Genetics and Public Health in the Twenty-first Century: Using Genetic Information to Improve Health and Prevent Disease*, New York: Oxford University Press.

Kumar, Satinder and Gantley, Madeleine (1999) 'Tensions between policy makers and general practitioners in implementing new genetics: grounded theory interview study', *British Medical Journal* 319: 1410–13.

Lambert, Helen and Rose, Hilary (1996) 'Disembodied knowledge? Making sense of medical science', in Alan Irwin and Brian Wynne (eds) *Misunderstood Science? The Public Reconstruction of Science and Technology*, Cambridge: Cambridge University Press, pp. 65–83.

Lewontin, Richard C. (1991) *The Doctrine of DNA. Biology as Ideology*, London: Penguin.

Lippman, Abby (1992) 'Led (astray) by genetic maps: the cartography of the human genome and health care', *Social Science and Medicine* 35 (12): 1469–76.

—— (1993) 'Worrying – and worrying about the geneticization of reproduction and health', in *Misconceptions* 1: 39–65 (eds G. Basen, M. Eichler, A. Lippman). Quebec: Voyageur Publisher.

Lowrance, William W. (2001) 'The promise of human genetic databases', *British Medical Journal* 322: 1009–10.

Macintyre, Sally (1995) 'The public understanding of science or the scientific understanding of the public? A review of the social context of the "new genetics"', *Public Understanding of Science* 4: 223–32.

Marteau, Theresa and Lerman, Caryn (2001) 'Genetic risk and behavioural change', *British Medical Journal* 322: 1056–9.

Mulkay, Michael (1976) 'The mediating role of the scientific elite', *Social Studies of Science* 6: 445–70.

Nelkin, Dorothy (1994) 'Promotional metaphors and their popular appeal', *Public Understanding of Science* 3: 25–31.

Nelkin, Dorothy and Lindee, Susan M. (1995) *The DNA Mystique. The Gene as a Cultural Icon*, New York: Freeman.

Nuffield Council on Bioethics (1993) *Genetic Screening Ethical Issues*, London: Nuffield Council on Bioethics.

Oliver, M. (1990) *The Politics of Disablement*, London: Macmillan.

Parsons, Evelyn and Atkinson, Paul (1992) 'Lay constructions of genetic risk', *Sociology of Health and Illness* 14: 437–55.

—— (1993) 'Genetic risk and reproduction', *The Sociological Review* 41: 679–706.

Paul, Diane (1992) 'Eugenic anxieties, social realities, and political choices', *Social Research* 59 (3): 663–83.

Petersen, Alan (1998) 'The new genetics and the politics of public health', *Critical Public Health* 8 (1): 59–71.

—— (1999) 'Counselling the genetically "at risk": the poetics and politics of "non-directiveness"', *Health, Risk and Society* 1 (3): 253–66.

Rapp, R. (2000) *Testing Women, Testing the Fetus. The Social Impact of Amniocentesis in America*, London and New York: Routledge.

Rose, Hilary (1994) *Love, Power and Knowledge. Towards a Feminist Transformation of the Sciences*, Cambridge: Polity Press.

—— (2001) *The Commodification of Bioinformation: The Icelandic Health Sector Database*, London: The Wellcome Trust.

Rose, Steven (1998) 'Neurogenetic determinism and the new euphrenics', *British Medical Journal* 317: 1707–8.

Savill, John (1997) 'Molecular approaches to understanding disease', *British Medical Journal* 314: 126–9.

Shakespeare, Tom (1995) 'Back to the future? New genetics and disabled people', *Critical Social Policy* 44: 7–21.

—— (1999) 'Losing the plot? Medical and activist discourses of contemporary genetics and disability', *Sociology of Health and Illness* 21 (5): 669–88.

Shuster, Evelyne (1992) 'Determinism and reductionism: A greater threat because of the Human Genome Project?' in G. J. Annas and E. Sherman (eds) *Gene Mapping. Using Law and Ethics as Guides*, Oxford: Oxford University Press.

Stone, D. and Stewart, S. (1996) 'Screening and the New Genetics: A public health perspective on the ethical debate', *Journal of Public Health Medicine*, 18: 3–5.

Tauber, Alfred I., and Sarkar, Sahotra (1992) 'The Human Genome Project: has blind reductionism gone too far?', *Perspectives in Biology and Medicine*, 35 (2): 220–35.

Turney, Jon (1995) 'The public understanding of genetics – where next?' *European Journal of Genetics and Society* 1: 5–20.

Willis, Evan (1998) 'Public health, private genes: the social consequences of genetic biotechnologies', *Critical Public Health* 8 (2): 131–9.

Yates, John R. W. (1996) 'Medical Genetics', *British Medical Journal* 312: 1021–5.

Zimmern, R. and Cook, C. (2000) *Genetics and Health: Policy Issues for Genetic Science and their Implications for Health and Health Services*, London: HMSO.

Zimmern, Ron, Emery, Jon, Richards, and Tessa (2001) 'Putting genetics in perspective', *British Medical Journal* 322: 1005–6.

Glossary

This glossary is intended only as a guide to defining terms; readers should refer to appropriate texts for fuller explanations. All definitions are given as they relate to and are understood in health promotion theory and practice

Acceptance variables

(*Innovation-diffusion theory*) These variables influence the degree or rate to which an innovation is taken up and may be divided into structural and individual variables.

Alma Ata Declaration

A declaration of the World Health Assembly at Alma Ata in the Soviet Union in 1977. The declaration committed all members of the World Health Organization to the principles of Health For All 2000 (HFA 2000).

Approach

(*Theoretical debate*) A term favoured by those shy of conceptual work – typically pragmatists (who focus on practicalities) and electicists (who mix ideas arbitrarily). Has connotations of a tentative movement.

At risk group

A group vulnerable to certain diseases or ill health because of their economic, social, or behavioural characteristics or environment. (*See Risk behaviour.*)

Audience segmentation

(*Social marketing*) The breakdown of an audience into discrete groups that show homogeneity within and heterogeneity between them. The process by which these groups are identified is arbitrary, but usually focuses on socio-economic characteristics such as social class, income, education, age, and ethnic group. Enables those marketing a message to direct it to those for whom it is intended, the target audience. (*See Target audience.*)

Bio-medical model

(*Sociology*) Focuses on the causes and treatment of ill health and disease in terms of biological cause and effect. This approach does not refer to the social, psychological, or economic conditions that may have influenced the health of the individual. (*See Health equity.*)

Causal attribution

(*Psychology*) The reason given for an event; to whom or to what we attribute the cause of an event. According to attribution theory, the nature of attributions made shapes future action. (*See Learned helplessness.*)

Change agent

(*Innovation-diffusion theory*) Used in relation to innovation-diffusion theory, it is defined as an individual who influences the client's innovation decision in a direction considered desirable by the change agency.

Channel gatekeepers

(*Social marketing*) Those who control the movement of messages through a communication channel, who act as intermediaries between those marketing a product or message and those it is directed at, for example, the personnel manager of a large organization. These individuals play an important part in the success or otherwise of health promotion campaigns.

Cohort

(*Epidemiology*) A component of the population born during a particular time period and identified by period of birth, so that the characteristics of this group at different points in time can be identified. More generally used to describe any group of people who are followed or traced over time. (*See Longitudinal study.*)

Communitarian(ism)

(*Politics*) Philosophy that highlights the importance of community and shared values to maintain social order and stability. This has been the subject of much recent research in public health and health promotion, particularly in the area of its relationship to social capital.

Conflict theory

(*Sociology*) The analysis of groups within society competing to serve their own conflicting interests. Fundamental to this type of analysis is the identification of inequalities between groups.

Consensus theory

(*Sociology*) The analysis of society as a whole, identifying the function of different groups in maintaining the equilibrium of the whole. This theory suggests that society tends to conservatism and the maintenance of the status quo.

Consequentialism

(*Ethics*) Theories that suggest that actions are right or wrong according to the balance of good or bad consequences. (*See Utilitarianism.*)

Cost-benefit analysis

(*Economics*) A means of evaluating a health promotion programme by comparing costs with benefits. If benefits outweigh costs, the programme is considered efficient in cost-benefit terms. This type of analysis is limited by the problems of placing values on costs and benefits, such as the value of life or the cost of passive smoking. (*See Cost-effectiveness analysis.*)

Cost-effectiveness analysis

(*Economics*) Similar to cost-benefit analysis, but compares units of effectiveness to cost in order to determine the most cost-effective way of achieving programme aims. For example, if prevention of cervical cancer is the aim of a programme, a unit of effectiveness could be defined as the detection of a positive smear test, rather than the numbers of women examined. (*See Cost-benefit analysis.*)

Cross-sectional study

(*Epidemiology*) A study that examines the relationship between disease, ill health, and other variables of interest as they exist in a defined population at one particular point in time. This study provides a snapshot of the characteristics of the population at one point in time. (*See Longitudinal study.*)

Deontology

(*Ethics*) Ethical theory which considers duty as the basis of morality. Some actions are obligatory regardless of their consequences.

DNA (deoxyribonucleic acid)

(*Genetics*) The genetic blueprints for all living things are made up of deoxyribonucleic acid (DNA). DNA carries the genetic instructions for making living organisms.

Empowerment

(*Ethics*) Situation in which individuals have a high degree of power. Empowerment is important in order to enable individuals and communities to make healthy choices.

Epidemiology

(*Epidemiology*) The study of the distribution and determinants of health-related states and events in populations, and the application of this study to the control of health problems.

Ethnomethodology

(*Sociology*) A method of enquiry in which the researcher's beliefs, attitudes, and values are accounted for in the process of research. As such it questions the notion of scientific objectivity.

Eugenics: (Gr. *eu* – well; *genos* – birth)

(*Genetics*) The science that deals with all the influences that improve the inborn qualities of the human race or develops them to the utmost advantage. Can be of the positive or negative variety.

Formative research

(*Social marketing*) Research conducted prior to full implementation of a social marketing strategy. It may include studies of the characteristics and needs of different audiences and pilot testing of the message or service to determine its acceptability.

Genotype

(*Genetics*) A characteristic of an organism is said to have two aspects: genotype and phenotype. Genotype is the make up of the gene itself – its code, or an individual's genetic make-up or constitution underlying a specific trait or constellation of traits. (*See phenotype.*)

Globalization

(*Politics*) Process in which different people, religions, and countries become linked economically, politically, and environmentally on a global scale. This has become a *cause célèbre* in health promotion recently with many commentators linking it to the global burden of disease.

Gross Domestic Product

(*Economics*) A measure of the total flow of goods and services produced by the economy over a specified time period, normally a year or a quarter. GDP is one measure of the total economic value of a country.

Health belief model

(*Psychology*) A model of action describing and predicting health behaviour in terms of beliefs and perceptions about illness, the costs, and benefits of action related to health and the available cues for action. It combines links with behaviour and belief with cost-benefit analysis. (*See Cost-benefit analysis.*)

Health equity

(*Sociology*) Implies that ideally everyone should have a fair opportunity to attain their full health potential and that no one should be disadvantaged from achieving this potential, if it can be avoided. Equity is therefore concerned with creating equal opportunities for health and with bringing health differentials down to the lowest level possible.

Healthy public policy

(*Social policy*) Healthy public policy is characterized by an explicit concern for health and equity in all areas of policy and by accountability for health impact. Clarified at the Adelaide 2nd International Conference on Health Promotion (WHO 1988), the concept anticipates a new culture of public policy that is pluralistic and looks beyond state administrative planning structures to develop and implement policy, calling for multi-sectoral, multi-level, and participative initiatives.

Hegemony

(*Politics*) Domination of one group, in this case one culture, over others through a combination of political and ideological means.

Heterophily

(*Communications theory*) The degree to which pairs of individuals who interact are different with regard to certain attributes. (*See Homophily.*)

Homophily

(*Communications theory*) Used in innovation-diffusion theory in relation to the characteristics of the change agent and his or her client group. When they share certain characteristics they are said to be homophilous and it is argued that under these conditions more effective communication occurs.

Iatrogenesis

The occurrence of illness as a result of earlier treatment by a doctor, or other health care worker, for a previous illness.

Innovation-diffusion theory

(*Communications theory*) A theory in which the process by which an innovation spreads through society is identified. Typically this follows an 'S' curve, slowly at first, then more rapidly, and finally slowing down again. It is useful to health promotion as different social groups play different roles in the uptake of an innovation, and their identification and allegiance can play an important role in the eventual success of a programme. (*See Innovation; Change agent; Pro-innovation bias; Acceptance variables.*)

Intermittent reinforcement

(*Psychology*) An unpredictable schedule of reinforcement (rewards) which may exert a powerful effect on behaviour. For example, when the discomfort and unpleasant consequences of binge drinking are interspersed with occasional euphoric and enjoyable experiences, drinking may be perceived as enjoyable and repeated.

Lay beliefs

(*Sociology*) Non-professional interpretations of the causes and treatment of ill health and disease and the reasons for susceptibility. They are frequency inconsistent, differing with the level of explanation required (contrasts with biomedical model).

Learned helplessness

(*Psychology*) A learnt response to unpleasant experiences beyond individual control. It is characterized by apathy and inability to avoid further unpleasant experiences. Generalization to other situations may occur and the behaviour may persist over time. This depends on the causal attribution made for the experience. (*See Causal attribution.*)

Longitudinal study

(*Epidemiology*) Sometimes called a cohort study. A study in which the same group of people are observed at different points in time.

Marketing mix

(*Social marketing*) The relative emphasis placed on the product, place, promotion, and price in a given marketing strategy. The different importance given to these factors is determined by the characteristics of the target audience. An effective marketing mix optimizes the communication of the message, service, or product being marketed.

Model

(*Theoretical debate*) A misused word – sometimes interchanged with theory, perspective, approach, and position. Refers to temporary conceptual constructions used to assist our thinking, more primitive than theories but perhaps embodying propositions, hypotheses, etc.

Morbidity

(*Epidemiology*) Any departure from a state of health or well-being, whether physiological or psychological. It can be measured by the numbers in a population who are ill, the periods of illness these people experienced, and the types of illness that these people suffered.

Multivariate analysis

(*Epidemiology*) A set of techniques used when the variation in several variables has to be measured at the same time. In statistics it is any analytical method that allows the simultaneous study of two or more dependent variables.

Networked organization

(*Politics*) Organization in which independent people and groups link across boundaries, to work together for a common purpose. There is no agreed and binding common policy. Each network participant is usually part of another team, based in a different place.

Normative

(*Ethics and Sociology*) Attempts to answer specific moral questions about what people should do or believe. The word 'normative' means guidelines or norms. Normative ethical theories are associated with Kantian ethics, virtue ethics, and utilitarian ethics.

Opinion leaders

(*Communications theory*) A social group playing a central role in the uptake of innovations. They are characteristically respected, with good communication systems. Their behaviour has an impact on their community, and they are identifiable as the key movers in the early uptake of new ideas, actions, and technology. (*See Innovation-diffusion theory.*)

Opportunity cost

(*Economics*) The cost of production judged by what has been forgone by not using resources in another way. In health promotion the cost could be a service, a new behaviour, or a product. For example, the opportunity cost of taking exercise would include the loss of benefits from using the time for other activities.

Paradigm

(*Theory, philosophy*) A wider concept than theory. It constitutes the agreed upon way of looking at and interpreting the world, or a particular field of study, and predicts the course of further investigation and study. A theoretical paradigm refers to the context within which a theory exists; two rival theories may share the same paradigm. For example, psychoanalysis and transactional analysis are both part of the psychodynamic paradigm, as they share fundamental similarities in their understanding of emotional life and how emotional problems may be cured.

Paradigm shift

(*Theory, philosophy*) Refers to the way in which one paradigm is replaced by another (Kuhn 1970). According to Kuhn, there are three stages in this process of scientific development: a pre-paradigm stage when several theories compete for dominance, then a period of normal science when a single paradigm has gained wide acceptance and provides structure for the field. This is followed by a period of crisis, when the accepted paradigm is replaced by another. This is called the paradigm shift; it is a revolution in thinking and in knowledge.

Paternalism

(*Ethics*) Authority in the manner of a father through the distribution of rewards and punishments to those subject to authority.

Perspective

(*Theoretical debate*) A term favoured by theorists to describe the unique qualities of their work. Best thought of as describing their epistemological basis (core assumptions about how their theoretical knowledge is generated).

Phenotype

(*Genetics*) How a gene manifests itself as an observable phenomenon (e.g. a visible characteristic of an organism). The expressed characteristics, or an expressed character of an organism. Not all phenotypic traits are genetic. (*See Genotype.*)

Polygenic

(*Genetics*) Controlled by or associated with more than one gene.

Position

(*Theoretical debate*) A term favoured by activists (who see theorizing as wasteful effort). Usually associated with a 'defence' of a position or developing a 'sound' position (meaning ideologically acceptable).

Process tracking

(*Social marketing*) Systematic measurement of effectiveness, in reaching and delivering a message to the target audience of a social marketing programme. It provides a means of assessing whether or not the aims and objectives of the programme are being met and the impact of the programme as a whole. (*See Target audience.*)

Pro-innovation bias

(*Communications theory*) The assumption by those researching or promoting an innovation that it is beneficial before it has been proven to be so. This usually occurs when alternatives have not been examined and can be remedied by the use of control groups and different experimental conditions for testing the innovation. Fosters a victim-blaming view if the innovation is not adopted. (*See Victim blaming.*)

Reference population

(*Epidemiology*) Equivalent to a control group (a group who have not been exposed to the conditions manipulated for study) or comparison group in studies observing populations.

Reflexive modernity

(*Social policy*) Social theorists have suggested that modern lifestyles at the turn of the twenty-first century can be characterized by a newer, more 'reflexive modernity' in which many traditional and familiar aspects of our lives are open to reflexive consideration, change, negotiation, and choice. As the pace of social and technological change has increased, individuals are presented with less certainty in most areas of their lives. Aspects of life that once seemed constant such as one's class and gender, are open to negotiation and change. (*See Risk society also.*)

Relativist

(*Ethics and politics*) Theories and values are considered relative to time and place. They can only be considered in the context that produced them.

Risk behaviour

Specific forms of behaviour known to be associated with increased susceptibility to certain diseases or ill health. In health promotion, changes to risk behaviour are a major goal in disease prevention. (*See At risk group.*)

Risk society

(*Social Policy, Sociology and Politics*) Sociologists such as Ulrich Beck (1992) and Anthony Giddens (1991) have argued that we now live in a 'risk society' in which we must increasingly reflect upon, choose, and construct our lifestyles and our identities. Traditional identities, based around relations of production, such as class relationships, are less binding, as employment patterns are less predictable and stable. Individuals increasingly experience life as characterized by risk and uncertainty. As the pace of social and technological change has increased, individuals and social institutions are presented with less certainty in most areas of their lives and increased risk calculation.

Saliency

(*Communications theory*) In the context of innovation adoption, the more salient or obvious the advantage, adoptability, or accessibility of an innovation, then the more likely it is that the innovation will be taken up. (*See Innovation-diffusion theory.*)

Self-regulation theory

(*Psychology*) Suggests the regulation of health-threatening behaviour occurs by active recall of the long-term consequences of the behaviour. This theory may be used in developing training programmes, such as alcohol counselling services, as it enables individuals to self-regulate their own health behaviour.

Sensitivity analysis

(*Economics*) Used to determine the sensitivity of cost-benefit analysis to changes in the assumptions on which it is based. It identifies those conditions around which most uncertainty exists, then alters their values. The analysis gives an indication of the degree of confidence one can have in the results of the cost-benefit analysis. (*See Cost-benefit analysis.*)

Social stratification

(*Sociology*) Persistent divisions identified in society that are resistant to change and are usually characterized by socio-economic factors, such as level of skill in employment. income, and education. The stratification of society may be said to be a structural characteristic as it is resistant to change.

Stages of change model

(*Psychology*) Identifies five major stages in effecting behavioural change: pre-contemplation, contemplation, ready for action, action, and maintenance. The model is dynamic and it is possible to move back and forth between stages. Different processes are involved at different stages, enabling health promoters to provide appropriate support. For example, awareness raising at the pre-contemplation stage, coping skills for those ready for action, and positive reinforcement and continued encouragement for those maintaining a behavioural change.

Statistical lives

(*Economics*) A term used to describe lives that do not exist, but are used in forecasting the future for statistical purposes, for example, the probable number of eyes lost in road accidents next year or the number of children whose lives could be saved through screening pregnant women for certain diseases.

Structuralism

(*Sociology*) An examination of the constraints placed on behaviour and social action by the environment in which the action occurs. Its areas of concern are, for example, local and national government, laws, taxation, and the planning of the built environment.

Subsidiarity

(*Politics*) Subsidiarity is a basic democratic principle that decisions are made at the lowest level of society, for example at local authority or regional level. The authority to deal with a particular problem is only passed on to a higher level if it cannot be solved at a lower level.

Target audience

(*Social marketing*) The group to whom a marketing programme is being directed. It is separated from the audience as a whole by identifying it by key characteristics, for example, age, sex, and social class.

Taxonomies

(*Theoretical debate*) Categorical classifications of elements into different species or groups.

Theories

(*Theoretical debate*) Organized or integrated sets of propositions, better thought of as a 'theoretical system' in contrast to the above terms. Synonymous with explanatory system. Retains etymology of 'composition' and 'speculation' (same origin as spectator, spectacle, etc., meaning viewpoint or perspective).

Typologies

(*Theoretical debate*) Dimensional classification with a continuously graded array of elements. Typological labels usually given to the extremes or polarities.

Utilitarianism

(*Ethics*) Theory of personal morality. Often associated with Jeremy Bentham's phrase 'the greatest happiness for the greatest number'. (*See Consequentialism.*)

Vicarious learning

(*Psychology*) Learning by observing others without direct experience. For example, smoking in children may be learnt vicariously as it is portrayed as an enjoyable or desirable activity by the media or by contemporaries at school.

Victim blaming

Health-promoting activities based on the belief that problems with health are the responsibility of the individual and not the social or economic environment in which the individual finds him or herself. (*See Pro-innovation bias.*)

Xenotransplantation

(*Genetics*) Animal to human organ transplants or xenografts. Their association with gene technology is because the animals will have to be genetically modified so that their organs when removed will 'look' sufficiently like human organs to the recipient's immune system that they will not be rejected.

Index